T0260261

The Spirit of Recovery

The scope of this book focuses on how information technology may assist in achieving goals and in providing solutions to problems such as a pandemic. Research on the Internet and on technology has been done, and the findings have applications in various sectors that rely on interdisciplinary knowledge. This book explores and describes state-of-the-art research conducted during the COVID-19 pandemic. Topics covered include the IT viewpoint and the rules governing digital transformation throughout the pandemic. The Digital Revolution sped up by a decade during COVID-19, which impacted both the user experience and that of software developers. As a component of the digital transformation process, this book explores the experiences of both the user and developer when attempting to change and adapt while utilizing an information technology program. This book includes five topics: (1) multidisciplinary artificial intelligence, (2) Smart City and Internet of Things applications, (3) game technology and multimedia applications, (4) data science and business intelligence, and (5) IT hospitality and information systems. Each topic is covered in several book chapters with some application in several countries, especially developing countries. The chapters provide insight from contributors with different perspectives and several diverse fields who present new ideas and approaches to solving problems associated with the worldwide pandemic.

Aji Prasetya Wibawa was awarded a doctoral degree in Electrical and Information Engineering from the University of South Australia (UniSA). He was formerly the head of the Electrical Engineering Department at Universitas Negeri Malang (UM) in Indonesia. He is currently head of the Academic Publication Center at UM. He is the leader of a research group that focuses on knowledge engineering and data science (KEDS). His research interests include artificial intelligence, data mining, machine translation, and social informatics. These research interests are reflected in the journals he edits, such as *Knowledge Engineering and Data Science (KEDS)* and *Bulletin of Social Informatics Theory and Application (BUSINTA)*.

The Spirit of Recovery
IT Perspectives, Experiences, and Applications during the COVID-19 Pandemic

Edited by
Aji Prasetya Wibawa

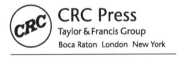

CRC Press
Taylor & Francis Group
Boca Raton London New York

CRC Press is an imprint of the
Taylor & Francis Group, an **informa** business

First edition published 2024
by CRC Press
2385 NW Executive Center Drive, Suite 320, Boca Raton FL 33431

and by CRC Press
4 Park Square, Milton Park, Abingdon, Oxon, OX14 4RN

CRC Press is an imprint of Taylor & Francis Group, LLC

ISBN: 9781032363837 (hbk)
ISBN: 9781032363844 (pbk)
ISBN: 9781003331674 (ebk)

DOI: 10.1201/9781003331674

Typeset in Times
by KnowledgeWorks Global Ltd.

Contents

Chapter 17   Food Security Clustering in Indonesia around the
                 COVID-19 Pandemic 205

*Imam Mukhlis, Aji Prasetya Wibawa, Agung Winarno,
and Özlem Sökmen Gürçam*

Chapter 18   Support Vector Machine for Sentiment Analysis
                 of COVID-19 Vaccine 217

*Poetri Lestari Lokapitasari Belluano, Audi Faathirmansyah
Mashar, Andi Widya Mufila Gaffar, Abdul Rachman Manga,
and Purnawansyah*

Chapter 19   Seasonal and Trend Forecasting of COVID-19 Cases
                 Using Deep Learning 225

*Agung Bella Putra Utama, Haviluddin, Andri Pranolo,
Xiaofeng Zhou, and Yingchi Mao*

Esther Irawati Setiawan, Joan Santoso, Julius Sugianto,
Alvin Sucita, Michael Tenoyo, Mitchell Arthur,
and Willyanto Dharmawan

Contributors

Ashri Shabrina Afrah
Universitas Islam Negeri Maulana
    Malik Ibrahim Malang, Malang,
    Indonesia

Rayner Alfred
Universiti Malaysia Sabah, Kinabalu,
    Malaysia

Desi Anggreani
Universitas Muslim Indonesia,
    Makassar, Indonesia

Mo Raymond A. P.
Institut Sains dan Teknologi Terpadu
    Surabaya, Surabaya, Indonesia

Yunifa Miftachul Arif
Universitas Islam Negeri Maulana
    Malik Ibrahim Malang, Malang,
    Indonesia

Mitchell Arthur
Institut Sains dan Teknologi Terpadu
    Surabaya, Surabaya, Indonesia

I Nyoman Gede Arya Astawa
Politeknik Negeri Bali, Badung,
    Indonesia

I Made Ari Dwi Suta Atmaja
Politeknik Negeri Bali, Badung,
    Indonesia

Huzain Azis
Universitas Muslim Indonesia,
    Makassar, Indonesia

Okta Qomarudin Aziz
Universitas Islam Negeri Maulana Malik
    Ibrahim Malang, Malang, Indonesia

Poetri Lestari Lokapitasari Belluano
Universitas Muslim Indonesia,
    Makassar, Indonesia

Putu Indah Ciptayani
Politeknik Negeri Bali, Badung,
    Indonesia

Herdianti Darwis
Universitas Muslim Indonesia,
    Makassar, Indonesia

Kadek Cahya Dewi
Politeknik Negeri Bali, Badung,
    Indonesia

Willyanto Dharmawan
Institut Sains dan Teknologi Terpadu
    Surabaya, Surabaya, Indonesia

Rafał Dreżewski
AGH University of Science and
    Technology, Kraków, Poland

Felix Andika Dwiyanto
AGH University of Science and
    Technology, Kraków, Poland

Johan Ericka
Universitas Islam Negeri Maulana
    Malik Ibrahim Malang, Malang,
    Indonesia

Muhamad Faisal
Universitas Islam Negeri Maulana
    Malik Ibrahim Malang, Malang,
    Indonesia

Farniwati Fattah
Universitas Muslim Indonesia,
    Makassar, Indonesia

FX. Ferdinandus
Institut Sains dan Teknologi Terpadu
  Surabaya, Surabaya, Indonesia

Erry Fuadillah
Universitas Pendidikan Indonesia,
  Bandung, Indonesia

Andi Widya Mufila Gaffar
Universitas Muslim Indonesia,
  Makassar, Indonesia

Gunawan
Institut Sains dan Teknologi Terpadu
  Surabaya, Surabaya, Indonesia

Özlem Sökmen Gürçam
Igdir University, Iğdır, Turkey

Jehad Abdelhamid Hammad
Al-Quds Open University, Abu Dis,
  Palestine

Eisuke Hanada
Saga University, Saga, Japan

Anik Nur Handayani
Universitas Negeri Malang, Malang,
  Indonesia

Fajar Rohman Hariri
Universitas Islam Negeri Maulana
  Malik Ibrahim Malang, Malang,
  Indonesia

Haviluddin
Universitas Mulawarman, Samarinda,
  Indonesia

Arya Tandy Hermawan
Universitas Negeri Malang, Malang,
  Indonesia

Leonel Hernández
Corporación Universitaria Reformada,
  Barranquilla, Colombia

Dolly Indra
Universitas Muslim Indonesia,
  Makassar, Indonesia

I Nyoman Eddy Indrayana
Politeknik Negeri Bali, Badung,
  Indonesia

Hartarto Junaedi
Institut Sains dan Teknologi Terpadu
  Surabaya, Surabaya, Indonesia

Ahmad Fahmi Karami
Universitas Islam Negeri Maulana
  Malik Ibrahim Malang, Malang,
  Indonesia

Meidya Koeshardianto
University of Trunojoyo Madura,
  Bangkalan, Indonesia

Yosi Kristian
Institut Sains dan Teknologi Terpadu
  Surabaya, Surabaya, Indonesia

Fachrul Kurniawan
Universitas Islam Negeri Maulana Malik
  Ibrahim Malang, Malang, Indonesia

Gulsun Kurubacak
Anadolu University, Eskişehir, Turkey

Aisyah Larasati
Universitas Negeri Malang, Malang,
  Indonesia

Abdul Rachman Manga
Universitas Muslim Indonesia,
  Makassar, Indonesia

Yingchi Mao
Hohai University, Nanjing, China

Audi Faathirmansyah Mashar
Universitas Muslim Indonesia,
  Makassar, Indonesia

Imam Mukhlis
Universitas Negeri Malang, Malang,
    Indonesia

Andrew Nafalski
University of South Australia, Adelaide,
    Australia

Fresy Nugroho
Universitas Islam Negeri Maulana
    Malik Ibrahim Malang, Malang,
    Indonesia

Hani Nurhayati
Universitas Islam Negeri Maulana
    Malik Ibrahim Malang, Malang,
    Indonesia

I Ketut Parnata
Politeknik Negeri Bali, Badung,
    Indonesia

I Putu Bagus Arya Pradnyana
Politeknik Negeri Bali, Badung,
    Indonesia

Edwin Pramana
Institut Sains dan Teknologi Terpadu
    Surabaya, Surabaya, Indonesia

Andri Pranolo
Hohai University, Nanjing, China
    and Universitas Ahmad Dahlan,
    Yogyakarta, Indonesia

Yuliana Melita Pranoto
Universitas Negeri Malang, Malang,
    Indonesia

Deni Prastyo
Universitas Negeri Malang, Malang,
    Indonesia

Putu Manik Prihatini
Politeknik Negeri Bali, Badung,
    Indonesia

Agus Rachmad Purnama
Universitas Nahdlatul Ulama Sidoarjo,
    Sidoarjo, Indonesia

Purnawansyah
Universitas Muslim Indonesia,
    Makassar, Indonesia

Andreas Adi Purwanto
Institut Sains dan Teknologi Terpadu
    Surabaya, Surabaya, Indonesia

Nastiti Susetyo Fanany Putri
Universitas Negeri Malang, Malang,
    Indonesia

Afrijal Rizqi Ramadan
Universitas Islam Negeri Maulana
    Malik Ibrahim Malang, Malang,
    Indonesia

Lala Septem Riza
Universitas Pendidikan Indonesia,
    Bandung, Indonesia

Harits Ar Rosyid
Universitas Negeri Malang, Malang,
    Indonesia

Yulita Salim
Universitas Muslim Indonesia,
    Makassar, Indonesia

Joan Santoso
Institut Sains dan Teknologi
    Terpadu Surabaya, Surabaya,
    Indonesia

Ong, Hansel Santoso
Institut Sains dan Teknologi
    Terpadu Surabaya, Surabaya,
    Indonesia

Ni Gusti Ayu Putu Harry Saptarini
Politeknik Negeri Bali, Badung,
    Indonesia

Herman Thuan To Saurik
Universitas Negeri Malang, Malang,
  Indonesia

Esther Irawati Setiawan
Institut Sains dan Teknologi Terpadu
  Surabaya, Surabaya, Indonesia

Eka Rahayu Setyaningsih
Institut Sains dan Teknologi Terpadu
  Surabaya, Surabaya, Indonesia

Chow Shean Shyong
Institut Sains dan Teknologi Terpadu
  Surabaya, Surabaya, Indonesia

Robert Subianto
Institut Sains dan Teknologi Terpadu
  Surabaya, Surabaya, Indonesia

Alvin Sucita
Institut Sains dan Teknologi Terpadu
  Surabaya, Surabaya, Indonesia

Julius Sugianto
Institut Sains dan Teknologi Terpadu
  Surabaya, Surabaya, Indonesia

Putu Wijaya Sunu
Politeknik Negeri Bali, Badung,
  Indonesia

Triyo Supriyatno
Universitas Islam Negeri Maulana Malik
  Ibrahim Malang, Malang, Indonesia

Supriyonoe
Universitas Islam Negeri Maulana Malik
  Ibrahim Malang, Malang, Indonesia

Michael Tenoyo
Institut Sains dan Teknologi Terpadu
  Surabaya, Surabaya, Indonesia

Fitriyani Umar
Universitas Muslim Indonesia,
  Makassar, Indonesia

Agung Bella Putra Utama
Universitas Negeri Malang, Malang,
  Indonesia

Shoffin Nahwa Utama
Universitas Islam Negeri Maulana
  Malik Ibrahim Malang, Malang,
  Indonesia

Roman Voliansky
Dniprovsky State Technical University,
  Kamianske, Ukraine

Aji Prasetya Wibawa
Universitas Negeri Malang, Malang,
  Indonesia

Agung Winarno
Universitas Negeri Malang, Malang,
  Indonesia

Ni Wayan Wisswani
Politeknik Negeri Bali, Badung,
  Indonesia

Ilham Ari Elbaith Zaeni
Universitas Negeri Malang, Malang,
  Indonesia

Xiaofeng Zhou
Hohai University, Nanjing, China

1 Automatic HTML Generator from Sketch Using Deep Learning to Speed Up Web Developing Post-COVID-19

Yosi Kristian, Robert Subianto,
and Eka Rahayu Setyaningsih
Institut Sains dan Teknologi Terpadu Surabaya
Surabaya, Indonesia

Anik Nur Handayani
Universitas Negeri Malang
Malang, Indonesia

1.1 INTRODUCTION

The COVID-19 pandemic triggered the acceleration of the shift in economic activity from traditional to digital. In the digital era, the acceleration of web and mobile platform development is the right option to support the buying and selling process in the community. Based on a report by the Indonesian National Bureau of Statistics [1], it was recorded that 10.58% growth in the Information and Communication Technology (ICT) sector in 2020 resulted from the rapid transition from a traditional to a digital economy, which was also accompanied by an increase in demand for telecommunications and gadget services. Attempting to help micro- to small-sized software developers develop rapid web applications, this study seeks to utilize the deep learning algorithm to be able to translate sketches written by ordinary people into HTML automatically.

Web applications are one of the options as a medium to support the digital economy. These days, many businesses need a website as their face to the public, thus increasing demand for a fast and affordable solution. This is where micro- and small-sized software developers fill in. One of the problems with website creation is that it takes a great deal of time [2]. One can accelerate website development by automatically converting a webpage sketch image into a webpage in HTML. In this chapter,

DOI: 10.1201/9781003331674-1

1

we elaborate on methods that can automatically convert a webpage sketch image into a similar looking webpage.

Our experiment used convolutional neural network (CNN)-based deep learning models, namely, Xception, DeeplabV3+, and Unet, to make a segmentation of the sketch image. We also experimented with five backbones for the three models we used. We then applied computer vision techniques, mainly contour detection, to get elements inside the segmentation result and construct a webpage.

The main contribution of this chapter is a deep learning-based system that can take an image of a webpage sketch and automatically convert it into a webpage that looks similar to the sketch image. The model has 20 classes to distinguish HTML elements, each with a distinct implemented color as one of the class features.

1.2   RELATED WORK

Numerous tries to convert a sketch image into an interface have been done before. SILK [3] attempted to make interfaces from sketches using hand gestures to recognize the component drawn. REMAUI [4] attempted to make an interface for a mobile application from screenshots using computer vision techniques such as contour detection, corner detection, and line detection. Pix2code [5] attempted to make an interface using a deep learning model based on long short-term memory (LSTM) architecture.

Image segmentation using deep learning has shown considerable success, which led to our approach to segment webpage sketch images [6]. Each pixel of the sketch image needs to be classified as an HTML element to explain the sketch image segmentation problem. Some approaches use ResNet-50 [2], LSTM [5], and ResNet-50 [6] models to accomplish this task.

Previous work divided HTML elements into two categories, elements and containers [6]. In both categories there are five classes of HTML elements making up 10 HTML elements. Those 10 classes are image, paragraph, input, title, button, stack, row, form, footer, and header. Each class has its sketch representation, with black and white as the primary color. In that previous work, there were two approaches to segmenting webpage sketch images [6]. The first approach used computer vision, and the second used a deep learning model. The second approach was better at classifying elements, whereas the first approach was better at classifying containers. In this chapter, the deep learning approach seems more applicable because we used color to represent the container elements.

In this chapter, we doubled the HTML element class to 20 classes, which are title, paragraph, image, video, progress bar, carousel, form, dropdown, input, button, radio button, checkbox, header, navigation, footer, list group, column, row, table, and pagination. We gave every element a different representation and used colors other than black and white for the nine elements. Colors are mainly used to differentiate the container element and make the element easier to detect. For extracting elements inside the segmentation result, we followed the method from [6], which consisted of postprocessing segmentation results using erosion and dilation, then applying contour detection to get elements inside the segmentation result, and using those elements to construct a webpage.

1.3   THE AUTOMATIC HTML GENERATOR FROM SKETCH

In this chapter, there are two tasks to accomplish. The first task is segmentation, which creates segmentation of a webpage sketch image based on the HTML element inside the image. The second task is element extraction, which extracts elements from the segmentation's result and constructs a webpage using the element extracted. The sketch's overview of the automatic HTML generator is shown in Figure 1.1.

From Figure 1.1, the sketch image within the input image is detected, cropped, and enhanced, then segmented into a probability mask using the DeeplabV3+ model. The model output will go through the postprocess phase, and then the element inside will be extracted using contour detection. Using those elements, the program will construct a webpage.

1.3.1 DATASET

To make a dataset, we used the program provided in [7]. The dataset generator generates an HTML structure and then makes a normalized webpage using this structure. A normalized webpage represents each element inside it with a square color that corresponds to the element. The generator detects each element and replaces them with the corresponding sketch image using the normalized webpage. Figure 1.2 shows sample images from the generated dataset.

There are two problems when using this program. First, we classified HTML elements using 20 classes, and the program only classifies HTML elements using 11 classes, 9 of which are the same as our classes. Second, the program does not

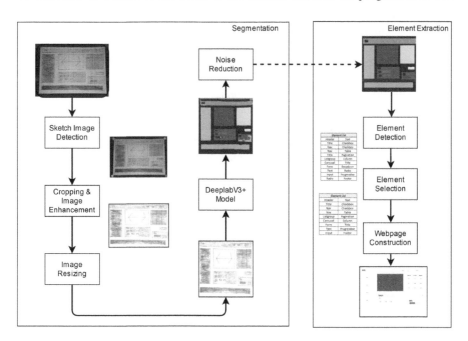

FIGURE 1.1   Automatic HTML generator from sketch.

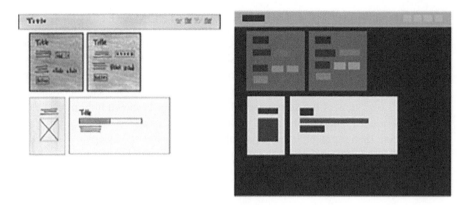

FIGURE 1.2   Sample images from our generated dataset.

make a class for each pixel we need as ground truth. To address this problem, we modified the program by adding 11 more HTML element classes and a function to give a class for each pixel in the image. Using the modified dataset generation program, we generated 1500 webpage sketches as a dataset.

1.3.2 INPUT

The input image is an image that contains a webpage sketch inside it. We limited the input image to only one sketch image that covers 80% of the input image, and it is drawn on white media. With those limitations, we know that the sketch might not be as big as the image size. We also have problems such as the image might be too dark or have a variety of sizes. To address this problem, we preprocessed the input image.

The preprocessing phase will first detect the sketch image inside the input image. To detect the sketch image, we turned the input image colorspace into grayscale, increase the brightness, then applied the image processing technique called dilation. By turning colorspace and increasing brightness, we can reduce the content inside the paper used to draw the sketch and reduce it by dilation.

We applied thresholding and contour detection to get contours inside the input image. Because of the limitation that the sketch image needs to cover 80% of the input image, we can safely assume that the most extensive contour obtained is the sketch image. Using the most prominent contour, we can get the four corners of the sketch image.

We can crop the input to the sketch image using the four corners, using a computer vision technique called perspective warping. We then increased the image brightness and contrast using the image processing technique contrast limited adaptive histogram equalization (CLAHE). Finally, we resized the image size to the desired input size by the model.

1.3.3 SEGMENTATION

We experimented with three deep learning models in the segmentation task: Xception, DeeplabV3+, and Unet. The architecture of this segmentation model is introduced in Figures 1.3, 1.4, and 1.5, respectively. In this section, we will explain

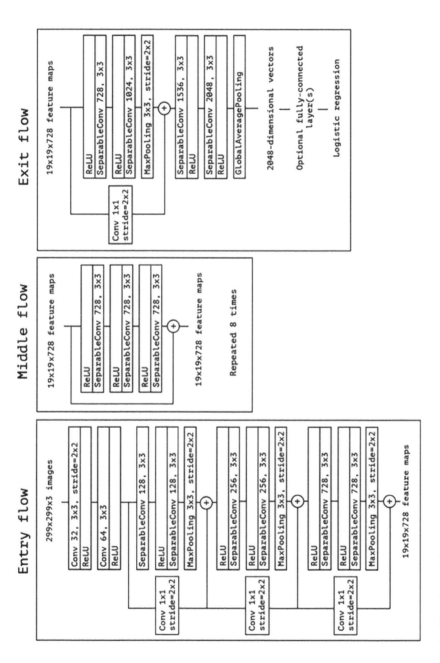

FIGURE 1.3 Xception architecture.

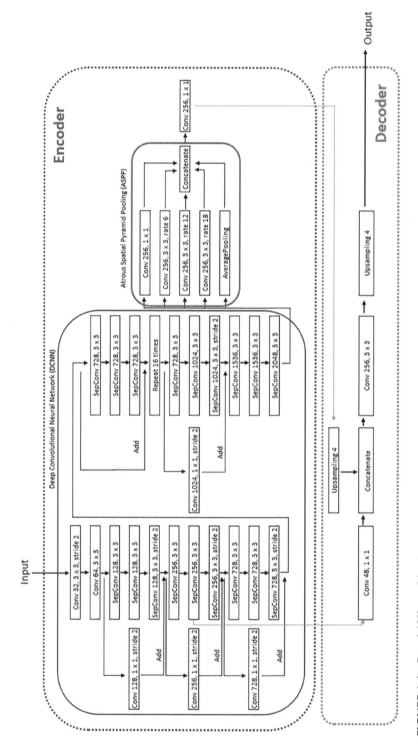

FIGURE 1.4 DeeplabV3+ architecture.

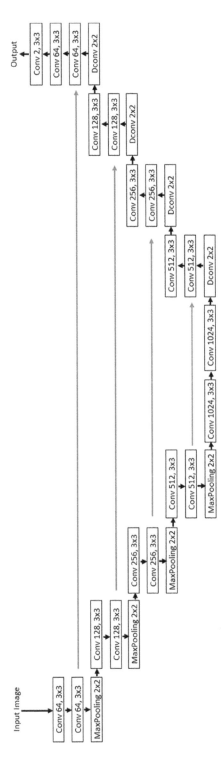

FIGURE 1.5 Unet architecture.

each model used and also the implementation of the models. All of our model implementations are done in Python using the Tensorflow library.

1.3.3.1 Xception

Xception is a model invented by François Chollet, who also is the creator of Python's deep learning library, Keras. Xception architecture is based entirely on depthwise separable convolution layers [8] (a layer that does depthwise and point-wise convolution). Depthwise convolution is a convolution operation where each channel from input has an $n \times n$ kernel of its own. Each channel is then convoluted using each kernel, and each result will be stacked together after depthwise convolution becomes pointwise convolution, which uses a 1×1 kernel to reduce the number of channels.

Depthwise separable convolution is used because it separates operations for spatial correlation and cross-channel correlation, similar to the Inception V3 module. Xception experimented using depthwise separable convolution and it was found that it had a better result than the Inception V3 module.

There are 36 layers in Xception used for the feature extraction base of the network. These layers are structured into 14 modules, all of which have linear residual connections, except the first and last modules. In short, Xception architecture is a linear stack of depthwise separable convolution layers with residual connections [8]. We experimented using the Xception model because it has high accuracy on the ImageNet dataset [8]. We implemented the Xception model using the Keras library.

1.3.3.2 DeeplabV3+

DeeplabV3+ is a model invented by Liang-Chieh Chen et al. [9]. The DeeplabV3+ model mainly used atrous convolution to extract features. Atrous convolution is a convolution that uses a kernel that has spacing for each value in the kernel. The spacing of the kernel is called the atrous rate. Atrous convolution is used because it is a powerful tool that can control the resolution of features computed by deep CNNs (DCNN) and adjust the filter's field of view to capture multiscale information [9].

The DeeplabV3+ model has an encoder-decoder architecture. The encoder part of DeeplabV3+ extracts features from an image using a DCNN and atrous spatial pyramid pooling (ASPP) module to extract features from the DCNN result. ASPP is an image segmentation module that applies atrous convolution using different atrous rates to extract features. ASPP solves the problem of different object sizes in an image. The decoder part of DeeplabV3+ upsamples encoder features and then concatenates it with low-level features obtained from DCNN.

In DeeplabV3+, there is a particular variable called output stride. This variable controls the resolution of extracted encoder features by atrous convolution to trade off precision and runtime [9]. We experimented using the DeeplabV3+ model because our referred paper in [6] also used the same model to perform the same task, which obtained good accuracy. We implemented DeeplabV3+ using the GitHub repository at github.com/bonlime/keras-deeplab-v3-plus created by Emil Zakirov [10]. This DeeplabV3+ implementation has two backbones, Xception and MobileNetV2, and we experimented with both of them.

1.3.3.3 Unet

Unet was developed by Olaf Ronnerberg et al. [11] for biomedical image segmentation. Unet architecture contains two paths: the contracting path, which works as the encoder, and the expanding path, which works as the decoder. The contracting path and expanding path both have steps or stages.

The contracting path aims to capture the context in the input image. It contains convolutional layers and pooling layers. The expanding path aims to restore the image size from the contracting path. It contains transposed convolution layers. Unet also has skip connections that deliver contracting path features to expanding paths for each step.

We experimented using the Unet model because, in [12], the Unet-based generative adversarial network (GAN) was implemented with human segment clothes and obtained better accuracy than regular CNN. We implemented Unet using Python library segmentation models [13]. This Unet implementation provides many backbones. We used three of the backbones provided, which included Inception V3, ResNet-152, and ResNeXt-101.

1.3.4 NOISE REDUCTION

The segmentation result shows many noises from the wrongly classified pixel. To reduce the amount of noise, we applied noise reduction techniques. We used erosion and dilation techniques and image processing methods to remove or add pixels on object boundaries. We first applied erosion to reduce the small noises, followed by dilation to restore the object's size from erosion.

1.3.5 ELEMENT EXTRACTION

This phase aims to extract HTML elements from the segmentation result and construct a webpage from the elements obtained. There are three steps to element extraction: element detection, element selection, and webpage creation, as shown in Figure 1.6. In element detection, we used a computer vision technique called contour detection. The contours of the objects inside the segmentation can be obtained from the contour detection results. Each contour obtained is considered an HTML element. Each element of information, such as size, position, and parent-child relationship, can be obtained by getting the four corners from the contour points. The system can also detect the table's column and row by cropping each detected table and applying canny and Hough lines. After receiving each element's information, we obtained a list of HTML elements.

Inside the element, the list contains all of the HTML elements detected from the contour detection, but probably not all are segmented correctly. To address this problem, element selection is performed, which selects the elements inside the element list to decide which element should be used to create the webpage. To select the element, we checked three things about the element. The first check is to see if the element has a width or height lower than 7 pixels. If so, the element will be categorized as a wrongly segmented element. The second check is to see if the

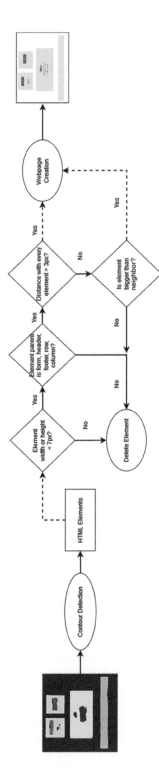

FIGURE 1.6 Detailed overview of the element extraction steps.

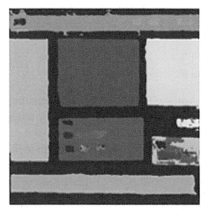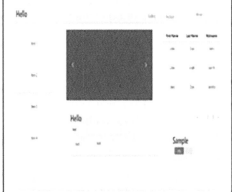

FIGURE 1.7 Result of element extraction.

element parent is not one of the proposed elements (form, header, footer, column, or row). If this happens then the element will be categorized as a wrongly segmented element. The last check is to see if the element is near another element with a distance of only 3 pixels or less. The minor element will be categorized as a wrongly segmented element if this occurs.

After the element selection, we obtained the elements necessary to build the webpage. We created a function to give each element its corresponding HTML tags to build the webpage. We then gave the HTML tags styling to adjust the position and size of the element. We also created bootstrap styling to make the webpage look better. The result of element extraction can be seen in Figure 1.7.

1.3.6 EVALUATION METRICS

There are two tasks to evaluate: segmentation and element extraction. The segmentation task evaluation assesses how well the model segments sketch images, and the element extraction evaluation gauges how well the program can extract HTML elements from segmentation and construct a webpage.

For segmentation evaluation, we used two metrics: the $F1$ and Jaccard scores. We used the $F1$ score, a metric that calculates precision and recall, to measure how well the model segments each element. The mathematical definition of the $F1$ score can be seen in Equation (1.1).

$$F1\ score = \frac{2 \times precision \times recall}{precision + recall} \tag{1.1}$$

We also use the Jaccard score, or intersection over union (IoU), which is a metric to measure similarity between two sets, to measure how good the model segmentation is as a whole. The Jaccard score measures similarity by searching the intersection of two sets and dividing it by the union of the two sets. This metric can also be converted into a loss function by subtracting 1 from the Jaccard score, also known as the Jaccard distance. The mathematical definition of the Jaccard score can be seen in Equation (1.2).

$$J(A,B) = \frac{A \cap B}{A \cup B} \tag{1.2}$$

We used the structural similarity index measure (SSIM) for element extraction evaluation. SSIM is a metric that compares the similarity of two images by using image aspects such as luminance, contrast, and structure. There are mathematical formulas to obtain these three aspects, and the three formulas combined result in the SSIM formula [Equation (1.3)].

$$\text{SSIM}(x,y) = \frac{\left(2\mu_x\mu_y + c_1\right)\left(2\sigma_{xy} + c_2\right)}{\left(\mu_x^2 + \mu_y^2 + c_1\right)\left(\sigma_x^2 + \sigma_y^2 + c_2\right)} \tag{1.3}$$

1.4   EXPERIMENTS AND RESULTS

In this section, we will outline our approaches to creating segmentation of sketch images and approaches to extracting HTML elements and constructing a webpage from the segmentation result. We will first explain the approaches for both tasks and then show the results from our experiments.

In the segmentation task, we trained three deep learning models with different backbones, resulting in a total of six different architectures. To train these models, we used a dataset obtained from dataset generation and split it into training data (80%) and validation data (20%). We one-hot encoded the ground truth and trained all of our models in Google Colaboratory. We trained the Xception model on GPU and DeeplabV3+ and Unet models on TPU, because they require more memory.

Each model was trained using pre-trained weight. The Xception and Unet models were trained using ImageNet pre-trained weight and DeeplabV3+ was trained using Cityscapes pre-trained weight. Even though ImageNet and Cityscapes do not contain sketch images inside them, it is known from ref. [6] that by using pre-trained weight, the model already learned basic features such as edges and corners, which gives the model a head start to learn more abstract features.

All models were trained using Jaccard distance as its loss function. We used five batches of images for training. We also used an EarlyStopping callback to stop the training if the validation loss did not go down for a particular epoch.

In element extraction, we used contour detection to detect elements from segmentation results, selected the element, and created a function to construct the webpage. To evaluate the accuracy of our methods, we tested them by extracting HTML elements from ground truth in test data and creating webpage normalization from the element obtained.

We tested the data ground truth, so we could obtain the evaluation of element extraction that is not dependent on the segmentation result. In this evaluation, we also made webpage normalization instead of a webpage, because there are many representations of a single HTML element. There is only one representation for each HTML element using the normalization webpage.

TABLE 1.1

Element Occurrence in Data Test

Element	Occurrence	Element	Occurrence
Title	52	Radio Button	31
Paragraph	60	Checkbox	28
Image	28	Header	27
Video	19	Navigation	41
Progress bar	16	Footer	23
Carousel	11	List group	15
Form	21	Column	29
Dropdown	33	Row	37
Input	32	Table	17
Button	48	Pagination	12

We obtained two types of test data: webpage sketch images and normalized webpage images. We used webpage sketch images to test the segmentation task and a normalized webpage image to test the element extraction task.

To obtain the sketch image, we manually drew 40 webpage sketch images. To obtain the normalized webpage image, we manually edited the sketch image we had drawn by giving each element its representative color. Each HTML element occurrence inside the test data can be seen in Table 1.1.

We trained six model configurations: Xception, DeeplabV3+ with Xception backbone, DeeplabV3+ with MobileNetV2 backbone, Unet with Inception V3 backbone, Unet with ResNet-152 backbone, and Unet with Resnext101 backbone. We evaluated each model using 40 webpage sketches using the $F1$ and Jaccard scores. The $F1$ and Jaccard score calculation is a pixel-based calculation in which the system calculates between the pixel in the ground truth and the pixel in the segmented sketch image.

From our experiments as in Figure 1.8, we found that the Xception model does not have a proper image size restoration module and did not perform well, but when Xception was used as a feature extractor or backbone in the DeeplabV3+ model, it could create segmentation of the sketch image quite well.

The other DeeplabV3+ backbone, MobileNetV2, does not perform that well, with a Jaccard score nearly the same as the base Xception model.

From experimenting with the Unet model, we found that all three backbone we used performed exceptionally well at segmentation sketch image. The performance of each backbone did not differ much with the Inception V3 backbone with the highest Jaccard score of 0.75, followed by the ResNet-152 backbone, which had a Jaccard score of 0.72, and followed by Resnext101, which had a Jaccard score of 0.66.

Comparing the three models we experimented with, the DeeplabV3+ model with Xception backbone performed the best at segmenting sketch images with a Jaccard score of 0.82 and could detect 18 of 20 classes of elements used as in Figure 1.9. While compared with the Unet model, the DeeplabV3+ model had a better Jaccard score of 0.07 and could detect one more HTML element class. Compared with the Xception model, the DeeplabV3+ model had a better Jaccard score of 0.56 and could detect seven more HTML element classes.

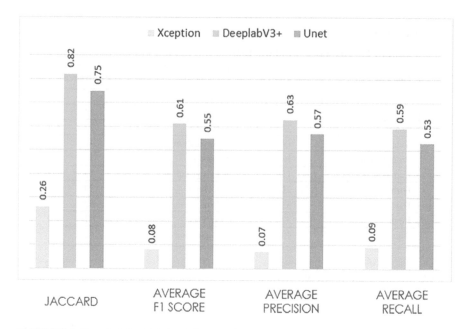

FIGURE 1.8 Performance comparison.

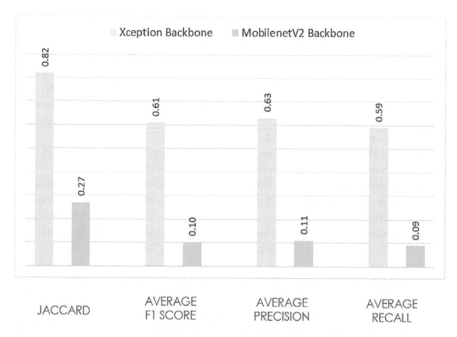

FIGURE 1.9 Performance comparison between DeeplabV3+ backbones.

TABLE 1.2
Element Extraction Results

Image	SSIM	Image	SSIM	Image	SSIM	Image	SSIM
1	0.93	11	0.91	21	0.91	31	0.91
2	0.9	12	0.93	22	0.95	32	0.92
3	0.88	13	0.92	23	0.95	33	0.92
4	0.89	14	0.94	24	0.93	34	0.93
5	0.88	15	0.9	25	0.88	35	0.89
6	0.87	16	0.82	26	0.91	36	0.91
7	0.92	17	0.9	27	0.93	37	0.9
8	0.88	18	0.92	28	0.91	38	0.93
9	0.91	19	0.93	29	0.92	39	0.92
10	0.91	20	0.91	30	0.85	40	0.96

The results for element extraction can be seen in Table 1.2. The element extraction method we used had an average SSIM of 0.91 and had the lowest SSIM score of 0.82 when tested in our testing image. The element extraction method performed exceptionally well in extracting elements and constructing a webpage.

Our work is not without drawbacks or limitations. First, because we used CNNs, the memory needed to train the model is relatively high.

Second, as we used 20 classes of the HTML element, some elements have the same features. Because of this, the model could not detect some elements. Another problem with element representation is the color. As we used color on containers and some elements do not have color, the segmentation had many noises from the wrongly classified pixel, especially elements inside a container. The segmentation results shown in Table 1.3.

The element detection method we used also had drawbacks. We obtained the element corner by using the minimum and maximum values for the x- and y-axis inside the contour of that element. By doing this, we did not obtain the element corner accurately. This can create a problem of incorrect element size and position. Incorrect element size and position can trigger the third noise checking in element selection, which will delete a small-sized element with a distance 3 pixels or less from another element. The example of program result to convert sketch image into a webpage represents in Figure 1.10.

1.5 CONCLUSION

We compared three models: Xception, DeeplabV3+, and Unet. We found that the DeeplabV3+ model using the Xception backbone performs well on segmenting sketch images, had a Jaccard score of 0.82, and can detect 18 of 20 classes of the HTML element. The Unet model with the Inception V3 backbone also performed exceptionally well compared with the DeeplabV3+ model, which has a different Jaccard score of 0.6 and can detect one less class. The technique we used to extract elements and construct the webpage also performed well, with an average SSIM of 0.91 on the data test.

TABLE 1.3

Segmentation Results

Element	Xception –	DeeplabV3+ Xception	DeeplabV3+ MobileNetV2	Unet Inception V3	Unet ResNet-152	Unet ResNeXt-101
Title	0.01	0.55	0.05	0.25	0.36	0.24
Paragraph	0.01	0.56	0	0.22	0.31	0.48
Image	0.04	0.58	0	0.71	0.67	0.52
Video	0.05	0	0.19	0.14	0.23	0.17
Progressbar	0	0.46	0	0.68	0.39	0.24
Carousel	0.04	0.78	0.24	0.93	0.88	0.73
Form	0	0.85	0.30	0.55	0.75	0.63
Dropdown	0	0.57	0	0	0	0
Input	0	0.67	0	0.21	0.29	0
Button	0	0.57	0	0.42	0.48	0
Radio Button	0	0	0	0	0	0
Checkbox	0	0.02	0	0	0	0
Header	0.07	0.92	0.29	0.87	0.61	0.80
Navigation	0	0.53	0	0.26	0	0
Footer	0.34	0.94	0.56	0.91	0.93	0.89
List group	0.12	0.82	0.37	0.96	0.64	0.57
Column	0.13	0.86	0	0.81	0.83	0.63
Row	0.31	0.92	0	0.85	0.73	0.64
Table	0.03	0.92	0	0.89	0.88	0.86
Pagination	0	0.72	0	0.36	0	0.25
Jaccard	*0.26*	*0.82*	*0.27*	*0.75*	*0.72*	*0.66*

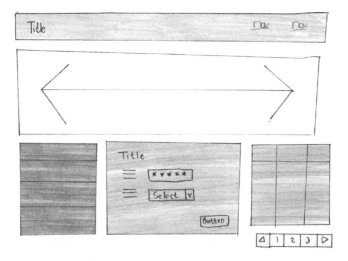

FIGURE 1.10   Example of the program result to convert sketch image into a webpage.

Our results might be slightly lower than previous research, but it should be noted that we used double the class used in the referenced paper. The element representation we used also affects the model's accuracy because there are two elements that the model cannot predict because of similar features. Using color as a feature on all container elements also hinders the model from correctly classifying elements inside the container, especially the one that does not have color.

REFERENCES

1. David Nugent, "Covid positive: The technological upside to the pandemic," 2022 [Online]. Available: https://www.forbes.com/sites/forbesbusinesscouncil/2022/11/15/covid-positive-the-technological-upside-to-the-pandemic/?sh=4d15e21e633b [Accessed 01-12-2022].
2. V. Jain, P. Agrawal, S. Banga, R. Kapoor, and S. Gulyani, "Sketch2Code: Transformation of sketches to UI in real-time using deep neural network," pp. 1–15, 2019 [Online]. Available: http://arxiv.org/abs/1910.08930.
3. J. A. Landay, and B. A. Myers, "Sketching interfaces: Toward more human interface design," *Computer (Long. Beach. Calif)*, vol. 34, no. 3, pp. 56–64, 2001, doi: 10.1109/2.910894.
4. T. A. Nguyen, and C. Csallner, "Reverse engineering mobile application user interfaces with REMAUI," *Proc. 2015 30th IEEE/ACM Int. Conf. Autom. Softw. Eng. ASE 2015*, pp. 248–259, 2016, doi: 10.1109/ASE.2015.32.
5. T. Beltramelli, "pix2code: Generating code from a graphical user interface screenshot," *Proc. ACM SIGCHI Symp. Eng. Interact. Comput. Syst. EICS 2018*, pp. 1–9, 2018, doi: 10.1145/3220134.3220135.
6. A. Robinson, "Sketch2code: Generating a website from a paper mockup," May, 2019 [Online]. Available: http://arxiv.org/abs/1905.13750.
7. A. Abdelhamid, "Sketched-webpages-generator," *Github Repos.*, 2019, [Online]. Available: https://github.com/Dev-Tarek/sketched-webpages-generator.
8. F. Chollet, "Xception: Deep learning with depthwise separable convolutions," *Proc. - 30th IEEE Conf. Comput. Vis. Pattern Recognition, CVPR 2017*, vol. 2017-Jan, pp. 1800–1807, 2017, doi: 10.1109/CVPR.2017.195.
9. L. C. Chen, Y. Zhu, G. Papandreou, F. Schroff, and H. Adam, "Encoder-decoder with atrous separable convolution for semantic image segmentation," Lect. Notes Comput. Sci. (Including Subser. Lect. Notes Artif. Intell. Lect. Notes Bioinformatics), vol. 11211 LNCS, pp. 833–851, 2018, doi: 10.1007/978-3-030-01234-2_49.
10. E. Zakirov, "Keras implementation of Deeplabv3+," *Github Repos.*, 2018 [Online]. Available: https://github.com/bonlime/keras-deeplab-v3-plus.
11. O. Ronneberger, P. Fischer, and T. Brox, "U-net: Convolutional networks for biomedical image segmentation," Lect. Notes Comput. Sci. (Including Subser. Lect. Notes Artif. Intell. Lect. Notes Bioinformatics), vol. 9351, pp. 234–241, 2015, https://arxiv.org/abs/1505.04597.
12. T. Tirtawan, E. K. Susanto, P. C. S. W. Lukman Zaman, and Y. Kristian, "Batik clothes auto-fashion using conditional generative adversarial network and U-net," *3rd 2021 East Indones. Conf. Comput. Inf. Technol. EIConCIT 2021*, pp. 145–150, 2021, doi: 10.1109/EIConCIT50028.2021.9431867.
13. P. Yakubovskiy, "Segmentation models," *Github Repos.*, 2019 [Online]. Available: https://github.com/qubvel/segmentation_models.

2 Dealing with COVID-19 Using Deep Learning for Computer Vision

Felix Andika Dwiyanto and Rafał Dreżewski
AGH University of Science and Technology
Kraków, Poland

Aji Prasetya Wibawa
Universitas Negeri Malang
Malang, Indonesia

2.1 INTRODUCTION: OVERVIEW OF DEEP LEARNING FOR COVID-19

According to the World Health Organization (WHO), coronavirus disease 2019 (COVID-19) is an infectious respiratory illness caused by the SARS-CoV-2 virus [1]. The name "coronavirus" is due to its visual appearance to the Solar Corona. Since its emergence in Wuhan, China, in December 2019, COVID-19 has become a global pandemic [2]. The virus spreads through coughing and sneezing droplets that are released into the air [3]. The battle against COVID-19 has inspired scientists worldwide to investigate, comprehend, and develop novel diagnostic and treatment methods to eliminate this threat. Computer vision (CV) is one of the interdisciplinary scientific fields that have potential to fight COVID-19. CV is a branch of computer science that examines how computers may derive high-level knowledge from digital images or videos [4, 5]. Therefore, this chapter explores how the CV environment is combating COVID-19 by suggesting new techniques and enhancing method performance.

From an engineering point of view, CV tries to comprehend and automate operations performed by the human visual system. Tasks associated with CV include acquiring, processing, analyzing, and understanding digital images and extracting high-dimensional data from the real world to provide numerical or symbolic information [6, 7]. In this discussion, *understanding* refers to the process through which visual images are converted into descriptions of the environment that are comprehensible to thinking processes and have the potential to trigger appropriate behavior. This picture comprehension can be understood as the untangling of symbolic information from visual data by utilizing models developed with the assistance of geometry, physics, statistical analysis, and learning theory. Moreover, CV investigates the theoretical underpinnings of artificial systems designed to derive information from pictures. The visual data may be presented in various formats, including video sequences, images obtained from several cameras, multi-dimensional data obtained

DOI: 10.1201/9781003331674-2

from a three-dimensional (3D) scanner or medical scanning device, and so on. The technological field known as CV aims to implement the theories and models it develops in building CV systems.

Moreover, deep learning as a subfield of machine learning has mainly been responsible for its rapid development over the past couple of decades [8]. CV techniques have demonstrated immense potential in various application areas such as robotics [9], self-driving cars [10], manufacturing [11], agriculture [12], and healthcare [4, 13]. Particularly in healthcare and medical research, CV approaches include disease diagnosis, prognosis, surgery, therapy, medical image analysis, and drug discovery. Therefore, in the COVID-19 era, many researchers contributed to developing CV applications for prevention, control, treatment, and management purposes [14–16].

Several CV techniques were proposed to address the COVID-19 pandemic from various angles. In general, CV techniques apply medical imaging to promote a faster and more reliable diagnosis of COVID-19. They can also categorize the characteristic conditions as bacterial, viral, COVID-19, or pneumonia. CV approaches also allow us to learn from imaging data collected from disease survivors to assess critically and noncritically ill individuals. In other ways, CV can be utilized to implement social separation and early screening of sick individuals. Three-dimensional CV can assist in maintaining the supply of medical equipment and the creation of a COVID-19 vaccine.

2.2 DATA SOURCE

2.2.1 COMPUTED TOMOGRAPHY SCAN

The common image data used for CV approaches in COVID-19 cases is computed tomography (CT). A CT scan, previously known as a computed axial tomography or CAT scan, is a medical imaging technique that is used in radiology (x-ray) to obtain internal images of the body that are detailed and noninvasive for diagnostic purposes. Radiographers or radiology technicians are medical professionals qualified to carry out CT scans. A revolving x-ray tube and a row of detectors are used in CT scanners to quantify the x-ray attenuations produced by the various tissues in the body. To make tomographic (cross-sectional) images of a body, many x-ray measurements are first made of the body from a variety of angles. Then the data from those measurements are input into a computer and processed using reconstruction methods. Due to the potentially harmful effects of ionizing radiation, there are occasions when its application is limited. On the other hand, CT can be used on individuals who have metallic implants or pacemakers, but magnetic resonance imaging (MRI) cannot be utilized on these people.

CT imaging can also be used during a radiological examination. A patient can have a chest CT scan to obtain a precise image of their chest. It is an advanced sort of x-ray technology that, compared with a regular x-ray, may produce images of the chest that are richer in depth. Because it creates images containing bone, fat, muscles, and organs, a CT scan gives doctors a better view, which is essential to give the correct diagnosis.

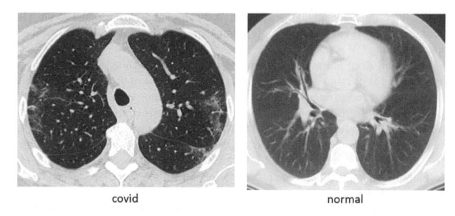

covid   normal

FIGURE 2.1   Images of CT scans for COVID-19 identification.

High-resolution and spiral CT scans are two varieties of chest CT scans. In a single revolution of the x-ray tube, the high-resolution chest CT scan can provide more than one slice, or image. In the spiral chest CT scan, a table travels in a circular motion through a passage that resembles a tunnel while an x-ray tube moves in a spiral motion. Spiral CTs produce a 3D image of the lungs, which is an advantage over the traditional CT. An example of CT scans for COVID-19 and normal lungs can be seen in Figure 2.1.

Important CT characteristics include ground-glass opacity (GGO), consolidation, reticulation or thickened interlobular septae, nodules, and lesion distribution (left, right, or bilateral lungs). In CT scans of patients with COVID-19 pneumonia, the most prominent characteristics are bilateral subpleural GGO and consolidation affecting the lower lobes [17, 18]. During the intermediate stage, which occurs between days 4 and 14 following the onset of symptoms, the crazy-paving pattern and the halo sign become essential if apparent. Even for seasoned radiologists, identifying disease symptoms is a time-consuming endeavor. Moreover, CV can automate this technique, reducing time and enhancing precision.

2.2.2   X-Ray Image

Radiography is a method of imaging that can be used to observe the inside structure of an object by employing x-rays, gamma rays, or other forms of comparable ionizing radiation and nonionizing radiation. Radiography has a variety of uses, particularly in the medical field, such as diagnostic and therapeutic radiography. In conventional radiography, a picture is formed by sending an x-ray beam that an x-ray generator creates in the target item's direction. The density and the structural makeup of the object play a role in the number of x-rays and other types of radiation that are absorbed by the object. A detector placed behind the object picks up any x-rays that make it through the object. This method generates two-dimensional (2D) images in a flat format, which is known as projection radiography. An x-ray source and the detectors that are associated with it rotate around the subject during a CT, while the subject itself moves through the conical x-ray beam that is produced.

At any one place within the subject, multiple distinct beams traveling at varying speeds will intersect that spot from a variety of directions. Information pertaining to the attenuation of these beams is collated and then calculated to provide 2D images in three planes (axial, coronal, and sagittal), which can then be further processed to construct a 3D image.

Ionizing and nonionizing radiation can be used to reveal the body's internal structure on an image receptor. This is done by emphasizing the differences between the substances that make up the body through attenuation, or ionizing radiation, through the absorption of x-ray photons by the denser substances (like calcium-rich bones). Radiographic anatomy is a subfield of anatomy that uses radiographic images to study human anatomy. The acquisition of images through medical radiography is often made by radiographers, whereas radiologists are typically responsible for performing image analysis. Image interpretation is a specialty that some radiographers have developed. Radiography in medicine encompasses various techniques that can generate many disparate kinds of images; each of these images can be utilized in a specific clinical setting.

One of the drawbacks of adopting CT imaging is the requirement for a high patient dose, which also increases expense. As a result, digital chest x-ray (CXR) radiography has become the imaging modality of choice for diagnosing chest pathology because of its reduced cost and wider availability. Computerized diagnosis of COVID-19 traits in a CXR is an extremely effective diagnostic tool in the fight against the disease [19, 20]. Different disorders, such as osteoporosis, cancer, and cardiovascular disease, can be diagnosed with the assistance of computer-aided diagnosis (CAD) using digital x-ray imagery. Enhancing contrast is a pre-processing step because it is extremely difficult to differentiate between different types of soft tissue when the x-ray image has a low contrast. Segmenting the lungs on CXRs is one of the most critical and vital steps to identify lung nodules. Several different segmentation procedures have been described in the medical literature. Image samples of chest x-ray for a COVID-19 and normal chest can be seen in Figure 2.2.

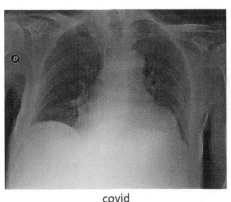
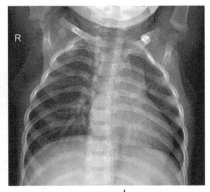

covid   normal

FIGURE 2.2   Images of a chest x-ray for COVID-19 identification.

Consolidation has been observed on CXR exams performed on COVID-19 patients. In a study conducted in Hong Kong, three patients were given daily CXRs [21]. Of these patients, two showed advancements in the lung consolidation over 3–4 days. CXR exams performed on subsequent days revealed an improvement in the patients' condition. Over 8 days, the third patient displayed no discernible pattern of change. On the other hand, a study that was quite similar to the previous one showed that the GGOs seen in the right lower lobe peripheral on the CT were not detectable on the chest radiograph that was done 1 hour after the first study [22]. CXR is still advised in conjunction with CT for improved radiological analysis. Several automated methods connected to CXR are currently under consideration.

2.3   DEEP LEARNING FOR COVID-19 IMAGE PROCESSING TASKS

2.3.1   CONVOLUTIONAL NEURAL NETWORKS

In deep learning, a convolutional neural network (CNN) is an artificial neural network (ANN) typically employed to evaluate visual pictures [23]. Contrary to common sense, most CNNs are equivariant rather than invariant to translation. In addition to image and video recognition, they can be utilized for recommender systems, image classification, image segmentation, medical image analysis, natural language processing, brain–computer interfaces, and financial time series. CNNs are regularized versions of multilayer perceptrons (MLPs).

Typically, when people talk about MLPs, they refer to completely linked networks; this means that every neuron in one layer is connected to all neurons in the following layer. These networks have a full connection, making it more likely to overfit the data. Regularization, also known as the prevention of overfitting, often involves either reducing connectivity or penalizing parameters during training (in the form of weight decay, for example, skipped connections, dropout, etc.). CNNs employ a distinct approach to regularization. They use the hierarchical pattern in the data and assemble increasingly complex patterns by embossing smaller and simpler patterns in their filters. In other words, CNNs take advantage of the hierarchical pattern in the data. As a result, they are located toward the bottom of the scale that measures connectedness and complexity. The architecture of CNN can be seen in Figure 2.3.

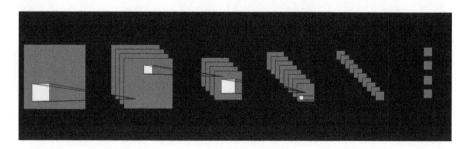

FIGURE 2.3   CNN architecture.

The connectivity pattern between neurons in CNNs is similar to the arrangement of the visual cortex in animal brains, which served as the source of inspiration for the design of these networks. The term "receptive field" refers to a certain part of the visual field that is the only one in which individual neurons in the cortex are able to respond to inputs. Because the receptive fields of several neurons partially overlap, it is possible to say that they cover the entire visual field. Compared with other image classification methods, CNNs require minimal preprocessing to function. This indicates that the network learns to optimize the filters (or kernels) through automatic learning, whereas in traditional methods these filters are hand-engineered. This is in contrast to the fact that the network learns to optimize the filters itself. One of the most significant benefits is that feature extraction can be done without requiring prior knowledge or the involvement of humans.

Based on CXR image categorization, a deep CNN architecture has been proposed for COVID-19 diagnosis. The experiment from Reshi et al. [19] showed a 99.5% overall accuracy for the suggested CNN model in the current application domain. Chakraborty et al. [24] classified COVID-19, pneumonia, and healthy cases using the pretrained VGG-19 architecture and transfer learning. The research achieved an accuracy of 97.11%, average precision of 97%, and average recall of 97% on a public dataset of 3797 x-ray pictures, including COVID-19 (1184), pneumonia (1294), and healthy images (1319). Many countries used containment and mitigation to battle COVID-19, but Dash et al. [25] removed the fully connected layers of a proven model VGG-16 and added a new simplified fully connected layer set with random weights on top of the CNN, which had already learned discriminative features such as edges, colors, geometric changes, shapes, and objects. To avoid damaging rich features, they warmed up the fully connected head by freezing all network layers, then unfreezing them to fine-tune. The suggested classification model identified COVID-19 with 97.12% accuracy, 99.2% sensitivity, and 99.6% specificity. Elaziz et al. [26] suggested classifying COVID-19 images using deep learning and swarm-based techniques.

CNN MobileNetV3 was used to extract relevant visual representations as a deep learning model. Experiments illustrated the proposed framework's strong classification accuracy and dimensionality reduction during feature extraction and selection. GoogleNet, a CNN architecture called Inception V1 for image classification, predicted COVID-19 from CXRs [27]. The model-classified photos which showed 99% training accuracy and 98.5% testing accuracy emphasized transfer learning models in illness prediction. Gour and Jain [28] proposed an uncertainty-aware CNN model, UA-ConvNet, for the automatic detection of COVID-19 disease from CXR pictures. The suggested method used a fine-tuned EfficientNetB3 model and Monte Carlo (MC) dropout. The proposed UA-ConvNet model obtained a G-mean of 98.02% confidence interval [CI]: 97.99–98.07, and a sensitivity of 98.15% on the COVID-19CXr dataset. The study from Heidari et al. [29] developed and tested a new CAD scheme of CXR images to detect COVID-19 pneumonia. Their research revealed that adding two image preprocessing steps and generating a pseudo-color picture played a crucial role in developing a deep learning CAD system for CXR images to improve pneumonia detection. By classifying three classes, the CNN-based CAD scheme achieves an overall accuracy of 94.5% (2404/2544) with a 95%

CI: 0.93–0.96]. Another study used CNN with many architectures to detect COVID-19 disease from CXR images. Hira et al. [30] employed nine CNN-based architectures (AlexNet, GoogleNet, ResNet-50, Se-ResNet-50, DenseNet121, Inception V4, Inception ResNet V2, ResNeXt-50, and Se-ResNeXt-50). Experimental results showed that the pre-trained model Se-ResNeXt-50 has the highest binary and multi-class classification accuracy. In addition to using CXR data, there was also research on the classification of COVID-19 by CNN using CT scan data. Based on research conducted by Feng et al. [31], COVIDx-classification CT's accuracy is 96.7%, which is greater than CNN (ResNet-152) and Transformer (Deit-B) (95.2% and 75.8%, respectively). Jia et al. [32] combined CXR and CT data using a MobileNet-modified CNN. The proposed approaches achieved 99.6% test accuracy on the five-category CXR dataset and 99.3% on the CT dataset.

2.3.2 GENERATIVE ADVERSARIAL NETWORKS

In June 2014, Ian Goodfellow and colleagues came up with the concept for a class of machine learning frameworks called generative adversarial networks (GANs). This method learns to produce new data with the same statistics as the training set when it is provided with a training set as input. For instance, a GAN trained on images can produce new photographs that, at least to human observers, appear to be superficially legitimate and have many realistic properties [33, 34]. GANs were first proposed as a form of generative model for unsupervised learning; however, they have been shown to be helpful for other types of learning, including semi-supervised learning, fully supervised learning, and reinforcement learning. The fundamental concept of a GAN is built on the concept of "indirect" training through the discriminator, which is another neural network that is able to determine the degree to which an input is "realistic." This neural network is also dynamically updated. This simply indicates that the generator is not trained to minimize the distance to a particular image; rather, it is trained to deceive the discriminator into thinking that the image is closer than it actually is. Because of this, the model is able to learn in a way that is not supervised. In evolutionary biology, mimicry is analogous to GANs, and both types of networks engage in an evolutionary arms race with one another. The architecture of GAN can be seen in Figure 2.4.

While the discriminative network assesses the candidates, the generative network creates new potential candidates. The competition is run according to the distribution of data. In most cases, the discriminative network is responsible for separating

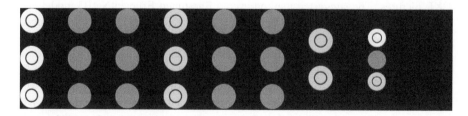

FIGURE 2.4   GAN architecture.

candidates that were produced by the generator from the actual data distribution, whereas the generative network is responsible for learning how to map from a latent space to a data distribution of interest. The goal of the training for the generative network is to enhance the error rate of the discriminative network by providing unique candidates that it believes are not synthesized. The initial training data for the discriminator is taken from an already known dataset. Training requires providing it with examples taken from the dataset that it will use and continue to use until it reaches an acceptable level of accuracy. The generator will improve its performance depending on how well it can trick the discriminator.

In most cases, the generator is "seeded" with random input that is taken from a predetermined latent space (e.g., a multivariate normal distribution). The discriminator will next make judgments based on the candidates that were generated. Both networks undergo their own unique backpropagation techniques so that the generator can produce higher quality samples and the discriminator may become more adept at identifying synthetic samples. When a neural network is used to generate images, the discriminator is often a CNN, but the generator is typically a deconvolutional neural network (DNN).

GANs frequently experience what is known as mode collapse, which is when they fail to generalize correctly and leave out entire modes from the input data. For instance, a GAN trained on the MNIST dataset, which has many examples of each digit, may be too hesitant to include a portion of those digits in its output. While some researchers believe that an insufficiently discriminative network is at fault for the issue because it fails to recognize the pattern of omission, others believe that a poor selection of objective function is to blame. There are many potential answers to this problem. There is currently no solution to the issue of GAN convergence. GANs are examples of implicit generative models. They do not explicitly model the likelihood function nor provide a means for finding the latent variable corresponding to a given sample. This contrasts with other models, such as the flow-based generative model, which is an example of an explicit generative model.

Using GAN, researchers improved COVID-19 detection data. Waheed et al. [35] developed an auxiliary classifier GAN model dubbed CovidGAN to generate synthetic CXR images with 95% accuracy compared with CNN's 85% accuracy. Shah et al. [36], using deep convolutional GAN, generated synthetic images for all classes (Normal, Pneumonia, and COVID-19). The trained EfficientNetB4 used the generated dataset. The experiments achieved 95% area under the curve (AUC) to validate that their network had learned lung x-ray features used Grad-CAM to visualize the underlying pattern. GAN for Enhancing Automated COVID-19 Chest X-Ray Diagnosis by Image-to-Image GAN Translation was another comparable study by Liang et al. [37]. His research concluded that the GAN-based data enhancement technique is appropriate for most medical image pattern recognition tasks and solves the typical expertise reliance issue in the medical arena with 97.8% classification accuracy. COVID-19 detection research can also be done with deep transfer learning on a restricted dataset. Khalifa et al. [38] found that GAN improves the proposed model's robustness, makes it immune to overfitting, and generates more images from the dataset. Using GAN and deep transfer models confirmed its accuracy. The research showed that ResNet-18 is the best deep transfer model based on testing accuracy and obtained 99% in precision, recall, and F1 score while utilizing GAN as an image augmenter. Mehta and Mehendale [39] researched COVID-19, pneumonia, and tuberculosis utilizing GAN with fine-tuned deep transfer learning models. The suggested model achieved 98.20% training and 94.21% validation accuracy. The GAN models helped enhance the training dataset and reduce overfitting.

2.3.3 MULTILAYER PERCEPTRONS

An ANN that belongs to the feedforward type is known as a multilayer perceptron (MLP) [40, 41]. A minimum of three layers of nodes is required to construct an MLP. These are referred to as the input, hidden, and output layers. Every node in the network is a neuron that employs a nonlinear activation function, except for the nodes that serve as inputs. Training in MLP is accomplished with a supervised learning method known as backpropagation. Compared with a linear perceptron, an MLP is distinguished by its nonlinear activation and numerous layers. It can differentiate between data that cannot be separated linearly.

The MLP was once employed in CV, but the CNN has since replaced it. MLP is no longer considered adequate for performing complex CV tasks. It has fully connected layers, meaning that each perceptron is linked to every other perceptron in the network. One potential drawback is that there may be an excessively high number of total parameters. Because there is duplication in such high dimensions, this approach is inefficient. It also does not consider any information about the surrounding space. As inputs, it accepts vectors that have been flattened. The architecture of MLP can be seen in Figure 2.5.

During the COVID-19 outbreak, masks in public were regulated. Using a camera and a detection algorithm, the entrance of a venue or a building determined whether or not someone is wearing a mask. MLP research classifies mask use with 83.85% accuracy [42]. Apart from being independent, using MLP for COVID-19 image classification is often combined with other methods. In research conducted by Rajasekar et al. [43], hybrid MLP and CNN were proposed to detect COVID-19 in CT scans. CNN extracts features and MLP classifies. This hybrid model was 94.89% accurate compared with CNN and MLPs (86.95 and 80.7%, respectively). Hybrid MLP and CNN were also used for COVID-19 image classification in CXRs with

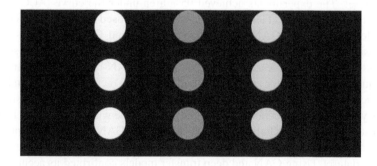

FIGURE 2.5 MLP architecture.

three different optimizations: Adam, SGD, and RMSprop [44]. A model trained with Adam can distinguish COVID-19 and non-COVID-19 patients with 96.3% accuracy.

2.3.4 DEEP BELIEF NETWORKS

Deep belief networks (DBNs) are generative graphical models or a class of deep neural networks employed in machine learning. They consist of many layers of latent variables, also referred to as hidden units, and contain linkages between the layers but not between the units included inside each layer [45, 46]. A DBN can learn to probabilistically reconstruct its inputs after being trained on a set of examples without any human intervention. Following this, the layers operate as feature detectors. A DBN may continue training under the supervision of an instructor to perform classification after completing this part of the learning process. DBNs can be viewed as a combination of simple, unsupervised networks, such as restricted Boltzmann machines (RBMs) or autoencoders, in which the hidden layer of one subnetwork serves as the visible layer for the next subnetwork in the chain. An RBM is an undirected and generative energy-based model. It consists of a visible input layer, a hidden layer, and connections between the layers but not inside the layers themselves. This composition results in a layer-by-layer, unsupervised training method that is executed rapidly. In this procedure, contrastive divergence is applied to each subnetwork in turn, beginning with the "lowest" pair of layers. One of the earliest successful deep learning algorithms was developed because of the discovery that DBN may be taught greedily, one layer at a time. In general, there are numerous appealing applications and uses of DBNs in real-life scenarios and applications, and this trend is expected to continue (e.g., electroencephalography and drug discovery). The architecture of DBN can be seen in Figure 2.6.

Abdulrahman and Salem [47] used DBN for detection of COVID-19, and the results showed that the proposed system identifies the COVID-19 cases with an accuracy of 90%. Vidhya et al. [48] classified COVID-19 for diabetics. The study examined the effects of COVID-19 on diabetic patients with the most prevalent COVID-19 indications and diabetes well-being characteristics using DBN, resulting in 98.86% accuracy during training and 97.81% accuracy during validation. DBN also works together to reach other algorithms to classify COVID-19 images. Mohammed et al. [49] employed a Corner-based Weber Local Descriptor (CWLD) for COVID-19 CXR

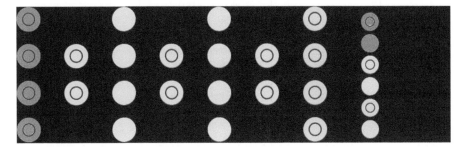

FIGURE 2.6 Deep belief network (DBN) architecture.

image analysis diagnostics. The Weber differential excitation and gradient orientation histogram was proposed to depict CXR image patterns. CWLD used DBN classifiers. Experiments on a genuine CXR database demonstrated that gradient orientation delivers 100% accuracy using the DBN classifier and CWLD size of 400. Gumpala et al. [50] conducted a study using a DBN whose hyperparameters were tuned using the cuckoo optimization algorithm. The results of his research showed 28.3 and 23.5% higher accuracy for Normal as well as 32.3 and 31.5% for COVID-19, 19.3 and 28.5% higher precision for Normal and 45.3 and 28.5% for COVID-19, 20.3 and 21.5% higher F1 score for Normal, and 40.3 and 21.5% for COVID-19. Govindharaju et al. [51] suggested a hybrid technique employing VGG-16 and DBN for feature extraction, classification, and prediction. Average classification accuracy, specificity, and sensitivity were 98.1, 98.6, and 98.3%, whereas multi-classification prediction rates were 98.6, 99.1, and 98.7%.

In general, a number of different deep learning approaches can be utilized in order to complete the COVID-19 image processing task. Table 2.1 provides a summary of deep learning applications, along with an analysis of their respective advantages and disadvantages.

TABLE 2.1

Summary of Deep Learning Applications and Their Advantages and Disadvantages

Method	Difference	Advantages	Disadvantages
CNN	• CNN is effective with 2D data [52] • Filters are utilized to transform 2D to 3D [52]	• The rapid learning model boosts performance [52, 53] • The capacity to internally depict a 2D image. This helps the model to learn the position and size of different data structures, which is crucial when working with images [54] • Pooling, a concept that makes CNN more resilient to changes in the position of the image feature, enables CNN to identify the identical pattern even if the item is slightly rotated or tilted [55]	• Numerous labeled data are necessary for image classification [52] • CNN does not encode the object's position and orientation [56]

(Continued)

TABLE 2.1 *(Continued)*

Summary of Deep Learning Applications and Their Advantages and Disadvantages

Method	Difference	Advantages	Disadvantages
MLP	• MLP employs one perceptron per input (e.g., pixel in an image), thus the number of weights quickly becomes unmanageable for huge images [57]	• They are highly adaptable and might be utilized generally to discover a mapping between inputs and outputs [58] • The pixels of an image can be condensed into a single data column and fed into an MLP [59]	• Consequently causing redundancy and inefficiency [60] • Difficulties develop during training, and overfitting might lead to a loss of generalizability [61] • MLPs respond differently to an input (image) and its translation; they are not translation invariant [62] • In an MLP, spatial information is lost when a picture is flattened (matrix to vector) [63]
GAN	• GANs are unsupervised; therefore, training them does not require labeled data [64]	• Extremely outstanding outcome in terms of generated material and realistic visual content [65] • Does not require additional preprocessing [66] • Can be modeled for image restoration and other applications [67]	• The model parameters oscillate, destabilize, and never converge [68] • Mode collapse: the generator fails, resulting in restricted sample variety [69] • Reduced gradient: the discriminator becomes so successful that the gradient of the generator vanishes and no new information is learned [70]

(Continued)

TABLE 2.1   *(Continued)*

Summary of Deep Learning Applications and Their Advantages and Disadvantages

Method	Difference	Advantages	Disadvantages
DBN	• DBN is employed for supervised and unsupervised learning [52] • Hidden layers function as visible layers for subsequent layers [52]	• DBN has specific classification robustness (size, position, color, view angle – rotation) [71] • DBN is efficient in the usage of hidden layers (higher performance gain by adding layers compared with MLP) [72] • Each layer employs a greedy method, and tractable inferences maximize the likelihood directly [52]	• Computational process initialization is expensive [73] • DBN has hardware specifications [74]

2.4   APPLICATIONS IN COVID-19

2.4.1   DIAGNOSIS

Within the context of the COVID-19 literature, the terms "detection" and "diagnosis" are frequently used interchangeably. On the other hand, the term "detection" is used differently in CV because this operation entails localizing an item. The image's object shape determines whether a bounding box (such as a rectangle, square, or contour) or interactive colors (heat maps) will be used to accomplish localization. This section focuses on approaches specifically specialized to identify COVID-19 and autonomously explore infected lung regions. However, we have noticed that only a relatively modest proportion of research articles have investigated CV-based detection for COVID-19 diagnosis. To cover a broader selection of relevant research, it included diagnostic approaches in which regions of interest (ROIs) or lesions are localized using contours, heat maps, bounding boxes, or interactive colors. These hybrid approaches, which also use graphical predictions, take segmentation and classification processes into account (heats maps, contours, or bounding boxes).

2.4.2   PREVENTION AND CONTROL

Guidelines for Infection Prevention and Control (IPC) strategies can be found on the WHO website. Coronavirus prevention aims to reduce the virus's spread in healthcare facilities through early detection and isolation of infectious sources, implementation of universal precautions for all patients, administrative and mana-gerial controls, and environmental and engineering safeguards. CV can help the implementation of IPC strategies.

The most common action to prevent any virus from spreading is using a mask. In the early stages of the progression of a disease, the use of masks and other personal protective equipment is an important technique for limiting the virus's transmission. During the COVID-19 pandemic, the use of masks as a disease control tool was applied in a number of different countries. The utilization of CV systems can signifi-cantly ease the process of its deployment.

With a dataset including only masked face photos, a masked face recognition method based on a multi-granularity masked face recognition model was 95% accu-rate. For research reasons, three distinct types of masked face datasets were made available to the public. The Masked Face Detection Dataset (MFDD) was trained and served as the foundation for the masked identification model. The Real-world Masked Face Recognition Dataset (RMFRD) was the largest masked face dataset in the world, consisting of 50,000 images of 525 people wearing masks and 90,000 photos of the same 525 people without masks. The sample image from the RMFRD dataset can be seen in Figure 2.7. On the other hand, the Simulated Masked Face Recognition Dataset (SMFRD) consisted of 500,000 photos of 10,000 distinct individuals.

Infrared thermography was a method of early detection used to identify peo-ple infected with COVID-19 as in Figure 2.8. This method was primarily utilized in public settings like airports and shopping malls. Infrared thermography widely applies to various medical purposes, including monitoring a patient's temperature. The utilization of a mobile platform for the purpose of performing an automatic fever screening based on the infrared temperature of the forehead is one technique. Systems that applied thermography and charge-coupled device (CCD) cameras for noncontact readings of vital signs can do infection screening with the help of feature

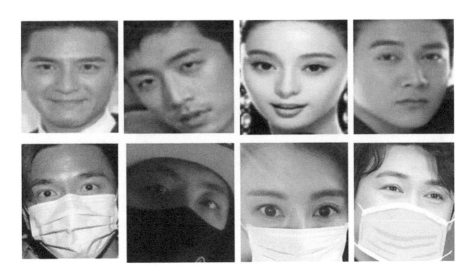

FIGURE 2.7   Images from RMFRD dataset: face images with and without a mask.

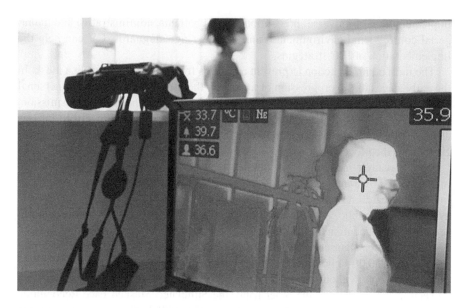

FIGURE 2.8   Infrared thermography application.

matching and MUSIC algorithms. The use of CV systems for fever screening in conjunction with thermography stations at entrances presented an opportunity for earlier Severe Acute Respiratory Syndrome (SARS) transmission control.

Moreover, pandemic drones designed specifically to combat and prevent pandemics were put into action as in Figure 2.9. Drones employed remote sensing and digital imaging to determine who in a population was infected. In the past, these kinds of technologies had been utilized in emergency management for remote monitoring of

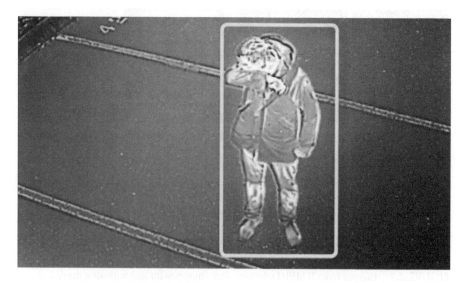

FIGURE 2.9   Pandemic drone application.

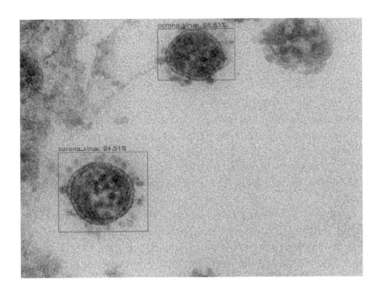

FIGURE 2.10   COVID-19 virus.

vital signs. One other application that was comparable to this is vision-guided robot control for 3D object detection. It is equipped with various sensors and cameras designed to detect potential health risks, such as symptoms of infectious diseases, in crowds. These drones can be used to monitor areas in which large groups of people gather, such as airports, train stations, and public events.

Germ scanning is possible as a weapon against COVID-19. A CNN for germ scanning, which includes the detection of bacteria using light-sheet microscopy image data as in Figure 2.10, obtained an accuracy of more than 90%. This process uses a particular technology to detect the presence of bacteria, viruses, or other microorganisms on surfaces, in the air, or on objects. This process is often used in healthcare settings, such as hospitals or clinics, to identify areas or items that contaminated with harmful pathogens. Machine learning can help identify potential sources of infection and enable healthcare professionals to take appropriate steps to prevent the spread of disease.

2.4.3   CLINICAL MANAGEMENT AND TREATMENT

There is no one-size-fits-all treatment available for the COVID-19 virus. On the other hand, several symptoms of the disease are treatable. Thus, the treatment is contingent on determining the patient's clinical status. Disease progression reflects the natural history of an illness: pain or a biomarker of therapeutic response such as blood pressure. The classification of patients according to the severity of their condition is one way that clinical treatment procedures can be made more effective. CV can be used by clinical institutions, for example, to identify individuals who are seriously ill and focus medical care toward them (critical patient screening).

The various types of afflicted individuals can be characterized using a score that quantifies the progression of the disease. The score is established using CT scan–derived assessments of polluted regions. This enables the measurement of patients' progress over time and the identification of those in the most critical state.

It has been demonstrated that depth cameras and deep learning can be utilized as a classifier for atypical respiratory patterns to carry out large-scale, accurate, and unobtrusive screenings for persons infected with the COVID-19 virus. The Respiratory Simulation Model (RSM) was initially projected to close the informational gap between the abundant training data and the limited real-world data.

Researchers have discovered that people infected with COVID-19 have a faster breathing rate. Considering this, the model uses a gated recurrent unit (GRU) neural network to classify six clinically relevant breathing patterns to identify severely unwell individuals. The program has an accuracy of 94.5% in classifying different breathing patterns.

Moreover, by adding 360-degree images of different chemical conformations into deep learning, the deep feature representation learning technique can be utilized for quantitative structure-activity relationship (QSAR) analysis. Deep learning, which is based on a unique method for the input of molecular images, can be used for QSAR analysis. This type of analysis can be applied to drug discovery, which can help assist the creation of vaccines.

2.5   CONCLUSION AND FUTURE DIRECTIONS

It is encouraging that the community working on CV research was called upon to help and played an important role in the COVID-19 pandemic. Data were gathered and disseminated in a relatively short period of time, and researchers presented a number of different strategies to address a variety of issues pertaining to disease control. Recent advances in the fields of deep learning and artificial intelligence have made CV a reality. Web repositories have contributed to the increased speed with which information is exchanged. However, due to a lack of scientific testing, objective evaluation, and sufficient imaging datasets, the relevance of this scientific study is restricted.

The research landscape presented during COVID-19 is fairly extensive, covering a wider range of topics than imaging and going outside the purview of CV research. The majority of research efforts focus on the problem of disease diagnosis, and because multiple performance indicators are being used and no clinical trials are being conducted, it is difficult to compare how well different methods function.

Since the beginning of the pandemic, numerous research datasets have been made available for further scientific investigation. Nevertheless, these datasets can only provide a restricted breadth and issue domains to work with. For the evolution of an illness, for instance, it is common practice to request many photos pertaining to a single patient together with the timeline. In a similar vein, to analyze several imaging modes, researchers require multimodal imaging data associated with the same patient, which is currently unavailable for use in research. Future work needs to include conducting an objective performance comparison of various methods, as well as collecting and benchmarking a large universal dataset.

REFERENCES

1. WHO, "Coronavirus disease (COVID-19) pandemic," 2020.
2. T. P. Velavan, and C. G. Meyer, "The COVID-19 epidemic," *Trop. Med. Int. Health.*, vol. 25, no. 3, pp. 278–280, 2020, doi: 10.1111/tmi.13383.
3. T. K. Koley, and M. Dhole, *The COVID-19 Pandemic*, London: Routledge India, 2020.
4. A. Esteva et al., "Deep learning-enabled medical computer vision," *NPJ Digit. Med.*, vol. 4, no. 1, p. 5, Dec. 2021, doi: 10.1038/s41746-020-00376-2.
5. A. Voulodimos, N. Doulamis, A. Doulamis, and E. Protopapadakis, "Deep learning for computer vision: A brief review," *Comput. Intell. Neurosci.*, vol. 2018, pp. 1–13, 2018, doi: 10.1155/2018/7068349.
6. R. Szeliski, *Computer Vision: Algorithms and Applications*, Springer Science & Business Media, 2010.
7. D. Forsyth, and J. Ponce, *Computer Vision: A Modern Approach*, 2nd edition, London, Dordrecht, Heidelberg, New York, NY: Springer, 2011.
8. Y. LeCun, Y. Bengio, and G. Hinton, "Deep learning," *Nature*, vol. 521, no. 7553, pp. 436–444, 2015, doi: 10.1038/nature14539.
9. C. Gonzalez Viejo, S. Fuentes, K. Howell, D. Torrico, and F. R. Dunshea, "Robotics and computer vision techniques combined with non-invasive consumer biometrics to assess quality traits from beer foamability using machine learning: A potential for artificial intelligence applications," *Food Control*, vol. 92, pp. 72–79, Oct. 2018, doi: 10.1016/j.foodcont.2018.04.037.
10. J. Janai, F. Güney, A. Behl, and A. Geiger, "Computer vision for autonomous vehicles: Problems, datasets and state of the art," *Found. Trends® Comput. Graph. Vis.*, vol. 12, no. 1–3, pp. 1–308, 2020, doi: 10.1561/0600000079.
11. L. Zhou, L. Zhang, and N. Konz, "Computer vision techniques in manufacturing," *IEEE Trans. Syst. Man, Cybern. Syst.*, pp. 1–13, 2022, doi: 10.1109/TSMC.2022.3166397.
12. D. I. Patrício, and R. Rieder, "Computer vision and artificial intelligence in precision agriculture for grain crops: A systematic review," *Comput. Electron. Agric.*, vol. 153, pp. 69–81, Oct. 2018, doi: 10.1016/j.compag.2018.08.001.
13. A. Esteva et al., "A guide to deep learning in healthcare," *Nat. Med.*, vol. 25, no. 1, pp. 24–29, Jan. 2019, doi: 10.1038/s41591-018-0316-z.
14. B. Zeeshan Hameed, V. Patil, D. Shetty, N. Naik, N. Nagaraj, and D. Sharma, "Use of artificial intelligence-based computer vision system to practice social distancing in hospitals to prevent transmission of COVID-19," *Indian J. Community Med.*, vol. 45, no. 3, p. 379, 2020, doi: 10.4103/ijcm.IJCM_366_20.
15. A. Ulhaq, J. Born, A. Khan, D. P. S. Gomes, S. Chakraborty, and M. Paul, "COVID-19 control by computer vision approaches: A survey," *IEEE Access*, vol. 8, pp. 179437–179456, 2020, doi: 10.1109/ACCESS.2020.3027685.
16. D. Khemasuwan, J. S. Sorensen, and H. G. Colt, "Artificial intelligence in pulmonary medicine: Computer vision, predictive model and COVID-19," *Eur. Respir. Rev.*, vol. 29, no. 157, p. 200181, 2020, doi: 10.1183/16000617.0181-2020.
17. P. Afshar et al., "COVID-CT-MD, COVID-19 computed tomography scan dataset applicable in machine learning and deep learning," *Sci. Data*, vol. 8, no. 1, p. 121, Dec. 2021, doi: 10.1038/s41597-021-00900-3.
18. L. Zieleskiewicz et al., "Comparative study of lung ultrasound and chest computed tomography scan in the assessment of severity of confirmed COVID-19 pneumonia," *Intensive Care Med.*, vol. 46, no. 9, pp. 1707–1713, Sep. 2020, doi: 10.1007/s00134-020-06186-0.
19. A. A. Reshi et al., "An efficient CNN model for COVID-19 disease detection based on X-ray image classification," *Complexity*, vol. 2021, pp. 1–12, May 2021, doi: 10.1155/2021/6621607.

20. S. Hassantabar, M. Ahmadi, and A. Sharifi, "Diagnosis and detection of infected tissue of COVID-19 patients based on lung X-ray image using convolutional neural network approaches," *Chaos Solitons Fractals*, vol. 140, p. 110170, Nov. 2020, doi: 10.1016/j.chaos.2020.110170.

21. M.-Y. Ng et al., "Imaging profile of the COVID-19 infection: Radiologic findings and literature review," *Radiol. Cardiothorac. Imaging*, vol. 2, no. 1, p. e200034, Feb. 2020, doi: 10.1148/ryct.2020200034.

22. H. Abdolrahimzadeh Fard et al., "Comparison of chest CT scan findings between COVID-19 and pulmonary contusion in trauma patients based on RSNA criteria: Established novel criteria for trauma victims," *Chinese J. Traumatol.-- English Ed.*, vol. 25, no. 3, pp. 170–176, 2022, doi: 10.1016/j.cjtee.2022.01.004.

23. L. Alzubaidi et al., "Review of deep learning: Concepts, CNN architectures, challenges, applications, future directions," *J. Big Data*, vol. 8, no. 1, p. 53, Dec. 2021, doi: 10.1186/s40537-021-00444-8.

24. S. Chakraborty, S. Paul, and K. M. A. Hasan, "A transfer learning-based approach with deep CNN for COVID-19- and pneumonia-affected chest X-ray image classification," *SN Comput. Sci.*, vol. 3, no. 1, p. 17, 2022, doi: 10.1007/s42979-021-00881-5.

25. A. K. Dash, and P. Mohapatra, "A fine-tuned deep convolutional neural network for chest radiography image classification on COVID-19 cases," *Multimed. Tools Appl.*, vol. 81, no. 1, pp. 1055–1075, 2022, doi: 10.1007/s11042-021-11388-9.

26. M. Abd Elaziz, A. Dahou, N. A. Alsaleh, A. H. Elsheikh, A. I. Saba, and M. Ahmadein, "Boosting COVID-19 image classification using MobileNetV3 and aquila optimizer algorithm," *Entropy*, vol. 23, no. 11, p. 1383, 2021, doi: 10.3390/e23111383.

27. D. Haritha, N. Swaroop, and M. Mounika, "Prediction of COVID-19 cases using CNN with X-rays," *2020 5th International Conference on Computing, Communication and Security (ICCCS)*, Oct. 2020, pp. 1–6, doi: 10.1109/ICCCS49678.2020.9276753.

28. M. Gour, and S. Jain, "Uncertainty-aware convolutional neural network for COVID-19 X-ray images classification," *Comput. Biol. Med.*, vol. 140, p. 105047, Jan. 2022, doi: 10.1016/j.compbiomed.2021.105047.

29. M. Heidari, S. Mirniaharikandehei, A. Z. Khuzani, G. Danala, Y. Qiu, and B. Zheng, "Improving the performance of CNN to predict the likelihood of COVID-19 using chest X-ray images with preprocessing algorithms," *Int. J. Med. Inform.*, vol. 144, p. 104284, Dec. 2020, doi: 10.1016/j.ijmedinf.2020.104284.

30. S. Hira, A. Bai, and S. Hira, "An automatic approach based on CNN architecture to detect covid-19 disease from chest X-ray images," *Appl. Intell.*, vol. 51, no. 5, pp. 2864–2889, 2021, doi: 10.1007/s10489-020-02010-w.

31. X. Fan, X. Feng, Y. Dong, and H. Hou, "COVID-19 CT image recognition algorithm based on transformer and CNN," *Displays*, vol. 72, p. 102150, Apr. 2022, doi: 10.1016/j.displa.2022.102150.

32. G. Jia, H.-K. Lam, and Y. Xu, "Classification of COVID-19 chest X-ray and CT images using a type of dynamic CNN modification method," *Comput. Biol. Med.*, vol. 134, p. 104425, Jul. 2021, doi: 10.1016/j.compbiomed.2021.104425.

33. X. Yi, E. Walia, and P. Babyn, "Generative adversarial network in medical imaging: A review," *Med. Image Anal.*, vol. 58, p. 101552, Dec. 2019, doi: 10.1016/j.media.2019.101552.

34. A. Aggarwal, M. Mittal, and G. Battineni, "Generative adversarial network: An overview of theory and applications," *Int. J. Inf. Manag. Data Insights*, vol. 1, no. 1, p. 100004, 2021, doi: 10.1016/j.jjimei.2020.100004.

35. A. Waheed, M. Goyal, D. Gupta, A. Khanna, F. Al-Turjman, and P. R. Pinheiro, "CovidGAN: Data augmentation using auxiliary classifier GAN for improved COVID-19 detection," *IEEE Access*, vol. 8, pp. 91916–91923, 2020, doi: 10.1109/ACCESS.2020.2994762.

36. P. M. Shah et al., "DC-GAN-based synthetic X-ray images augmentation for increasing the performance of efficient net for COVID-19 detection," *Expert Syst.*, vol. 39, no. 3, Mar. 2022, doi: 10.1111/exsy.12823.

37. Z. Liang, J. X. Huang, J. Li, and S. Chan, "Enhancing automated COVID-19 chest X-ray diagnosis by image-to-image GAN translation," *2020 IEEE International Conference on Bioinformatics and Biomedicine (BIBM)*, Dec. 2020, pp. 1068–1071, doi: 10.1109/BIBM49941.2020.9313466.

38. P. M. Shah *et al.*, "DC-GAN-based synthetic X-ray images augmentation for increasing the performance of EfficientNet for COVID-19 detection," *Expert Syst.*, vol. 39, no. 3, Mar. 2022, doi: 10.1111/exsy.12823.

39. T. Mehta, and N. Mehendale, "Classification of X-ray images into COVID-19, pneumonia, and TB using cGAN and fine-tuned deep transfer learning models," *Res. Biomed. Eng.*, vol. 37, no. 4, pp. 803–813, 2021, doi: 10.1007/s42600-021-00174-z.

40. A. Rana, A. Singh Rawat, A. Bijalwan, and H. Bahuguna, "Application of multi-layer (Perceptron) artificial neural network in the diagnosis system: A systematic review," *2018 International Conference on Research in Intelligent and Computing in Engineering (RICE)*, Aug. 2018, pp. 1–6, doi: 10.1109/RICE.2018.8509069.

41. H. Taud, and J. F. Mas, "Multilayer perceptron (MLP)," in *Geomatic Approaches for Modeling Land Change Scenarios*, M. Camacho Olmedo, M. Paegelow, J. Mas, and F. Escobar, Eds. Springer, 2018, pp. 451–455.

42. T. Ladić, and A. Mandekić, "Face mask classification using MLP classifier," *Student Scientific Conference RiSTEM 2021*, 2021, pp. 77–80.

43. S. J. S. Rajasekar, V. Narayanan, and V. Perumal, "Detection of COVID-19 from chest CT images using CNN with MLP hybrid model," *Stud Heal. Technol Inf.*, Oct. 2021, doi: 10.3233/SHTI210617.

44. M. M. Ahsan, T. E. Alam, T. Trafalis, and P. Huebner, "Deep MLP-CNN model using mixed-data to distinguish between COVID-19 and non-COVID-19 patients," *Symmetry (Basel)*, vol. 12, no. 9, p. 1526, 2020, doi: 10.3390/sym12091526.

45. M. Kaur, and D. Singh, "Fusion of medical images using deep belief networks," *Cluster Comput.*, vol. 23, no. 2, pp. 1439–1453, 2020, doi: 10.1007/s10586-019-02999-x.

46. Y. Rizk, N. Hajj, N. Mitri, and M. Awad, "Deep belief networks and cortical algorithms: A comparative study for supervised classification," *Appl. Comput. Informatics*, vol. 15, no. 2, pp. 81–93, 2019, doi: 10.1016/j.aci.2018.01.004.

47. S. A. Abdulrahma, and A.-B. M. Salem, "An efficient deep belief network for detection of coronavirus disease COVID-19," *Fusion Pract. Appl.*, vol. 2, no. 1, pp. 05–13, 2020, doi: 10.54216/fpa.020102.

48. K. Vidhya, V. Rasikha, T. C. Kumar, and S. Fowajiya, "Deep belief network (DBN) approach for classification of COVID-19 impact on people with diabetes," *Turkish Online J. Qual. Inq.*, vol. 12, no. 3, pp. 28–40, 2021.

49. S. N. Mohammed, A. K. Abdul Hassan, and H. M. Rada, "COVID-19 diagnostics from the chest x-ray image using corner-based weber local descriptor," in *Studies in Big Data*, Springer Cham,, 2020, pp. 131–145.

50. V. Gampala, K. Rathan, C. N. S, F. H. Shajin, and P. Rajesh, "Diagnosis of COVID-19 patients by adapting hyperparameter tuned deep belief network using hosted cuckoo optimization algorithm," *Electromagn. Biol. Med.*, vol. 41, no. 3, pp. 257–271, 2022, doi: 10.1080/15368378.2022.2065679.

51. A. M., K. Govindharaju, J. A., S. Mohan, A. Ahmadian, and T. Ciano, "A hybrid learning approach for the stage-wise classification and prediction of COVID-19 X-ray images," *Expert Syst.*, vol. 39, no. 4, May 2022, doi: 10.1111/exsy.12884.

52. R. Selvanambi, J. Natarajan, M. Karuppiah, S. H. Islam, M. M. Hassan, and G. Fortino, "Lung cancer prediction using higher-order recurrent neural network based on

glowworm swarm optimization," *Neural Comput. Appl.*, vol. 32, no. 9, pp. 4373–4386, 2020, doi: 10.1007/s00521-018-3824-3.

53. Y. Ning, S. He, Z. Wu, C. Xing, and L.-J. Zhang, "A review of deep learning based speech synthesis," *Appl. Sci.*, vol. 9, no. 19, p. 4050, 2019, doi: 10.3390/app9194050.

54. A. Geetha, and P. Sharmila, "Advanced driver assistance system using convolutional neural network," *Turkish J. Comput. Math. Educ.*, vol. 12, no. 2, pp. 896–905, Apr. 2021, doi: 10.17762/turcomat.v12i2.1098.

55. S. Bharati, P. Podder, and M. R. H. Mondal, "Hybrid deep learning for detecting lung diseases from X-ray images," *Informatics Med. Unlocked*, vol. 20, p. 100391, 2020, doi: 10.1016/j.imu.2020.100391.

56. G. Merlin Linda, N. V. S. Sree Rathna Lakshmi, N. S. Murugan, R. P. Mahapatra, V. Muthukumaran, and M. Sivaram, "Intelligent recognition system for viewpoint variations on gait and speech using CNN-CapsNet," *Int. J. Intell. Comput. Cybern*, vol. 15, no. 3, pp. 363–382, 2022, doi: 10.1108/IJICC-08-2021-0178.

57. G. V. Sivanarayana, K. Naveen Kumar, Y. Srinivas, and G. V. S. Raj Kumar, "Review on the methodologies for image segmentation based on CNN," in *Communication Software and Networks, Lecture Notes in Networks and Systems*, 2021, pp. 165–175.

58. O. Odebiri, J. Odindi, and O. Mutanga, "Basic and deep learning models in remote sensing of soil organic carbon estimation: A brief review," *Int. J. Appl. Earth Obs. Geoinf.*, vol. 102, p. 102389, Oct. 2021, doi: 10.1016/j.jag.2021.102389.

59. K. T. Butler, M. D. Le, J. Thiyagalingam, and T. G. Perring, "Interpretable, calibrated neural networks for analysis and understanding of inelastic neutron scattering data," *J. Phys. Condens. Matter*, vol. 33, no. 19, p. 194006, 2021, doi: 10.1088/1361-648X/abea1c.

60. Y. Zeng, X. Wang, J. Yuan, J. Zhang, and J. Wan, "Local epochs inefficiency caused by device heterogeneity in federated learning," *Wirel. Commun. Mob. Comput.*, vol. 2022, pp. 1–15, Jan. 2022, doi: 10.1155/2022/6887040.

61. M. B. Mayhew et al., "A generalizable 29-mRNA neural-network classifier for acute bacterial and viral infections," *Nat. Commun.*, vol. 11, no. 1, p. 1177, Dec. 2020, doi: 10.1038/s41467-020-14975-w.

62. A. Khotanzad, and J.-H. Lu, "Classification of invariant image representations using a neural network," *IEEE Trans. Acoust.*, vol. 38, no. 6, pp. 1028–1038, 1990, doi: 10.1109/29.56063.

63. W. R. Moskolaï, W. Abdou, A. Dipanda, and Kolyang, "Application of deep learning architectures for satellite image time series prediction: A review," *Remote Sens.*, vol. 13, no. 23, p. 4822, 2021, doi: 10.3390/rs13234822.

64. D. Lin, K. Fu, Y. Wang, G. Xu, and X. Sun, "MARTA GANs: Unsupervised representation learning for remote sensing image classification," *IEEE Geosci. Remote Sens. Lett.*, vol. 14, no. 11, pp. 2092–2096, 2017, doi: 10.1109/LGRS.2017.2752750.

65. J. Lee, N. H. Goo, W. B. Park, M. Pyo, and K. Sohn, "Virtual microstructure design for steels using generative adversarial networks," *Eng. Rep.*, vol. 3, no. 1, Jan. 2021, doi: 10.1002/eng2.12274.

66. W. Lin et al., "Bidirectional mapping of brain MRI and PET with 3D reversible GAN for the diagnosis of Alzheimer's disease," *Front. Neurosci.*, vol. 15, Apr. 2021, doi: 10.3389/fnins.2021.646013.

67. J. Pan et al., "Physics-based generative adversarial models for image restoration and beyond," *IEEE Trans. Pattern Anal. Mach. Intell.*, vol. 43, no. 7, pp. 2449–2462, Jul. 2021, doi: 10.1109/TPAMI.2020.2969348.

68. T. Rahman, Y. Du, L. Zhao, and A. Shehu, "Generative adversarial learning of protein tertiary structures," *Molecules*, vol. 26, no. 5, p. 1209, 2021, doi: 10.3390/molecules26051209.

69. Z. Wu, Z. Wang, Y. Yuan, J. Zhang, Z. Wang, and H. Jin, "Black-box diagnosis and calibration on GAN intra-mode collapse: A pilot study," *ACM Trans. Multimed. Comput. Commun. Appl.*, vol. 17, no. 3s, pp. 1–18, 2021, doi: 10.1145/3472768.

70. C. Wang, C. Xu, X. Yao, and D. Tao, "Evolutionary generative adversarial networks," *IEEE Trans. Evol. Comput.*, vol. 23, no. 6, pp. 921–934, 2019, doi: 10.1109/TEVC. 2019.2895748.

71. H. Yalcin, "Plant recognition based on deep belief network classifier and combination of local features," *29th Signal Processing and Communications Applications Conference (SUI)*, 2021, doi: 10.1109/SIU53274.2021.9477879.

72. M. Titos, A. Bueno, L. Garcia, and C. Benitez, "A deep neural networks approach to automatic recognition systems for volcano-seismic events," *IEEE J. Sel. Top. Appl. Earth Obs. Remote Sens.*, vol. 11, no. 5, pp. 1533–1544, 2018, doi: 10.1109/JSTARS. 2018.2803198.

73. Y. Pan, G. Zhang, and L. Zhang, "A spatial-channel hierarchical deep learning network for pixel-level automated crack detection," *Autom. Constr.*, vol. 119, p. 103357, Nov. 2020, doi: 10.1016/j.autcon.2020.103357.

74. C.-C. Chung, Y.-Z. Lee, and H.-X. Zhang, "Design of a DBN hardware accelerator for handwritten digit recognitions," *2019 IEEE International Conference on Consumer Electronics - Taiwan (ICCE-TW)*, May 2019, pp. 1–2, doi: 10.1109/ICCE-TW46550.2019.8991890.

3 Real-Time Detection of COVID-19 Protocol Implementation Using Convolutional Neural Networks and Inverse Perspective Mapping

Yosi Kristian, Mo Raymond A. P.,
FX. Ferdinandus and Gunawan
Institut Sains dan Teknologi Terpadu Surabaya
Surabaya, Indonesia

Arya Tandy Hermawan and
Ilham Ari Elbaith Zaeni
Universitas Negeri Malang
Malang, Indonesia

Jehad Abdelhamid Hammad
Al-Quds Open University
Abu Dis, Palestine

3.1 INTRODUCTION

In 2020, scientists found a new type of coronavirus called COVID-19 in Wuhan, China. This virus spreaded fast and infected people around the globe in a short amount of time. On May 11 2020, there were more than 118,000 cases in 114 countries and 4291 people died. Therefore, the World Health Organization (WHO) declared this virus as a pandemic [1]. At that time, several countries imposed total lockdowns to reduce the number of virus transmissions; however, this had become a drastic impact on the global community.

Various research was being done to find a cure or vaccine to kill this deadly virus, but there were still no effective results. The situation forces the global community to look for an alternative way to stop the virus from spreading. Maintaining physical distance between people had been reported effectively to "flatten the curve" of viral transmission [2, 3]. It aimed at reducing the physical contact between possibly

DOI: 10.1201/9781003331674-3

infected individuals and healthy persons in public places. This method also helped the economy to keep going but in limited ways.

On the other hand, wearing a face mask in public places helped to decrease the virus transmission rate. As shown in [4], wearing a mask in public places can reduce the virus transmission rate and mortality by up to 65%. In Indonesia, the COVID-19 regulation [5] also proposed implementing these two things in citizen's daily lives. There had been several studies conducted to create a deep learning-based method to monitor the implementation of physical distancing [6, 7] and wearing a face mask [8, 9]. This method had been reported to work effectively.

In 2020, Hou et al. in [6] introduced a deep learning-based method to monitor COVID-19 social distancing using camera surveillance video as the input. They utilized a pre-trained YOLOv3 model to perform object detection of people. The camera view was first calibrated in their approach to set up the camera's Region of Interest (ROI). They calculated the distance between people using the Euclidean distance; however, their proposed works could not run in real-time and needed recorded surveillance footage to be processed. In the same year, Punn et al. [7] proposed a similar method for monitoring real-time-COVID-19 physical distancing. They utilized a fine-tuned YOLOv3 model to perform object detection of people and track their location. These two approaches were only able to monitor COVID-19 physical distancing.

In 2020, several studies also detected the use of face masks. First, Loey et al. [8] introduced a deep learning-based COVID-19 face mask detection approach using YOLOv2 architecture with ResNet-50 as its backbone. This approach generated a good result, but it could not run and monitor the protocol in real-time. They input a real-life person image, resulting in face mask usage detection. Susanto et al. [9] introduced their face mask detection approach, which also utilized the deep learning method. They used the YOLOv4 model to detect the use of face masks in real-time, and the result was pretty good. Their approach only detected the use of face masks in two classes, correctly used and without a face mask.

However, most approaches were specific; some focused on monitoring the use of face masks, and some focused on monitoring physical distancing. Most of them were not running in real-time, so they were required to input in the form of a video or footage that had already happened and could not report the violation in real-time. Moreover, they mostly did not support multiple Internet Protocol (IP) cameras.

Motivated by those works, this chapter aimed to create a real-time monitoring system for COVID-19 physical distancing and face mask usage detection. The real-time system simultaneously gathered input from multiple IP cameras streaming via a Real-Time Streaming Protocol (RTSP) connection. The input frame was then processed using a Convolutional Neural Network (CNN) and Inverse Perspective Mapping (IPM). This system detected face mask usage in three classes: correctly used face mask, incorrectly used face mask, and no face mask. Furthermore, while the COVID-19 protocol was violated, the system sent a message to the administrator via the Telegram chatbot with the evidence. A web interface enabled the administrator to manage the system and monitor the situation simultaneously.

In addition, the system could be used for smart city issues, such as management, security, and public awareness.

3.2   RELATED WORKS

The approaches employed in this study are based on numerous efficient and effective research forms.

3.2.1 FACE OBJECT DETECTOR

In the past few decades, there have been many studies on face object detection tasks. One of the well-known detectors is the Viola-Jones detector, which can run in real-time conditions [10]. This method extracts features by using the Haar feature descriptor.

On the other hand, in the past few years, a few deep learning-based face object detectors have performed excellently. This method is preferred because of its robustness and feature extraction capability. In 2017, Jiang et al. [11] tried to make a face detection model using Faster R-CNN network architecture. Faster R-CNN is fast because it has a region proposal that decreases the computational cost. Faster R-CNN does not have to feed all region proposals to CNN every time; it is general object detection that can perform excellently in a face detection task. However, Faster R-CNN still has a two-stage object detector. Later in 2019, Deng et al. [12] proposed a single-stage face object detector. They also combined it with several methods like three-dimensional (3D) face reconstruction and multi-task loss, which outstandingly increase the model's performance in face detection.

3.2.2   PERSON OBJECT DETECTOR

The person detection task is one of the famous tasks in object detection problems. The Viola-Jones detector performs well in the traditional object detection method and can run in real time, but it is still computationally expensive. A few deep learning-based object detectors have shown excellent performance in the past few years. There are two popular categories in object detectors: one-stage and two-stage. These approaches still need to be applied in real-time applications. In 2016, Redmon et al. [13] proposed a single-stage object detector called You Only Look Once (YOLO) that can outperform two-stage approaches. The base model of YOLO can achieve real time at 45 frames per second (fps). The smaller version of the network, Fast YOLO, can process 155 fps while achieving double the mean average precision (mAP) score of earlier object detectors, such as two-stage object detectors.

3.2.3   INVERSE PERSPECTIVE MAPPING

There have been many studies about distance estimation using camera footage. One promising use is IPM or bird's eye view transformation. In 1991, Mallot et al. [14] proposed an image transformation technique. This technique can modify the geometrical image, resulting in a top-down perspective of the image. This technique can simplify the optical flow computation.

In 2010, Luo et al. [15] proposed a technique to implement this transformation for on-vehicle cameras. Their paper focused on the low-cost implementation of IPM so that the transformation process can run faster. Later in the same year, Tuohy et al. [16] proposed a method for estimating actual distance using IPM. Their approach had a good result, and the system can run in real time and achieve 30 fps.

3.3 RESEARCH METHOD

The workflow of the proposed method is shown in Figure 3.1. The system's input is a real-time frame gathered from the IP cameras. We put the image into the preprocessing stage from the IP cameras, which resulted in the preprocessed image. The preprocessed image was taken into two processes: the person detection model and the face mask detection model. First, the person detection model resulted in a person object position, which was taken to the IPM calculation. We got the transformed person object position used for the distance calculation between the person object detected. Second, the face mask detection model took input from the preprocessed frame and the person object position from the person detection model. The face mask detection model used the person object position to look for facial objects only in the region of the person object detected. This process resulted in an encoded vector that contained the face mask usage classification of the detected face object. Then the last step was the violation detection, which gained input from the calculated distance vector and the face mask model encoded vector result to produce the overall detection output.

Figure 3.2 shows the system's four modules: API, frontend, streamer, and mask and person detection. Each module will be explained in the following paragraphs.

The API module handles requests from the frontend module. This module provides all activities, such as storing, retrieving data, login process, master user settings, master camera settings, and violation report data. A WebSocket connection is used to connect this module with the streamer and frontend modules. The WebSocket connection synchronizes real-time data changes such as violation reports

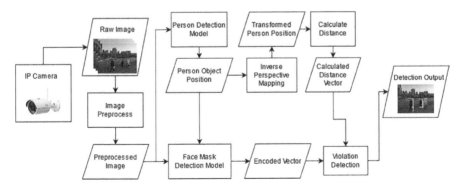

FIGURE 3.1 The system workflow.

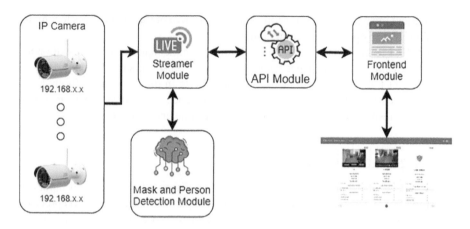

FIGURE 3.2   The system architecture.

and notifications. This module is also connected to the Telegram bot and handles all
messages and commands in the Telegram chat.

The admin uses the frontend module to configure the system and perform administrative tasks. The API module provides the system interface, for example, the login
page. The camera configuration setting is provided by the master camera page, while
the master user page sets up all users in the system. The dashboard page monitors
cameras in real-time, and the report page shows the violation report.

The streamer module is used for streaming raw image frames from the IP cameras. On implementing multithread for the camera streaming process, ensure each
step will have a different thread. Therefore, it is possible to stream and process each
camera frame at once. This module will retrieve the detection result from the mask
and person detection module and then perform the violation detection. If any violation happens, this module will take an image and record a video of the breach and
send the violation data to the API module to be broadcast to the frontend module and
the admin via the Telegram chatbot.

The mask and person detection module detects the person object and classifies the
face mask usage. This module will run inference on all explained machine learning
models. The result of the detection process is then sent back to the streamer module
to perform the violation detection process.

3.3.1   DATASETS

We trained the face mask detection model with our face mask usage dataset in this
system. To ensure our model, can classify different types of face mask usage (correctly used a face mask, incorrectly used a face mask, and no face mask), we collected
images from multiple face mask usage datasets: Masked Face-Net [17], Real-World
Masked Face Dataset (RMFD) [18], and Masked Face (MAFA) [19]. Those datasets
were combined into a single face mask dataset. A representative sample of our face
mask usage dataset is shown in Figure 3.3.

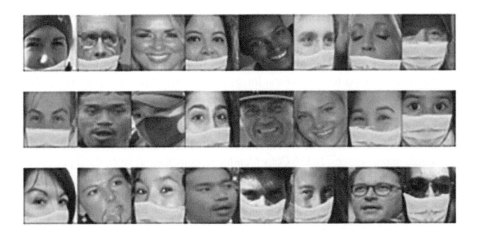

FIGURE 3.3   Example of face mask usage images.

3.3.2   FACE OBJECT DETECTOR

We used a pre-trained RetinaFace [12] model as the face object detector. RetinaFace is a single-shot multilevel face localization model. Three face localizations (face detection, two-dimensional [2D] face alignment, and 3D face reconstruction) were processed simultaneously with only a single shot. The face alignment and face reconstruction created excellent performance when detecting face objects at various angles. Moreover, the Single-Stage Detector (SSD) in this model made the model run lightweight and fast and can handle real-time frames in this system.

3.3.3   FACE MASK USAGE CLASSIFIER

In this system, we tested three object detection models to be used as face mask usage classifiers. These three models, MobileNetV2 [20], MobileNetV3 [21], and MnasNet [22], were proven to run lightweight and fast, but they were still fairly accurate. These models were used to classify face mask usage classes, which were correctly used a face mask, incorrectly used a face mask, and without a face mask. These will be explained in the following paragraphs.

First, MobileNetV2 is a mobile neural network architecture for object detection and classification. This model used a layer called an inverted residual block, which has a skip connection between the beginning and the end of the convolutional block. The network can access earlier activations not modified in the convolutional block and learn better.

Second, MobileNetV3 is an improved version of MobileNetV2. This model is faster and more accurate than MobileNetV2 regarding the classification task. This is because of the new H-Swish nonlinearity function, which has been proven [21]. This model also runs faster because of the layer removal in the last block compared with MobileNetV2.

Third, MnasNet is a mobile neural network architecture like MobileNet, but it runs 1.5 times faster than MobileNet while reaching the same ImageNet top 1 accuracy, which happens because it implements the reinforcement learning architecture. In the proposed system, we tested this architecture as the face mask usage classifier because it is reported to perform image classification faster than the MobileNet architecture.

Figure 3.4 shows the model architecture of MnasNet used in this chapter. MBConv (mobile inverted bottleneck convolution), layers are computationally efficient, allowing us to construct a deep network architecture that can run on devices with limited computational resources. In DWConv (depthwise convolution) layer, the input tensor is convolved using a set of filters; so instead of applying a single filter to the entire input tensor, different filters are applied to each input channel. This allows the network to learn spatial patterns within each channel independently while still considering the relationships between channels.

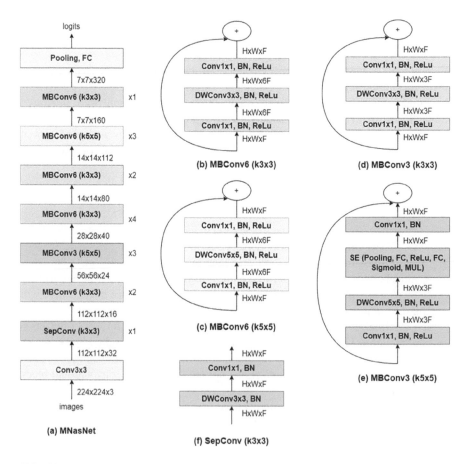

FIGURE 3.4 MnasNet architecture. BN, batch normalization; ReLu, rectified linear unit activation function.

3.3.4 PERSON OBJECT DETECTOR

YOLO architecture is a state-of-the-art real-time object detector. In this proposed system, we use YOLOv5 architecture as the person object detection model based on YOLOv1 until YOLOv4. We choose YOLOv5 [23] as the person object detector model for several reasons. First, it uses the Cross Stage Partial (CSP) networks [24] to extract rich, informative features from an input image. CSP Net also fixes the problems of repeated gradient information in the large-scale backbone, improving the inference's speed and accuracy. In this system, the speed and accuracy of object detection are essential because the system runs in real time. Second, the head of YOLOv5 is attached by a YOLO layer. This layer generates three different sizes of feature maps: small, medium, and big. In this system, this architecture is vital to improve the accuracy in person detection because the person object may come in various sizes.

3.3.5 INVERSE PERSPECTIVE MAPPING (IPM)

IPM is a method used to transform images to remove the perspective effect from a camera at a low altitude. This technique transforms a geometrical image to produce a top-view perspective of an image or bird's-eye view, as shown in Figure 3.5.

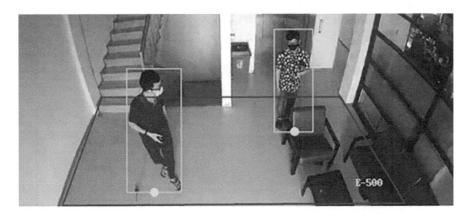

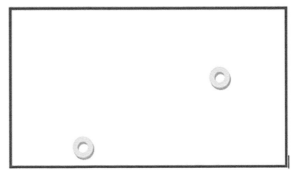

FIGURE 3.5 Inverse perspective mapping transformation.

The top image shows the original image, and the bottom is the result after IPM. In the past decade, there have been several kinds of research on this technique [25, 26] and estimating real-world distance from an image by using this technique [15, 16, 27], and it has been stated to work well. In this proposed system, IPM is used for transforming the person object position detected by the person object detector. We change the middle-bottom of each person object detected, which is then calculated to estimate the distance between persons.

3.4   EXPERIMENTS AND RESULTS

There are two major parts of the experiment. In the first part, we tried to build a face mask detector consisting of a face object detector and a face mask usage classifier. In the second part, we combine the whole parts and evaluated the result of the overall system.

3.4.1   FACE MASK DETECTOR

In this system, face mask detection consists of the face object detector and the face mask usage classifier. We use the pre-trained RetinaFace model as the face object detector. We trained all three models [20–22] from scratch using our face mask usage dataset for the face mask usage classifier. The face mask usage dataset was split into the train (80%) and the validation (20%) datasets. Each model was built and trained using the same scenario as [28] and [29]. Our models were built using PyTorch [30] and trained in Google Colaboratory [31] with an initial epoch set to 20 and early stopping. The training result comparison of all models is shown in Figure 3.6. From the result, we can see that all models learn well and could achieve more than 95% accuracy on the

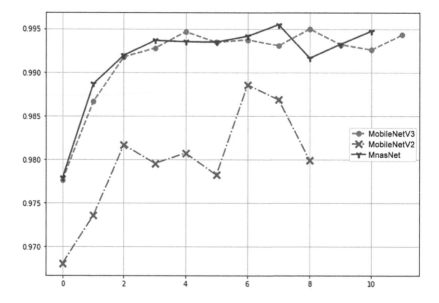

FIGURE 3.6   The face mask classifier accuracy comparison.

TABLE 3.1

Confusion Matrix of the Overall System Test

		Predicted	
		No Violation	**Violation**
Actual	No Violation	**115**	5
	Violation	3	**23**

validation dataset. The graph shows that MobileNet V3 and MnasNet have similar results. Still, when we tested the real-life situation with an actual camera, the MnasNet model performed much better than the MobileNet V3. So, we implement the MnasNet model as the face mask usage classifier on this system.

3.4.2 OVERALL SYSTEM

We tested the overall system in the hallway of Institut Sains dan Teknologi Terpadu Surabaya. We evaluated the system by running it for about 3.5 hours during the working hours on weekdays. After that, we cross-checked between the violation report generated by the system and the actual condition as the ground truth. The actual condition is made by watching the CCTV camera footage while the overall system test runs and manually validating the violation within the selected ROI. The confusion matrix in Table 3.1 shows the evaluation result of the overall system.

Table 3.1 shows that the overall system can achieve 94.52% accuracy with a 0.852 average F1 score. However, face mask detection is sometimes inconsistent and misclassifies the use of face masks for a second. However, it still shows the correct classification results for about 75% of the violation videos. Figure 3.7 shows the detailed footage result taken during the comprehensive system test. A red box means no face

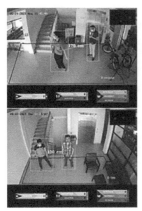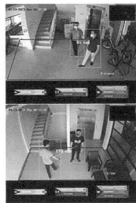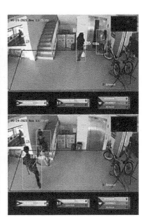

FIGURE 3.7 Output samples of the proposed system for monitoring physical distancing and face mask usage detection.

TABLE 3.2

Distance Measurement Test

Classroom			Hallway		
System's Measurement	Actual (mm)	Difference	System's Measurement	Actual	Difference
		16 cm			10 cm
		1 cm			25 cm
		2 cm			2 cm

mask detected, a blue box means incorrect face mask detected, and a green box means correctly used face mask detected.

We also performed a distance measurement test to measure the tolerance value of the system. This test took place in the hallway and classroom of Institut Sains dan Teknologi Terpadu Surabaya. This tolerance value represents the variance between the system distance measurement and the actual distance between people. We conducted the test using two people standing next to each other with various positions within the selected ROI. We measured the distance between those two people. Then we compared the actual measurement result with the measurement done by the system and calculated the difference.

The detail of the conducted distance measurement test is shown in Table 3.2. From those results, we calculated the average variance between the actual distance and the system's calculated distance. The average variance represents the tolerance value of the proposed method. From those images, we can see that the system can achieve a tolerance value of 11.9 cm, which is pretty good. We also provide a dashboard page for real-time monitoring of the actual condition.

As in Figure 3.8, the dashboard page provides a simultaneous preview of the camera and a summary of the violations that occurred in a single day. The dashboard page can preview up to three cameras simultaneously. Figure 3.9 shows an example of a violation reported via the Telegram chatbot. The message will contain the number of violations and the time they occurred. A photo of the violation is also provided as evidence.

We also provide a dashboard page for real-time monitoring of the actual condition. As shown in Figure 3.8, the dashboard page can preview up to three cameras

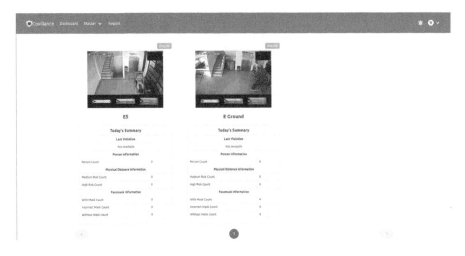

FIGURE 3.8 This system dashboard design.

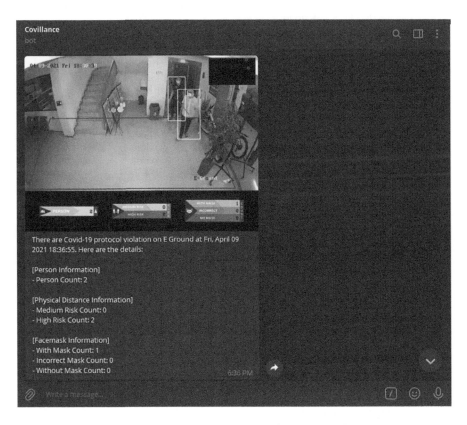

FIGURE 3.9 Example of a violation reported via the Telegram chatbot.

simultaneously. Figure 3.9 shows an example of a violation reported via the Telegram chatbot. The message will contain the number of violations and the time they occurred. A photo of the violation as evidence is also provided.

3.5   CONCLUSION AND FUTURE WORK

In this chapter, we had proposed a system that can monitor the implementation of the COVID-19 protocol, specifically in physical distancing detection and face mask usage detection tasks in real time, using a deep learning-based method. We achieve a reasonable distance prediction error of 11.9 cm and face mask usage detection with an accuracy of 94.52%. We have also shown that multithread and deep learning perform excellently when processing frames from multi-cameras simultaneously with high accuracy. For future work, we plan to add human pose and thermal detection system.

REFERENCES

1. "WHO Director-General's opening remarks at the media briefing on COVID-19 - 11 March 2020." Accessed: May 30, 2021. Available: https://www.who.int/director-general/speeches/detail/who-director-general-s-opening-remarks-at-the-media-briefing-on-covid-19—11-march-2020.
2. L. Matrajt, and T. Leung, "Evaluating the effectiveness of social distancing interventions to delay or flatten the epidemic curve of coronavirus disease," *Emerg. Infect. Dis.*, vol. 26, no. 8, pp. 1740–1748, Aug. 2020, doi: 10.3201/eid2608.201093.
3. C. M. Freeman, M. A. Rank, C. M. Bolster LaSalle, T. E. Grys, and J. C. Lewis, "Effectiveness of physical distancing: Staying 6 feet over to put respiratory viruses 6 feet under," Mayo Clin. Proc., vol. 96, no. 1, pp. 148–151, Jan. 2021, doi: 10.1016/j.mayocp.2020.10.040.
4. S. E. Eikenberry et al., "To mask or not to mask: Modeling the potential for face mask use by the general public to curtail the COVID-19 pandemic," Infect. Dis. Model., vol. 5, pp. 293–308, Jan. 2020, doi: 10.1016/j.idm.2020.04.001.
5. Kementerian Kesehatan Republik Indonesia, *Pedoman Pencegahan dan Pengendalian Serta Definisi Coronavirus Disease (COVID-19)*. Jakarta Selatan: Direktorat Jenderal Pencegahan dan Pengendalian Penyakit, 2020.
6. Y. C. Hou, M. Z. Baharuddin, S. Yussof, and S. Dzulkifly, "Social distancing detection with deep learning model," in 2020 8th International Conference on Information Technology and Multimedia (ICIMU), 2020, pp. 334–338, doi: 10.1109/ICIMU49871.2020.9243478.
7. N. S. Punn, and S. K. Sonbhadra,. Agarwal, and G. Rai, "Monitoring COVID-19 social distancing with person detection and tracking via fine-tuned YOLO v3 and Deepsort techniques," pp. 1–10, 2020.
8. M. Loey, G. Manogaran, M. H. N. Taha, and N. E. M. Khalifa, "Fighting against COVID-19: A novel deep learning model based on YOLO-v2 with ResNet-50 for medical face mask detection," Sustain. Cities Soc., vol. 65, p. 102600, Feb. 2021, doi: 10.1016/j.scs.2020.102600.
9. S. Susanto, F. A. Putra, R. Analia, and I. K. L. N. Suciningtyas, "The face mask detection for preventing the spread of COVID-19 at Politeknik Negeri Batam," in 2020 3rd International Conference on Applied Engineering (ICAE), 2020, pp. 1–5, doi: 10.1109/ICAE50557.2020.9350556.

10. P. Viola, and M. Jones, "Rapid object detection using a boosted cascade of simple features," Proc. IEEE Computer Society Conference on Computer Vision and Pattern Recognition, vol. 1, 2001, doi: 10.1109/CVPR.2001.990517.

11. H. Jiang, and E. Learned-Miller, "Face detection with the faster R-CNN," in 2017 12th IEEE International Conference on Automatic Face Gesture Recognition (FG 2017), 2017, pp. 650–657, doi: 10.1109/FG.2017.82.

12. J. Deng, J. Guo, Y. Zhou, J. Yu, I. Kotsia, and S. Zafeiriou, "RetinaFace: Single-stage dense face localisation in the wild." Accessed: May 11, 2021. [Online]. Available: https://github.com/deepinsight/.

13. J. Redmon, S. Divvala, R. Girshick, and A. Farhadi, "You only look once: Unified, real-time object detection," in 2016 IEEE Conference on Computer Vision and Pattern Recognition (CVPR), Jun. 2016, pp. 779–788, doi: 10.1109/CVPR.2016.91 Jun. 2016

14. H. A. Mallot, H. H. Bülthoff, J. J. Little, and S. Bohrer, "Inverse perspective mapping simplifies optical flow computation and obstacle detection," Biol. Cybern., vol. 64, no. 3, pp. 177–185, 1991, doi: 10.1007/BF00201978.

15. Lin-Bo Luo, In-Sung Koh, Kyeong-Yuk Min, Jun Wang, and Jong-Wha Chong, "Low-cost implementation of bird's-eye view system for camera-on-vehicle," in *2010 Digest of Technical Papers International Conference on Consumer Electronics (ICCE)*, Jan. 2010, pp. 311–312, doi: 10.1109/ICCE.2010.5418845

16. S. Tuohy, D. O'Cualain, E. Jones, and M. Glavin, "Distance determination for an automobile environment using Inverse Perspective Mapping in OpenCV," IET Irish Sign. Syst., vol. 2010, pp. 100–105, 2010, doi: 10.1049/cp.2010.0495.

17. A. Cabani, K. Hammoudi, H. Benhabiles, and M. Melkemi, "MaskedFace-Net – A dataset of correctly/incorrectly masked face images in the context of COVID-19," Smart Heal., vol. 19, Aug. 2020, doi: 10.1016/j.smhl.2020.100144.

18. Z. Wang et al., "Masked face recognition dataset and application." Accessed: May 04, 2021. [Online]. Available: https://github.com/X-zhangyang/.

19. S. Ge, J. Li, Q. Ye, and Z. Luo, "Detecting Masked Faces in the Wild with LLE-CNNs," in Proceedings of the IEEE Conference on Computer Vision and Pattern Recognition, 2017, pp. 2682–2690.

20. M. Sandler, A. Howard, M. Zhu, and A. Zhmoginov, and L.-C. Chen, "MobileNetV2: Inverted Residuals and Linear Bottlenecks," in 2018 IEEE/CVF Conference on Computer Vision and Pattern Recognition, Jun. 2018, pp. 4510–4520, doi: 10.1109/CVPR.2018.00474

21. A. Howard et al., "Searching for MobileNetV3," in 2019 IEEE/CVF International Conference on Computer Vision (ICCV), Oct. 2019, pp. 1314–1324, doi: 10.1109/ICCV.2019.00140

22. M. Tan et al., "MnasNet: Platform-aware neural architecture search for mobile." Accessed: May 12, 2021. [Online]. Available: https://github.com/tensorflow/tpu/.

23. G. Jocher et al., "ultralytics/yolov5: v5.0 - YOLOv5-P6 1280 models, AWS, Supervisely and YouTube integrations." Zenodo, Apr. 2021, doi: 10.5281/zenodo.4679653.

24. C.-Y. Wang, H.-Y. M. Liao, I.-H. Yeh, Y.-H. Wu, P.-Y. Chen, and J.-W. Hsieh, "CSPNet: A New Backbone that can Enhance Learning Capability of CNN," in 2020 IEEE/CVF Conference on Computer Vision and Pattern Recognition Workshops (CVPRW), Jun. 2020, pp. 1571–1580, doi: 10.1109/CVPRW50498.2020.00203

25. I. Kholopov, "Bird's Eye View Transformation Technique in Photogrammetric Problem of Object Size Measuring at Low-Altitude Photography," in 2017 International Conference Actual Issues of Mechanical Engineering (AIME 2017) 2017, doi: 10.2991/aime-17.2017.52

26. M. Venkatesh, and P. Vijayakumar, "A simple bird's eye view transformation technique," Int. J. Sci. Eng. Res., vol. 3, 2012, [Online]. Accessed: August 12, 2022. Available:

https://www.ijser.org/researchpaper/A-Simple-Birds-Eye-View-Transformation-Technique.pdf.

27. M. H. Tanveer, and A. Sgorbissa, "An Inverse Perspective Mapping Approach Using Monocular Camera of Pepper Humanoid Robot to Determine the Position of Other Moving Robot in Plane," in Proceedings of the 15th International Conference on Informatics in Control, Automation and Robotics, 2018, pp. 219–225, doi: 10.5220/0006930002190225

28. Y. Kristian, I Purnama, K. E. Sutanto, E. H. Zaman, L. Setiawan, and E. I. Purnomo, "Klasifikasi nyeri pada video ekspresi wajah bayi menggunakan DCNN autoencoder dan LSTM," Jurnal Nasional Teknik Elektro Dan Teknologi Informasi, vol. 7, no. 3, pp. 308–316, 2018.

29. S. E. Limantoro, Y. Kristian, and D. D Purwanto. Deteksi Pengendara Sepeda Motor Menggunakan Deep Convolutional Neural Networks. In Seminar Nasional Teknologi Informasi dan Komunikasi, 2017, pp. 79–86.

30. A. Paszke et al., "PyTorch: An Imperative Style, High-Performance Deep Learning Library," in 2019 33rd Conference on Neural Information Processing Systems (NeurIPS 2019), Apr. 2019.

31. E. Bisong, "Google Colaboratory," in Building Machine Learning and Deep Learning Models on Google Cloud Platform: A Comprehensive Guide for Beginners, Berkeley, CA: Apress, 2019, pp. 59–64.

4 Marketplace Product Image Grouping Using Transfer Learning of Deep Convolutional Neural Network in COVID-19 Post-Pandemic Situation

Yuliana Melita Pranoto and Anik Nur Handayani
Universitas Negeri Malang
Malang, Indonesia

Yosi Kristian
Institut Sains dan Teknologi Terpadu Surabaya
Surabaya, Indonesia

4.1 INTRODUCTION

The COVID-19 outbreak, which began at the end of December 2019, significantly impacted businesses, especially Small and Medium Enterprises (SMEs). SMEs must adapt their business model using digital technology [1]. On the other hand, the COVID-19 crisis had brought about essential changes in the business world, allowing a mature and adaptable business capability in digitalization and remote working [2].

In Indonesia, the e-commerce business has also increased 10-fold, with the addition of new customers reaching more than 50% during the pandemic [3]. The increase in new customers is accompanied by an increase in new online shops in the marketplace. The higher the traffic, the more products are added to e-commerce or the marketplace daily. This condition increases the dynamics of product categories, where the same products can fall into different categories in different stores. Therefore, a machine learning model is needed to recommend similar products, allowing customers to choose the right store to buy a specific product and reducing time in product search.

A large amount of visual data (images), both from the Web and social media, is an essential source of data for research. References [4–6] include a collection of datasets created by Google or Flickr by utilizing human intelligence to help improve research results. Before processing the product image, it is necessary to collect data

DOI: 10.1201/9781003331674-4

and identify predetermined categories [7]. The collected data needs to be analyzed and annotated to be grouped into the same category [8].

On the other hand, the standard approach used for product classification is by using price tag, color, and size features. This cannot be easy to implement in online shops because pictures often introduce the products. Sakamaki [9] performed categorization based on product pictures, where the product data to be categorized are taken from the Fashion MNIST database, and then attributes from those products are extracted with feature vectors using deep learning.

The problem today is that the number of product items in the marketplace is increasing daily. With so many offers for the same product from different sellers/ retailers, it becomes difficult for the buyer to find the best price [10].

In this chapter, we took a deep learning approach to similar group products based on predefined categories on 4634 product images and 281 groups. We modified a few pre-trained networks; customized the last layers; then conducted freezing, fine-tuning, and retraining on the combination that had been set.

4.2   RELATED WORK

Machine Learning has brought improvement in technology. A convolutional neural network (CNN) can recognize many visual representations, which has significantly improved the search result [11]. It is related to classification using a deep learning approach and performing classification on large-scale pictures, which are pictures in Facebook Marketplace [12]. A two-phase training approach using a deep CNN includes the first phase, which is to perform training to recognize visual representation, and the second phase, which is to perform categorization based on data [13].

Performing the classification process on product images using the CNN model [14] uses two CNN architectures to perform text and image classification. The CNN architecture used is the VGG model using a dataset from the online shop walmart. com with as many as 1.2 million products.

Our study uses deep learning models from Keras Applications [15]. These models have been pre-trained using ImageNet, which is an image dataset organized according to the WordNet hierarchy. Images of each concept are quality controlled and human annotated. Illustrating the usefulness of ImageNet is done through three simple applications: object recognition, image classification, and automatic object clustering [16].

Models used in this study were VGG-16, MobileNetV2, and EfficientNetV2M. The original performance for each model (trained with ImageNet) is displayed in Table 4.1. We altered the last layer, freezing and fine-tuning, then retrained the models.

Top-1 and top-5 accuracy refer to the model's performance on the ImageNet validation dataset. Depth refers to the topological depth of the network. This includes activation layers, batch normalization layers, etc. Depth counts the number of layers with parameters.

Performing transfer learning uses pre-trained VGG-16 models to overcome problems with classification, regression, and clustering [17]. Transfer learning is reusing

TABLE 4.1

Performance of Deep Convolutional Neural Network Models

Model	Size (MB)	Top-1 Accuracy	Top-5 Accuracy	Parameters	Depth
VGG-16	528	71.3%	90.1%	138.4M	16
MobileNetV2	14	71.3%	90.1%	3.5M	105
EfficientNetV2M	220	85.3%	97.4%	54.4M	–

a pre-trained model knowledge for another task. In [18] transfer learning to fine-tune the pre-trained network (VGG-19) parameters for the image classification task is used. Further, the performance of the VGG-19 architecture is compared with AlexNet and VGG-16. AlexNet, VGG-16, and VGG-19 are the famous CNN architectures introduced for the object recognition task.

Pre-trained models such as MobileNet, MobileNetV2, VGG-16, VGG-19, and ResNet-50 have been used for image classification and prediction [19]. The result shows that MobileNetV2 performance is relatively better than other pre-trained models. MobileNetV2 uses a smaller number of parameters compared with other trained models.

Li et al. [20] proposed an improved infrared target detection model I-CenterNet based on the anchor-free model CenterNet. The EfficientNetV2 with the channel attention mechanism is used instead of the traditional structure as the backbone network to enhance feature extraction.

4.3 RESEARCH METHODOLOGY

4.3.1 DATASET

In this study, we used the Kaggle dataset. Kaggle is an online community that allows its members to share ideas, learn, and even compete in data science and machine learning [21]. The dataset was taken from the e-commerce platform Shopee, containing 4634 data images with 281 product label groups.

Shopee is one of the major e-commerce platforms in Indonesia. Based on the study conducted by Ipsos regarding e-commerce competition in Indonesia in late 2021, Shopee is on the top of the list as the most used e-commerce platform in Indonesia [22].

Most online shops give different names for the same product categories. Figure 4.1 shows examples of hair treatment products belonging to the same label group. However, each shop gives a different title for the product, such as "hair tonic," "hair vitamin," "hair full treatment," "*paket perawatan rambut,*" "hair care series," "natural extract hair tonic," and "promo paket tonic."

Figure 4.2 shows examples of body lotion products belonging to the same label group. But each shop gives a different title for the product, such as "*cream pelembab,*" "baby day lotion," "lotion with shea butter," "baby day lotion calendula," "lotion face and body," "daily lotion 400 ml," and "*losion bayi murah.*"

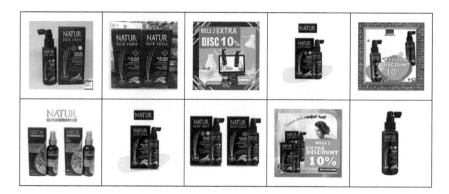

FIGURE 4.1   Examples of hair treatment products with the same group label.

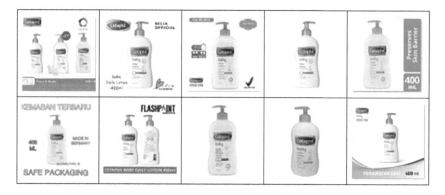

FIGURE 4.2   Examples of body lotion products with the same group label.

This is why specific keywords entered by users will not result in an expected product list. Therefore, we conclude that pictures play an important role in providing better search recommendations to users.

4.3.2 SYSTEM ARCHITECTURE

Figure 4.3 shows the system architecture used, whereas this study starts with reducing the pictures' dimension, which will be later processed with the CNN model. The expected dimension is 384 × 384, where every pixel consists of three values for the RGB channels. The 384 × 384 size is chosen to fasten the training process while maintaining a good detail of features.

We utilized the transfer learning method from pre-trained CNN models (VGG-16, MobileNetV2, and EfficientNetV2M) modifying the last few layers and then fine-tuning the models. Some layers will be frozen so that the retraining process will be quicker. Frozen layers are the early layers (close to input layers and store low-level information), whereas the last layers, which store higher-level information, are not frozen.

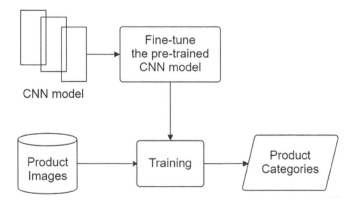

FIGURE 4.3 System architecture.

The output obtained here is the products classified according to labels prepared before. The 4634 product images were categorized into 281 product groups. The arrangement of data for training and validation is 80:20, a total of 3707 data are used for training, and 927 data are used for validation.

4.3.3 VGG-16 ARCHITECTURE

The modification we have done on the VGG-16 architecture model can be seen in Figure 4.4. The first 19 layers in our architecture are the original VGG-16 layers, consisting of convolution layers of a 3 × 3 filter with stride one and using the same padding and max pool layer of a 2 × 2 filter with stride 2. Conv-1 layer has 64 filters, Conv-2 has 128 filters, Conv-3 has 256 filters, and Conv 4 and Conv 5 have 512 filters.

The layer cut is performed before the dense layer. After the flatten process, the dense artificial layer was added, with the number of neurons adjusted to the number of categories, which was 281. The final activation function used is softmax.

Most layers are not retrained (freeze). Retraining is performed starting on the last six layers, starting on layer block5_conv3 (Conv2D) layer. From a total of 36,917,969 parameters, 24,563,089 parameters were retrained. We used 20 epochs and a batch size of 100.

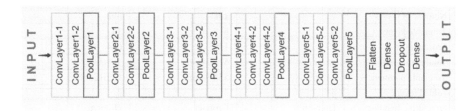

FIGURE 4.4 Our VGG-16 design.

4.3.4 MobileNetV2 Architecture

As for the previous model (VGG-16), images sent through MobileNetV2 will be resized to 384 × 384. We cut the last layer right before the output layer, adding several new layers at the back with dropout to prevent overfitting, and we used the softmax activation function.

Most of the layers are frozen. Retraining is performed starting from the last eight layers, starting on layer *block_16_project_BN (BatchNormalization)*. From a total of 57,638,865 parameters, 55,793,681 parameters will be retrained. We used 20 epochs and a batch size of 200.

4.3.5 EfficientNet2VM Architecture

Like the two previous architectures, we modified the pre-trained model of EfficientNetV2M by cutting the last layer before the output layer. After the flattening process (making the output one layer with size 184320), we added two dense layers and one dropout; the softmax activation function was used.

Most layers are not retrained. The retraining process is conducted from the last 14 layers, which starts on layer *block7e_project_conv (Conv2D)*. From a total of 108,531,269 parameters, there are 57,612,689 parameters retrained. We used 20 epochs and a batch size of 200.

4.4 RESULT DISCUSSION

Table 4.2 shows the resume of modification we have done to the three pre-trained models (VGG-16, MobileNetV2, and EfficientV2M), including the number of layers, trainable layers, frozen layers, trainable parameter, added layers, and overfitting handler.

VGG-16 architecture is simple, but its large size consumes many GPU resources during the training process. For the 20 epochs performed, validation accuracy kept increasing until the 20th epoch. The accuracy value of the F1 score is 70%, and the weighted average is 70%.

TABLE 4.2
Modification of Our CNN Models

Model	VGG-16	MobileNetV2	EfficientNetV2M
Number of layers	23	158	698
Trainable layers	6	8	14
Frozen layer	17	150	684
Total parameters	36,917,969	57,638,865	108,531,269
Trainable parameters	24,563,089	55,793,681	57,612,689
Added layers	4	4	4
Overfitting handler	Dropout	Dropout	Dropout

TABLE 4.3

Result Comparison

Model	VGG-16	MobileNetV2	EfficientNetV2M
Number of epochs	20	20	20
Time to train (minutes)	25	5	30
Accuracy	70%	57%	84%
Weighted average F1 score	70%	56%	84%

Although MobileNetV2 consists of many layers, the size of this architecture is small. It does not fit for large datasets, but in this study, we used this architecture anyway to see the possibility of using it as a recommender for mobile applications. For 20 epoch training, the accuracy gain in F1 score is 57%.

The last architecture is EfficientNetV2M, which has many more layers than the other two, so it takes more time to train the model, and the result is better. For 20 epochs, the accuracy increases starting from the 15th epoch, but it declines on the 16th. F1 score and weighted average are the same at 84%.

From several modifications on three pre-trained models, i.e., VGG-16, Mobile-NetV2, and EfficientV2M, Table 4.3 compares the results of the three models.

Based on the testing we have performed, the highest accuracy is given by EfficientNetV2M with 84%, followed by VGG-16 with 70%, and the last is MobileNetV2 with 57%. The time needed for completing the training process with 20 epochs is approximately 30 minutes for EfficientNetV2M, approximately 25 minutes for VGG-16, and MobileNetV2 approximately in 5 minutes. With the same number of epochs, the weighted average age for these three models is EfficientNetV2M at 84%, VGG-16 at 70%, and MobileNetV2 at 56%.

4.5 CONCLUSION AND FUTURE STUDIES

The main objectives of this study are to determine which of these three models (VGG-16, MobileNetV2, and EfficientNetV2M) achieves the best result of accuracy. The dataset we used in this research was taken from the e-commerce platform Shopee, containing 4634 data with 281 product label groups. We have utilized a transfer learning process, modified the architecture, and fine-tuned several deep CNNs.

Per the results, the EfficientNetV2M model provided the best accuracy, but it needed more learning time, considering the EfficientNetV2M consisted of more layers compared with the other models.

We plan for our future studies to improve our product matching by utilizing clustering-based matching and extracting features from multiple modalities. We also plan to implement hierarchical clustering so our model is not class-bound like in this paper and can be used for any product. We believe that the multi-modality approach will improve our product matching quality.

REFERENCES

1. Winarsih, Indriastuti, M., Fuad, K. 2021. Impact of Covid-19 on Digital Transformation and Sustainability in Small and Medium Enterprises (SMEs): A Conceptual Framework. In: Barolli, L., Poniszewska-Maranda, A., Enokido, T. (eds) Complex, Intelligent and Software Intensive Systems. CISIS 2020. *Advances in Intelligent Systems and Computing*, vol 1194. Springer, Cham. https://doi.org/10.1007/978-3-030-50454-0_48

2. Florina Pinzaru, Alexandra Zbuchea, and Lucian Anghel. October 2020. The impact of the Covid-19 pandemic on business, *Strategica (International Academic Conference)*, 8th edition, Bucharest, Pages 721–730.

3. Nurlela. 2021. E-Commerce, Solusi di Tengah Pandemi COVID-19, *Jurnal Simki Economic*, Volume 4, Issue 1, Pages 47–56, https://jiped.org/index.php/JSE.

4. O. Russakovsky *et al.* 2015. "ImageNet Large Scale Visual Recognition Challenge," *Int. J. Comput. Vis.*, Volume 115, Issue 3, Pages 211–252. doi: 10.1007/s11263-015-0816-y.

5. M. Everingham, L. VanGool, C. Williams, J. Winn, and A. Zisserman. 2015. The Pascal visual object classes (VOC) challenge. *International Journal of Computer Vision*, Volume 88, Issue 2, Pages 303–338, Jun. 2010. doi: 10.1007/s11263-009-0275-4.

6. T.-Y. Lin, *et al.* 2014. Microsoft' COCO: Common objects in context. in *Lecture Notes in Computer Science*, Springer Cham, 2014, pp. 740–755.

7. Yoshua Bengio, Jérôme Louradour, Ronan Collobert, and Jason Weston. 2009. Curriculum Learning, in Proceedings of the 26th Annual International Conference on Machine Learning, Jun. 2009, Pages 41–48, doi: 10.1145/1553374.1553380.

8. Yoshua Bengio, and Jean-Sébastien Senécal. 2008. Adaptive importance sampling to accelerate training of a neural probabilistic language model, *IEEE Transactions on Neural Networks*, Volume 19, Issue 4, Pages 713–722.

9. Yoshikazu Sakamaki. June 2022. A Study on product categorization using machine learning clustering of image data using convolutional processing, *Journal of Data Science and Modern Techniques*, Volume 1, Pages 1–18.

10. Robert-Aandrei Damian. 2022. Finding duplicate offers in the online marketplace catalogue using transformer based methods. CLNS – Cloud and Network Infrastructure, EIT Digital.

11. Corey Lynch, Kamelia Aryafar, and Josh Attenberg. 2016. Images Don't Lie: Transferring Deep Visual Semantic Features to Large-Scale Multimodal Learning to Rank. Proceedings of the 22nd ACM SIGKDD International Conference on Knowledge Discovery and Data Mining, Aug. 2016, San Francisco, CA, Pages 541–548, doi: 10.1145/2939672.2939728.

12. Yina Tang, and Fedor Borisyuk, et al., MSURU: Large scale E-commerce Image classification with weakly supervised search data, KDD '19: Proceedings of the 25th ACM SIGKDD International Conference on Knowledge Discovery & Data Mining, Pages 2518–2526, July 2019, https://doi.org/10.1145/3292500.3330696

13. Xinlei Chen, and Abhinav Gupta. 2015. Webly Supervised Learning of Convolutional Networks. in 2015 IEEE International Conference on Computer Vision (ICCV), Santiago, Chile, Pages 1431–1439, Dec. 2015. doi: 10.1109/ICCV.2015.168.

14. Tom Zahavy, Alessandro Magnani, Abhinandan Krishnan, and Shie Mannor. November 2016. Is a picture worth a thousand words? A deep multi-modal fusion architecture for product classification in e-commerce, arXiv:1611.09534v1. https://doi.org/10.48550/arXiv.1611.09534

15. ONEIROS (Open-ended Neuro-Electronic Intelligent Robot Operating System). 2022. Keras Applications. https://keras.io/api/applications/

16. J. Deng, W. Dong, R. Socher, L. Li, Kai Li, and Li Fei-Fei. 2009. ImageNet: A Large-Scale Hierarchical Image Database. in 2009 IEEE Conference on Computer Vision and

Pattern Recognition, Jun. 2009, Miami, FL, Pages 248–255. doi: 10.1109/CVPR.2009. 5206848.

17. Srikanth Tammina. October 2019. Transfer learning using VGG-16 with deep convolutional neural network for classifying images. International Journal of Scientific and Research Publications, Volume 9, Issue 10, Pages 143–150, Oct. 2019. doi: 10.29322/ IJSRP.9.10.2019.p9420.

18. Manali Shaha, and Meenakshi Pawar. March 2018. Transfer learning for image classification. 2018 Second International Conference on Electronics, Communication and Aerospace Technology (ICECA), Coimbatore, India.

19. J. Praveen Gujjar, H.R. Prasanna Kumar, and Niranjan N. Chiplunkar. 2021. Image Classification and Prediction Using Transfer Learning in Colab Notebook. Global Transitions Proceedings, Volume 2, Issue 2, Pages 382–385, Nov. 2021. doi: 10.1016/ j.gltp.2021.08.068

20. X. Li, Y. Qian, R. Guo, and N. Ao. 2022. "CenterNet: Road infrared target detection based on improved CenterNet," *IET Image Process.*, Volume 17, Issue 1, Pages 57–66, Jan. 2023. doi: 10.1049/ipr2.12616

21. Shopee. 2021. shopee-product-matching. https://www.kaggle.com/

22. Kompas, "Hasil Riset Ipsos: Shopee jadi E-Commerce yang Paling Banyak Digunakan pada 2021," *Kompas Magazine*, accessed on 20 June 2022, https://money.kompas.com/ read/2022/01/31/204500426/hasil-riset-ipsos-shopee-jadi-e-commerce-yang-paling-banyak-digunakan-pada?page=all.

5 The Chamber Monitoring Suspected COVID-19 Based on IoT Geographic Information Systems

Fachrul Kurniawan, Yunifa Miftachul Arif,
Afrijal Rizqi Ramadan, Shoffin Nahwa Utama,
Supriyonoe, Johan Ericka, Okta Qomarudin Aziz,
Fresy Nugroho, and Fajar Rohman Hariri
Universitas Islam Negeri Maulana Malik Ibrahim Malang
Malang, Indonesia

Meidya Koeshardianto
University of Trunojoyo Madura
Bangkalan, Indonesia

5.1 INTRODUCTION

The coronavirus had altered human behavior. The virus was known to be active and capable of inflicting rapid death which raised fears of widespread transmission among experts from diverse fields of science [1, 2]. Since this virus was identified in late 2019 in Wuhan, China, it is mainly referred to as coronavirus disease (COVID-19). COVID-19 was highly contagious and can infect infants [2], children [3], adults [4], and the elderly [5], with an equitable distribution worldwide. The COVID-19 virus invaded Indonesia around the end of March 2020 [6].

A COVID-19 virus is a group of viruses that infect the respiratory system of humans. This virus frequently caused respiratory system infections ranging from mild (flu) to severe, specifically lung infections (pneumonia) [7]. In the majority of cases, this virus caused mainly moderate respiratory infections, such as fever [8], runny nose [9], cough [10], sore throat [11], and headache [12] or severe respiratory infections, such as high fever [13], coughing up phlegm [14] and occasionally blood [15], shortness of breath [16], and chest pain [17]. However, when infected with the virus, the first signs are fever (body temperature greater than 38°C), coughing, and shortness of breath. The COVID-19 virus can be transmitted in a variety of ways, the most common of which are as follows:

- Accidentally inhaled saliva splashes from sneezing or coughing with COVID-19 sufferers.

DOI: 10.1201/9781003331674-5

- Touch the mouth or nose without washing hands first after grabbing an object that the saliva of a COVID-19 sufferer has splashed.
- Close contact with people with COVID-19, for example, touching or shaking hands.
- Join a crowd that does not follow strict health procedures.

The epidemic's epicenter was in the metropolis, where the population was highly mobile [18]. Dense urban community activities enabled active transmission. Resulting in a big, infected population that quickly filled hospitals [19]. Additionally, the population mortality rate was higher than before the COVID-19 epidemic. Along with treating and curing an infection, preventative steps were the most prudent course of action. This prevention can begin with monitoring, tracking, isolating, and giving adequate nutrition for the entire city population's body.

In South Asia, they built an Android-based application using the concept of the Internet of Things (IoT) for a COVID-19 monitoring system (IoT-based Smart Health Application). A portable device monitoring system had been introduced in Pakistan [20] to aid people in their fight against the COVID-19 pandemic. The system comprised a NodeMCU ESP8266 with a built-in Wi-Fi module and an Android application for both the user and the administrator (Doctor). DHT11 and a pulse sensor measured the main COVID-19 symptoms, such as temperature and heartbeat. The data were read and processed in the NodeMCU before being sent to the Firebase database. The system periodically notified the user by applying various conditions to the user's data. Using an Arduino Uno-based system, Bangladesh [21] used an IoT-based system to monitor the patient's body temperature, pulse rate, and oxygen saturation, which were the most important measurements required for critical care in real-time. In India [22], a monitoring system was built to help immediately inform the caretaker as soon as the patient's irregular health data occurs for emergency care by tracking the patient's location using a GPS module and sending alerts via Wi-Fi using IoT.

During the COVID-19 pandemic in South Africa, virtual healthcare services and digital health technologies for monitoring systems were deployed [23]. During the COVID-19 pandemic, South Africa used digital technologies like SMS-based solutions, mobile health apps, telemedicine and telehealth, WhatsApp-based systems, artificial intelligence and chatbots, and robotics to provide healthcare services. These cutting-edge technologies had been used for various purposes, including disease surveillance and monitoring, medication and treatment compliance, and raising awareness and communication. Remote monitoring systems, telemedicine, and video consultations were integrated into public health services in the UK and the United States [24]. During the COVID-19 pandemic in the United States, gamification was also used to improve an elderly monitoring system [25]. Many efforts had been made to prevent COVID-19 spread, such as using a COVID-19 monitoring system.

A monitoring system is software and hardware that helps monitor and track specific purposes. In the case of COVID-19, these tools monitor and track human traffic to collect basic information, such as their current physical condition regarding cough, sneezing, and fever. For example, in Japan, a chatbot-based healthcare system named COOPERA was developed using the LINE app to evaluate the current Japanese epidemiological situation. In Egypt, an integrated system that can ingest big data from different sources using Micro-Electro-Mechanical System (MEMS) IR sensors and display results in an interactive map or dashboard to track and control the spread of COVID-19 was used.

One of the possibilities discussed in this study is the use of technology to prevent the virus from becoming more widespread. Researchers study the IoT and Geographic Information Systems (GIS). Consistently recording human mobility data via sensors and storing the data in a prepared database are services discussed in this chapter. The combination may prove new in terms of assisting in the fight against the spread of the COVID-19 virus. Numerous prior studies had demonstrated how IoT technology was applied in a variety of industries [26, 27], including the use of a set of sensors to collect agricultural data to assist farmers in determining which crops were acceptable and swiftly harvested when planting season arrives [28]. IoT technology enabled real-time and continuous recording via assembled sensors. Using GIS was critical because it ensured that the mobility monitoring process was adequately documented and current. Previously researched GIS had been utilized for various purposes, including the identification and monitoring of sites where tools or individuals can be swiftly tracked and analyzed using this technology [29, 30]. Geolocation and geotagging were critical to adopting this technology. This chapter offers a prototype for a monitoring tool that uses IoT technologies and GIS to detect COVID-19 in the past.

5.2 DESIGN OF MONITORING CHAMBER

A monitoring chamber is a place where several pieces of equipment in the form of sensors are placed to detect human mobility from one place to another. By adopting the framework, this prototype chamber was made with several modifications. Figure 5.1 presents the schematic of making chamber monitoring hardware.

Figure 5.1 is the workflow of the monitoring chamber development, which starts with making a design and then recording material requirements. The material needed is mild steel and a transparent plastic cover with a minimum size of 2–5 mm. The choice of steel frame is intended to facilitate the mobility of moving the chamber. The chamber size, with a height of 2 m and a width of 1.5 m, is adjusted to the sensor's ability to detect human body temperature. Figure 5.2 presents the prototype of a monitoring chamber.

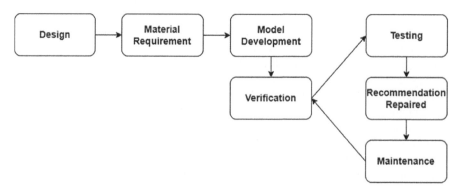

FIGURE 5.1 The workflow of the monitoring chamber.

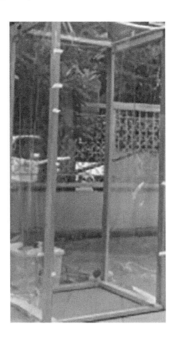

FIGURE 5.2 The monitoring chamber.

The function of the monitoring chamber is to detect human mobility, so it is important to place the chamber so that every citizen of the city will pass through it. Inside the chamber will be a body temperature sensor, a height sensor, and a location sensor.

5.3 RESULT AND DISCUSSION

GIS and interactive maps are critical tools for tracking and monitoring COVID-19. This chapter describes the first interactive page to visualize and track the daily reported real-time cases of COVID-19 in the past. The data was stored on the server and displayed on a webpage that provided the body temperature, date, and time information. The page also showed the number of people and classified their temperature as average (36–37.5°C) and fever (>37.5°C).

This developed dashboard, called the 3AS dashboard, according to the first letter of the authors' names, declared the location and number of confirmed COVID-19 cases, deaths, and recoveries in Egypt. Also, it helped researchers, scientists, and public health authorities to perform searches and used Artificial Intelligence (AI) models to create statistics. All data collected and displayed are available and taken from the Egyptian Health Ministry, World Health Organization (WHO) reports, and Google Sheets about COVID-19. These reported data displayed on the developed 3AS dashboard aligned with the daily and WHO situation reported within Egypt (Figure 5.3). Furthermore, the 3AS dashboard was particularly effective at capturing data about infected cases and deaths from COVID-19 in newly infected regions all over Egypt. The developed 3AS dashboard provided a great deal of information related to COVID-19 including the detailed reported data of each governate in Egypt, hotline links with the Egyptian Health Ministry, International link of COVID-19 for WHO, and statistics results of the

Live Chamber Position

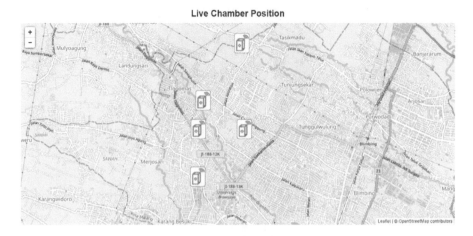

FIGURE 5.3   Dashboard aligns with the daily and WHO situation reports within Egypt.

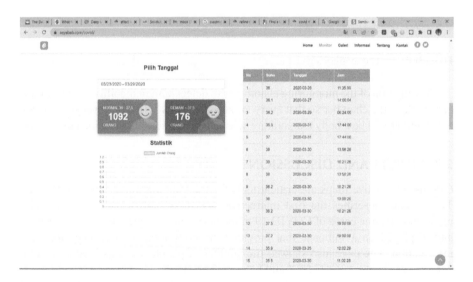

FIGURE 5.4   Statistics results of the AI model daily (accumulated).

AI model daily/accumulated (Figure 5.4). Also, the new confirmed cases can use the 3AS dashboard to find the nearest hospital that had empty intensive care beds.

5.4   CONCLUSION

This chapter describes developing an integrated IoT system to provide information on the potential spread of COVID-19. The system is composed of both hardware and software components. The hardware component is a chamber installed at specific locations, with temperature sensors, and integrated with the IoT. The hardware part is intended to take people's temperatures and transmit the data acquired to AI models to generate statistics about them. At the same time, the Web-based software component provides a variety of data regarding the temperature of individuals traveling through the chamber and a live chamber position.

REFERENCES

1. L. B. Sihombing, L. Malczynski, J. Jacobson, H. G. Soeparto, and D. T. Saptodewo, "An analysis of the spread of COVID-19 and its effects on Indonesia's economy: A dynamic simulation estimation," *SSRN Electron. J.*, 2020, doi: 10.2139/ssrn.3597004.

2. D. A. Schwartz, and A. L. Graham, "Potential maternal and infant outcomes from coronavirus 2019-nCoV (SARS-CoV-2) infecting pregnant women: Lessons from SARS, MERS, and other human coronavirus infections," *Viruses*, vol. 12, no. 2, p. 194, 2020, doi: 10.3390/v12020194.

3. K. M. Posfay-Barbe *et al.*, "COVID-19 in children and the dynamics of infection in families," *Pediatrics*, vol. 146, no. 2, Aug. 2020, doi: 10.1542/peds.2020-1576.

4. W. Xia, J. Shao, Y. Guo, X. Peng, Z. Li, and D. Hu, "Clinical and CT features in pediatric patients with COVID-19 infection: Different points from adults," *Pediatr. Pulmonol.*, vol. 55, no. 5, pp. 1169–1174, 2020, doi: 10.1002/ppul.24718.

5. G. Tiseo *et al.*, "What have we learned from the first to the second wave of COVID-19 pandemic? An international survey from the ESCMID study group for infection in the elderly (ESGIE) group," *Eur. J. Clin. Microbiol. Infect. Dis.*, vol. 41, no. 2, pp. 281–288, Feb. 2022, doi: 10.1007/s10096-021-04377-1.

6. R. Djalante *et al.*, "Review and analysis of current responses to COVID-19 in Indonesia: Period of January to March 2020," *Prog. Disaster Sci.*, vol. 6, p. 100091, Apr. 2020, doi: 10.1016/j.pdisas.2020.100091.

7. A. Al-Baadani, F. Elzein, S. Alhemyadi, O. Khan, A. Albenmousa, and M. Idrees, "Characteristics and outcome of viral pneumonia caused by influenza and middle East respiratory syndrome-coronavirus infections: A 4-year experience from a tertiary care center," *Ann. Thorac. Med.*, vol. 14, no. 3, p. 179, 2019, doi: 10.4103/atm.ATM_179_18.

8. Y. Liang *et al.*, "Prevalence and clinical features of 2019 novel coronavirus disease (COVID-19) in the Fever Clinic of a teaching hospital in Beijing: a single-center, retrospective study," *medRxiv*, p. 2020.02.25.20027763, 2020, [Online]. Available: https://doi.org/10.1101/2020.02.25.20027763.

9. M. Wujtewicz, A. Dylczyk-Sommer, A. Aszkiełowicz, S. Zdanowski, S. Piwowarczyk, and R. Owczuk, "COVID-19 – What should anaethesiologists and intensivists know about it?" *Anaesthesiol. Intensive Ther.*, vol. 52, no. 1, pp. 34–41, 2020, doi: 10.5114/ait.2020.93756.

10. B. M. Davis *et al.*, "Human coronaviruses and other respiratory infections in young adults on a university campus: Prevalence, symptoms, and shedding," *Influenza Other Respir. Viruses*, vol. 12, no. 5, pp. 582–590, Sep. 2018, doi: 10.1111/irv.12563.

11. M. W. El-Anwar, M. Eesa, W. Mansour, L. G. Zake, and E. Hendawy, "Analysis of ear, nose and throat manifestations in COVID-19 patients," *Int. Arch. Otorhinolaryngol.*, vol. 25, no. 3, pp. e343–e348, 2021, doi: 10.1055/s-0041-1730456.

12. T. Toptan, Ç. Aktan, A. Başarı, and H. Bolay, "Case series of headache characteristics in COVID-19: headache can be an isolated symptom," *Headache J. Head Face Pain*, vol. 60, no. 8, pp. 1788–1792, 2020, doi: 10.1111/head.13940.

13. L. Su *et al.*, "The different clinical characteristics of corona virus disease cases between children and their families in China – The character of children with COVID-19," *Emerg. Microbes Infect.*, vol. 9, no. 1, pp. 707–713, Jan. 2020, doi: 10.1080/22221751.2020.1744483.

14. N. Marwah, S. Naik, A. Al-Ehaideb, and S. Vishwananthaiah, "Primordial-level preventive measures for dental care providers against life-threatening corona virus disease (COVID-19)," *Int. J. Clin. Pediatr. Dent.*, vol. 13, no. 2, pp. 176–179, 2020, doi: 10.5005/jp-journals-10005-1735.

15. A. Mitra *et al.*, "Leukoerythroblastic reaction in a patient with COVID-19 infection," *Am. J. Hematol.*, vol. 95, no. 8, pp. 999–1000, Aug. 2020, doi: 10.1002/ajh.25793.

16. H. Liang, and G. Acharya, "Novel corona virus disease (COVID-19) in pregnancy: What clinical recommendations to follow?" *Acta Obstet. Gynecol. Scand.*, vol. 99, no. 4, pp. 439–442, 2020, doi: 10.1111/aogs.13836.

17. A. Jajodia, L. Ebner, B. Heidinger, A. Chaturvedi, and H. Prosch, "Imaging in corona virus disease 2019 (COVID-19)—A scoping review," *Eur. J. Radiol. Open*, vol. 7, p. 100237, 2020, doi: 10.1016/j.ejro.2020.100237.

18. A. Allibert *et al.*, "Residential mobility of a cohort of homeless people in times of crisis: COVID-19 pandemic in a European metropolis," *Int. J. Environ. Res. Public Health*, vol. 19, no. 5, p. 3129, Mar. 2022, doi: 10.3390/ijerph19053129.

19. B. Farahani, F. Firouzi, and K. Chakrabarty, "Healthcare IoT," in *Intelligent Internet of Things*, Cham: Springer International Publishing, 2020, pp. 515–545.

20. Z. Chen, S. Khan, M. Abbas, S. Nazir, and K. Ullah, "Enhancing healthcare through detection and prevention of COVID-19 using internet of things and Mobile application," *Mob. Inf. Syst.*, vol. 2021, pp. 1–11, Nov. 2021, doi: 10.1155/2021/5291685.

21. M. M. Khan, S. Mehnaz, A. Shaha, M. Nayem, and S. Bourouis, "IoT-based smart health monitoring system for COVID-19 patients," *Comput. Math. Methods Med.*, vol. 2021, pp. 1–11, Nov. 2021, doi: 10.1155/2021/8591036.

22. K. Reddy Madhavi, Y. Vijaya Sambhavi, M. Sudhakara, and K. Srujan Raju, "COVID-19 isolation monitoring system," in *Lecture Notes on Data Engineering and Communications Technologies*, Cham: Springer, 2021, pp. 601–609.

23. E. Mbunge, J. Batani, G. Gaobotse, and B. Muchemwa, "Virtual healthcare services and digital health technologies deployed during coronavirus disease 2019 (COVID-19) pandemic in South Africa: A systematic review," *Glob. Heal. J.*, Mar. 2022, doi: 10.1016/j.glohj.2022.03.001.

24. R. Ohannessian, T. A. Duong, and A. Odone, "Global telemedicine implementation and integration within health systems to fight the COVID-19 pandemic: A call to action," *JMIR Public Heal. Surveill.*, vol. 6, no. 2, p. e18810, 2020, doi: 10.2196/18810.

25. R. Leite Araujo, T. Da Silva Sena, and P. Takako Endo, "Gamification applied to an elderly monitoring system during the COVID-19 pandemic," *IEEE Lat. Am. Trans.*, vol. 19, no. 6, pp. 1074–1082, 2021, doi: 10.1109/TLA.2021.9451254.

26. M. Ge, H. Bangui, and B. Buhnova, "Big data for internet of things: A survey," *Futur. Gener. Comput. Syst.*, vol. 87, pp. 601–614, Oct. 2018, doi: 10.1016/j.future.2018.04.053.

27. H. Aly, M. Elmogy, and S. Barakat, "Big data on internet of things: Applications, architecture, technologies, techniques, and future directions," *Int. J. Comput. Sci. Eng.*, vol. 4, no. 6, pp. 300–3013, 2015.

28. S. Roy *et al.*, "IoT, big data science & analytics, cloud computing and mobile app based hybrid system for smart agriculture," in *2017 8th Annual Industrial Automation and Electromechanical Engineering Conference (IEMECON)*, 2017, pp. 303–304, doi: 10.1109/IEMECON.2017.8079610.

29. M. Jensen, J. M. Gutierrez, and J. M. Pedersen, "Vehicle data activity quantification using spatio-temporal GIS on modelling smart cities," 2015, doi: 10.1109/ICCNC.2015.7069359.

30. K.-T. Chang, "Geographic information system," in *International Encyclopedia of Geography: People, the Earth, Environment and Technology*, Oxford: John Wiley & Sons, Ltd, 2017, pp. 1–9.

6 Comprehensive Analysis of Information Technology Solutions and the Impact of the COVID-19 Pandemic on Human Life

Triyo Supriyatno and Fachrul Kurniawan
Universitas Islam Negeri Maulana Malik Ibrahim Malang
Malang, Indonesia

6.1 INTRODUCTION

The way people react to diverse circumstances and how society reacts to an individual's behavior have changed as humans evolved. An in-depth examination of an individual's potential impact on the environment and the community is necessary to grasp the significance of human existence. Every human reaction matters, particularly in response to disasters or difficult situations such as the COVID-19 pandemic [1]. Social connections generate a sense of community, and their absence makes people feel out-of-place. This can have a detrimental impact, particularly in situations like a pandemic. Even at the individual level, human behavior invariably produces broader consequences due to interconnections among people, with each action affecting the larger community.

Human behavior has an impact as a result of mental activity [2]. How seriously a person takes into account privacy and social connection depends on their beliefs and values. Thoughts and mental explanations frequently provide acute justifications for human behavior [3]. Furthermore, people and the environment have been affected by human behavior. When human thoughts and behavior hinder development, this prevents society from realizing its full potential. A barrier to human growth negatively impacts an individual's capacity to support themselves, which negatively affects their mental health [4] and sets off a chain reaction of negative outcomes.

For most people, their surroundings frequently include places of employment. As a result, their negative actions affect their coworkers and the workplace, eventually leading to loss of productivity. A positive work environment is built on the foundations of psychology [5], particularly social psychology, which includes concepts like accountability, motivation, teamwork, management, supervision, and leadership.

People react based on the type of instruction and information they are given from various sources. It is important that people are well informed about local, national, and international situations and changes to prevent widespread panic in difficult times [6]. Lack of knowledge can lead to mass hysteria when people face the unknown. Adaptability is key to effectively handling and overcoming any significant catastrophe. Every person is innately adaptable to their environment, but it can only help if this natural ability is developed. The better a problem is handled, the quicker humans adapt. Economic and financial changes may be triggered depending on how well people adjust and react to the changes impacting their livelihood [7].

Thus, human behavior and the acts influenced by it are subject to a wide range of variables including culture, age, nationality, environment, education, self-awareness, and knowledge. It is crucial to create a taxonomy that serves as a foundation for studying human psychology, behavior, and interpersonal connections, because such effects on behavior can lead to actions that impact society.

6.2   MOTIVATIONS AND THEORETICAL FRAMEWORK

Current literature offers a vertical classification of one of the aspects of life that COVID-19 affected. Most papers only discuss how COVID-19 affects people's lives in terms of psychology [8], education [9], healthcare [10], and economics [11]. There is little research on the interpersonal impact and behavioral and social consequences [12]. As a result, we felt the need to present a comprehensive analysis of the post-COVID-19 impact on several aspects of life and the various mitigation strategies used to address the issues that emerged post-pandemic.

In this chapter, we provide a horizontal classification of seven key areas of life impacted by post-COVID-19 and the gravity of the effects, both favorable and unfavorable. We thoroughly study the technological domains involved in the proposed or adopted post-COVID-19 solutions and the areas they adversely impacted. The study is carried out by considering each of the seven areas and the overall perspective of society. Finally, we discuss the difficulties, unresolved problems, and potential future research areas in the analyzed domains.

Figure 6.1 is a diagrammatic representation of our survey's organizational structure; it illustrates the horizontal nature of the survey information. The remainder of the chapter is structured as follows: Section 6.3 gives a thorough explanation of how the pandemic affected society, healthcare, economics, psychology, behavior, interpersonal interactions, and academics. Section 6.4 looks at how COVID-19 is being combated using significant technologies such as the Internet of Things (IoT), blockchain, Artificial Intelligence (AI), and Augmented Reality (AR)/Virtual Reality (VR), as well as the challenges they present and potential directions for further research. Conclusion and suggestions are presented in Section 6.5.

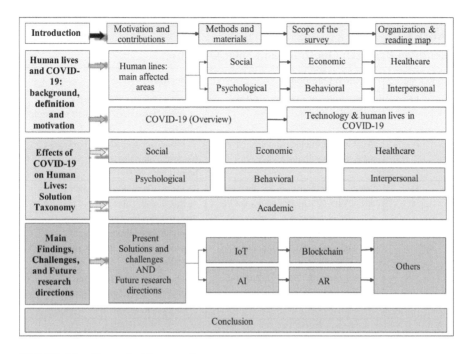

FIGURE 6.1 Theoretical framework.

6.3 SURVEY METHODOLOGY

6.3.1 EXAMINATION OF PLANNING

This section includes the planned format of review planning, research questions to help understand the review statement, relevant data sources, search criteria during the literature review, inclusion and exclusion criteria, and quality evaluation to carry out a systematic study and establish a structured approach. Many existing literature sources were discovered and cited for the study, including news stories, publications, and updates from international organizations. Before considering this study, the included sources were examined for quality.

The authors gathered and verified the literature pertinent to the statement regarding both COVID-19's impact on human life elements and the technical solutions that assisted in the impact mitigation to gain a clear grasp of the review statement. Identified research questions and their objectives are displayed in Table 6.1.

6.3.2 SOURCES OF DATA

A wide range of trustworthy and accurate data sources is necessary for an extensive study. We relied on journals, articles, and books from the medical and technical fields. We used standard peer-reviewed journal databases like IEEE Xplore Digital Library, ScienceDirect journals (Elsevier), University Digital Library, PubMed

TABLE 6.1

Identified Research Questions and Their Objectives

RQ No.	Research Question	Objective
1	What aspects of human life did the pandemic affect specifically?	To enumerate the various aspects of human life that the COVID-19 pandemic affected.
2	What impact did the pandemic have on these aspects of human life?	To investigate and address how the pandemic impacted various aspects of human life.
3	Which current literature has shed light on COVID-19's impact on human life, and what elements does it examine?	To identify currently published articles on this research question and to compare them to identify unmet objectives.
4	Which information technology has aided in reducing the negative effects of COVID-19?	To highlight the value of specific technological developments in reducing COVID-19.
5	What aspects of human life have the various technological breakthroughs benefited, and in what ways?	To present a thorough analysis of technological developments and their use in mitigating the COVID-19 effects.

journals, and SpringerLink, as well as electronic data sources for finding the literature on the impact of the pandemic and how technologies helped to address the issue. Technical publications (published on the IEEE, Elsevier, and Springer platforms), reports (from government and World Health Organization [WHO]), prediction agency websites, and online literature (pharmaceutical blogs, technical blogs, news articles)—all of which pertinent to the issue raised in a thorough survey—are additional data sources.

6.3.3 SEARCH PARAMETERS

The search criteria in the survey include terms like, "Information of Technologies and COVID-19," as well as the combination of technologies like, "AI, ML, IoT, AR-VR, and blockchain" along with "social, economic, psychological behavioral, interpersonal, healthcare, or pandemic," and other related terms, as shown in Figure 6.2. A manual search was carried out because many research papers and articles contain search strings that are not mentioned in the publication's title or abstract.

Potential Search Terms
Keywords: "Information of Technologies and COVID-19," "AI/ML for COVID," IoT in COVID," Effects of COVID," "Physical effects of covid," Psychology and covid," society and covid," "Economy in covid," "Human life and covid"

FIGURE 6.2 Potential search terms.

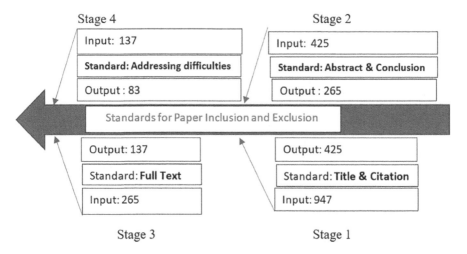

FIGURE 6.3 Standards of article inclusion and exclusion.

6.3.4 INCLUSION AND EXCLUSION STANDARDS

Because one of the main aims of the survey is to demonstrate how technology has contributed to the COVID-19 pandemic, the search terms "COVID-19" and "Information of Technologies" frequently generate results that are not relevant, making filtering difficult. We therefore used the search criteria specified in Section 6.3.3 to prevent this. We included early-access articles and the most current and pertinent publications from 2020. Survey papers, technical patents, books, news items, blogs, and other resources are also included for a broader perspective. The filtering of articles according to relevancy and other factors is shown in Figure 6.3. This filtration is broken down into several levels based on the title, abstract, body of the article, and research. Finally, we identified a few relevant papers and concentrated on those with many citations.

6.4 COVID-19 AND HUMAN LIVES: BACKGROUND, DEFINITION, AND MOTIVATION

Based on a thorough literature analysis, Table 6.2 displays the relative comparisons of the surveys we took into consideration. We found a great deal of literature that only focuses on the vertical sphere of social, psychological, academic, or economic aspects of human life in a pandemic. In this study, we try to cover all horizontal aspects of human life impacted by the pandemic. We determined that COVID-19 affected seven aspects of human life: healthcare, economic, social, psychological, behavioral, interpersonal, and academic.

The equilibrium that humans maintained in their lives prior to COVID-19 was upended. In the next section, the pandemic's impact on various aspects of human life is briefly covered.

TABLE 6.2

Main Areas of Human Lives Affected by COVID-19

Parameters	Brief Description	Relevance to COVID-19
Social	Social events such as weddings and family gatherings stopped. Daily interactions with people in all areas of life also stopped or were restricted.	With social distancing a norm during COVID-19, an individual's social life came to a halt, and in-person interactions turned virtual. Moreover, most countries observed lockdowns as a mitigation measure for the pandemic. So, daily social interactions were also reduced to a minimum. Hence, it is important to study how this change affected human lives.
Healthcare	Being healthy is essential to human life. From a healthcare aspect, different age groups were affected differently.	How COVID-19 affected a patient's health is of obvious relevance. Patients suffering from other preexisting diseases being at higher risk is an example.
Economic	An individual's life decisions revolve around the amount of money they have, which also determines their future. Further, so is the case for a nation's economy.	A pandemic such as COVID-19 affected most people's economic situations and changed the overall economy of nations. Hence, it is essential to study the effect of COVID-19 on the overall economic situation worldwide.
Psychological	Human psychology is inherently connected to other aspects of human lives, and changes in these aspects affect the human mind and response to life's situations.	COVID-19 brought out many changes in human psychology with large and lasting consequences. Hence, it is necessary to study the mental effects of COVID-19 on people.
Behavioral	Behavioral aspects of human life comprise every action an individual can perform. These include sleep cycles, dietary behaviors, workplace attitudes, buying habits, physical activities, behavior with friends, colleagues, and family, and personal hygiene habits.	A wide array of behavioral changes can be seen in people post-COVID-19. Due to stress, anxiety, depression, and changes in sleeping cycles, drug consumption and the suicide rate increased. People started hoarding things unnecessarily and thought twice before going to public places. Thus, it is important to study the effects of COVID-19 on human behavior.
Interpersonal	Interpersonal relations are the building blocks of society. As human beings are social animals, it is important to understand how individuals think about and act toward other people around them.	Lockdowns, social distancing, and working from home made people feel lonely and lack physical interaction and psychosocial support, which indirectly affected other aspects of an individual's life. Thus, it is crucial to understand this parameter.
Academic	Academics consists of an individual's overall learning and growing process irrespective of age. Academics helps people use their knowledge to contribute to society.	In-person learning shifted to online or virtual mode due to COVID-19. This shift brought a drastic change in teaching style, contents delivered, and way of delivery. This parameter is very important to study, as it affected the mental state of every individual who is part of educational systems worldwide.

6.4.1   HUMAN LIVES: PRIMARY AFFECTED AREAS

Humans are naturally social creatures and depend on their interactions with others to conduct themselves properly [13]. Restrictions on social connections, public gatherings, celebrations, group work, educational gatherings, and private meetings are just a few of the many alterations brought about by the shift in daily routine as a result of COVID-19 [14]. These social gatherings or activities impact people's lives to some extent.

Cultural gatherings are frequently seen as a regular practice in social norms and are effective at bringing people together. Daily religious gatherings or rituals serve as a social gathering place as well. These religious pursuits significantly occupy most people's lives. Humans are accustomed to social connection, even in the form of strangers or friends simply sharing space in silence. An abrupt end to the social aspect of a person's daily life might have extremely negative effects.

During COVID-19 in _the world,_a complete lockdown was implemented as an emergency response to the rapidly worsening health crisis. Retail shops and godowns were among the first private companies that shut down [15, 16]. Grocery and medical supply stores were among the few businesses that remained open. Banks and private international corporations cut back on staff hours or demanded that their presence be reported online rather than in person. Several people were stuck outside their hometowns and without jobs due to the quick decision made to lock down. Also, laborers could not reach their villages, and urgent transport routes were closed. As a result, people's economic situation became very difficult due to the country-wide crisis [17].

As to healthcare, people's health hang in limbo especially for those who needed special care and consideration [18]. The rapid spread of COVID-19 raised concerns about public health, particularly for children and the elderly. Young people may have had a better chance of recovering from the disease [19], but it did not mean they could not contract the virus and spread it to others. Major households had children, older people, or both. It was therefore important to limit outings, wear protective masks when going out [20], and isolate if one got sick with the virus.

From a psychological perspective, people's emotions flared [21] which unearthed psychological problems. People's minds are affected as their physical environments change [22]. Individual psychological reactions and group psychological responses can vary. These reactions may be more chaotic than usual when unexpected changes occur. Furthermore, with the unanticipated shift in other key elements of everyday life, such as social, economic [23–25], and healthcare-based situations, there are certain to be dramatic effects on mental health [26].

Finally, human behavior frequently changes due to a person's mental state and is closely related to their environment. The actions of other nearby people can have an impact on an individual's behavior [27].

6.4.2   INFORMATION TECHNOLOGY SOLUTIONS

The Internet of Things (IoT) has played a crucial role in technological advancements aimed at reducing the COVID-19 pandemic. Scalability challenges, bandwidth and spectrum restrictions, security and privacy concerns, and the need for massive data centers are a few of these areas [28].

Because a single IoT device may need numerous sensors, implementing IoT for wearables and IoT services has resulted in the utilization of a significant amount of IoT hardware, such as sensors. Scalability problems and energy needs are exacerbated by this, along with the volume of data circling IoT nodes [28].

Additionally, because of the permitted spectrum that the majority of IoT devices now use, their available bandwidth is currently constrained. With the increase of these devices, bandwidth problems and data delay now arise that could cause a data transfer error [28]. The quick and accurate conveyance of data is of the utmost importance in challenging real-time scenarios such as COVID-19.

In addition, big data storage centers are being employed to store the expanding data. Future factors must be identified to reduce some of these problems. Lightweight security techniques based on many metrics, such as the angle of arrival, time of arrival, phasor information, and received signal strand indications, could be introduced to address scalability difficulties.

To reduce scalability concerns and achieve a logically centralized control for data collecting and monitoring, another approach to the same problem might be to incorporate more and more software-defined IoT [29]. Additionally, attempts to improve security are increasingly focused on energy-efficient primitives that use less memory and have simpler computing requirements [29].

The proposed cognitive-radio-enabled IoT does not have a bandwidth problem [28, 30]. The devices can sense their surroundings and identify open frequencies on their own through the cognitive radio parameters. They can then choose the best spectrum based on their quality-of-service needs [28].

During COVID-19, blockchain was crucial in a variety of fields, including agriculture, supply chain management, and e-governance, as well as COVID-19 disaster assistance and insurance, and patient information sharing. Some difficulties have surfaced as a result of this varied utilization [31].

Lack of a specialized, skilled staff in the field of blockchain is a problem. Blockchain platforms demand a variety of talents, including engineering, app development, and security. Few people investigated blockchain further because there are so few experts in all of these sectors.

As a result, enterprises experienced a severe lack of competent workers because of COVID-19 making it difficult for businesses to train new personnel in blockchain-oriented technologies in the event of a pandemic. To make up for this, internal training programs and outsourcing was started [32].

Distributed databases used by the blockchain network enable decentralized automation. Decentralization also brings anonymity with it. The current legal standards, which demand that someone hold power in the event of any disagreements, are in conflict with this [33].

Scalability, throughput, and latency are a few more significant blockchain concerns. COVID-19 required real-time operation and response, but due to the high network traffic that blockchain encounters, the delay reached up to a few minutes. This could subsequently lead to a decrease in output, which would impact scalability [32, 33]. To reduce this, there are two scalability solutions [33, 34], the unique Versum technique [32, 35] and sharding [33, 36], among others.

Blockchain network privacy concerns are of the utmost importance. Because the blockchain nodes have access to the full database, this raises privacy concerns for sensitive information held by an organization or by users. Furthermore, the sensitivity of personal data is further heightened by various data processing and storage techniques used at various stages. Utilizing distributed off-chain storage to make the data both accessible and private is one way to guarantee the privacy of the user and the organization [33]. Along with this, new privacy techniques can be employed to offer an additional layer of security, like privacy-by-design and mixing, attribute-based encryption, and zero-knowledge proof, among others [33].

Even though blockchain is extremely secure, it is still possible for attacks to be mounted directly into the blockchain application. Whether it's malware targeting cryptocurrency theft or wallets, these attacks can exploit vulnerabilities without concern for the security of the underlying blockchain architecture, enabling swift execution within applications [33]. Additionally, as quantum computing develops, attacks may happen more frequently in the future. Better encryption methods have been developed as a result [33].

We employed AI to combat COVID-19, but we ran across several problems that were present in the existing solutions, such as a lack of data, noisy data with outliers, large data hubris, unorganized data, and algorithmic dynamics [37]. It is difficult to train AI-based models to detect and diagnose COVID-19 because of inconsistent and unreliable data.

Open-source data platforms can be used to address the problem of inadequate data. We can build public confidence in open data that can be utilized to train models because of reproducibility, openness, open science, and open research [38]. The conduct of scientific research in a cooperative and barrier-free environment speeds up the generation of new information, encourages discovery through open cooperation, and strengthens the reliability of findings through inclusive evaluation and peer review [39]. The World Health Organization has used open-source data-sharing activities. The Allen Institute of AI, Microsoft, and Facebook have provided 44,000 open-source articles that can be used for data mining.

Elsevier, ScienceDirect, The Lens, Google, and Amazon all offer carefully curated and current data pools [40]. This addresses the data shortage, but again, an abundance of data can lead to redundancy and large data noise, overfitting the model [39]. This can be resolved by algorithmic adjustments and content curation, which are now done manually by humans but can be carried out automatically by integrating machine learning and natural language processing. By thoroughly pre-processing data and applying a variety of data mining techniques on sizable datasets before using them for models, the problem of noisy data can be resolved in a few minutes. False forecasts are caused by problems with inconsistent and disorganized data. Data labeling, data segmentation, and data organization from various websites can be among these issues. Numerous datasets exist in various languages and formats; therefore, we must translate them into a single, universal language and format [41] for any predictions made by an AI-based model to be used anywhere. Other unrelated problems can be brought on by human mistakes, inaccurate sensor read-ings, falsified information in the global database, and a variety of other factors.

For instance, thermal camera sensors may struggle to accurately detect COVID-19 in individuals wearing eyeglasses, prevented COVID-19 detection from being done successfully [37]. Problems may also arise due to the resolution of the photos used for COVID-19 detection. Transfer learning can be utilized to gain benefits; however, over-parameterizing models reduces performance, necessitating the employment of more precise image processing methods [41]. Every reliable diagnostic or prognostic model must yield accurate results for each sample taken from the target population, not only the sampled population [41]. We still need more human interaction to apply and comprehend data before employing AI models to forecast the future; as a result, more automated solutions are needed to lessen human error.

6.5 DISCUSSION

This chapter offers a thorough analysis of technological approaches for analyzing the COVID-19 pandemic and its consequences. The absence of a comprehensive com-pilation that examined how the pandemic affected people's lives while also looking into potential technical remedies was the impetus for this chapter. Issues like intel-lectual and economic aspects are the topic of existing works [9, 11]. Literature like Goodwin et al. [1] offers a geographical overview of how COVID-19 affected social interactions. No literature examines the worldwide impact. While briefly touching on some of the characteristics, including the economy and healthcare-based components, Chamola et al. [8] focused more on the technical aspects. Furthermore, although they discussed various technical developments, it is unclear exactly how each one benefits human life. Consequently, this review study can fill this gap in the literature.

Through this review study, we now have a comprehensive understanding of the extent to which COVID-19 altered different aspects of people's lives—social, economic, interpersonal, psychological, behavioral, intellectual, and healthcare. COVID-19's negative effects manifested in various ways: people's social life suf-fered, economies of nations took a nose-dive (though they have gradually but not fully recovered), human interactions shifted from in-person to virtual settings, people suffered psychologically as a result of feeling afraid and isolated, and healthcare took a severe hit with medical professionals feeling overwhelmed and overworked.

Despite all of this, a few advantages have been associated with the pandemic. Many families had better opportunities to spend time together. Many businesses adopted a hybrid style of working from home, allowing employees to select the most practical choice. Technological development has given people a way to deal with the unanticipated change while reducing COVID-19. Testing and healthcare delivery was made more accessible, academics were enhanced, and data security was increased thanks to AI, blockchain, AR/VR, and IoT. The integration of arti-ficial intelligence (AI), blockchain, augmented reality/virtual reality (AR/VR), and Internet of Things (IoT) technologies has significantly contributed to the advance-ment of academic endeavors. These technologies have been crucial in enabling tailored learning experiences, expediting research processes, fostering interna-tional cooperation, facilitating immersive educational encounters, enhancing accessibility, streamlining administrative tasks, and providing vital insights based on data analysis.

6.6 CONCLUSION

In this chapter, we saw how COVID-19 impacted various aspects of human life and the ramifications that followed. We looked at the various information technologies currently in use and those that are being developed. We reflected on how human life has been affected by the pandemic and several real-life issues that can be solved by integrating technology. Technological fields like AI, blockchain, AR/VR, and IoT have significantly benefited.

These technological fields play a crucial role in creating information technology and instruments that support the social, medical, economic, psychological, behavioral, interpersonal, and intellectual aspects of human life. With these technologies, the equilibrium that was disrupted by COVID-19 can be partially restored, with even better outcomes in the future. Information technology has improved due to the COVID-19 pandemic, laying the groundwork for more substantial facilities and planning should another pandemic strike soon or on a bigger scale.

This timely study contributed significantly to the thorough investigation of COVID-19's impacts on human life, assisted in developing information technology solutions, and inspired interested researchers and practitioners to invest more time and resources in this exciting field.

REFERENCES

1. Goodwin, R.; Hou, W.K.; Sun, S.; Ben-Ezra, M. Quarantine, distress, and interpersonal relationships during COVID-19. Gen. Psychiatry. 2020, 33, e100385.
2. Serafini, G.; Parmigiani, B.; Amerio, A.; Aguglia, A.; Sher, L.; Amore, M. The psychological impact of COVID-19 on the mental health of the general population. QJM Int. J. Med. 2020, 113, 531–537.
3. Kuruppu, G.N.; Zoysa, A.D. COVID-19 and panic buying: An examination of the impact of behavioural biases. SSRN Electron. J. 2020, 1–15, doi: 10.2139/ssrn.3596101.
4. Boden, M.; Zimmerman, L.; Azevedo, K.J.; Ruzek, J.I.; Gala, S.; Abdel Magid, H.S.; Cohen, N.; Walser, R.; Mahtani, N.D.; Hoggatt, K.J.; et al. Addressing the mental health impact of COVID-19 through population health. Clin. Psychol. Rev. 2021, 85, 102006.
5. Passavanti, M.; Argentieri, A.; Barbieri, D.M.; Lou, B.; Wijayaratna, K.; Foroutan Mirhosseini, A.S.; Wang, F.; Naseri, S.; Qamhia, I.; Tangerås, M.; et al. The psychological impact of COVID-19 and restrictive measures in the world. J. Affect. Disord. 2021, 283, 36–51.
6. Tahir, M.B.; Masood, A. The COVID-19 outbreak: Other parallel problems. SSRN Electron. J. 2020, 1–12, doi: 10.2139/ssrn.3572258.
7. Ozili, P.K.; Arun, T. Spillover of COVID-19: Impact on the global economy. SSRN Electron. J. 2020, 1–27, doi: 10.2139/ssrn.3562570.
8. Chamola, V.; Hassija, V.; Gupta, V.; Guizani, M. A comprehensive review of the COVID-19 pandemic and the role of IoT, drones, AI, blockchain, and 5G in managing its impact. IEEE Access. 2020, 8, 90225–90265.
9. Arora, M.; Goyal, L.M.; Chintalapudi, N.; Mittal, M. Factors affecting digital education during COVID-19: A statistical modeling approach. In Proceedings of the 2020

5th International Conference on Computing, Communication and Security (ICCCS), Patna, India, 14–16 October 2020; pp. 1–5.

10. Kummitha, R.K.R. Smart technologies for fighting pandemics: The techno- and human-driven approaches in controlling the virus transmission. Gov. Inf. Q. 2020, 37, 101481.

11. Nicola, M.; Alsafi, Z.; Sohrabi, C.; Kerwan, A.; Al-Jabir, A.; Iosifidis, C.; Agha, M.; Agha, R. The socio-economic implications of the coronavirus pandemic (COVID-19): A review. Int. J. Surg. 2020, 78, 185–193.

12. Brown, E.; Gray, R.; Lo Monaco, S.; O'Donoghue, B.; Nelson, B.; Thompson, A.; Francey, S.; McGorry, P. The potential impact of COVID-19 on psychosis: A rapid review of contemporary epidemic and pandemic research. Schizophr. Res. 2020, 222, 79–87.

13. Verma, A.; Prakash, S. Impact of COVID-19 on environment and society. J. Glob. Biosci. 2020, 9, 7352–7363.

14. United Nations Department of Economic and Social Affairs. The impact of COVID-19 on sport, physical activity, and well-being and its effects on social development. 2020. Available online: https://www.un.org/development/desa/dspd/2020/05/covid-19-sport/ (accessed on 16 July 2022).

15. Salinas Fernández, J.A.; Guaita Martínez, J.M.; Martín, J. An analysis of the competitiveness of the tourism industry in a context of economic recovery following the COVID-19 pandemic. Technol. Forecast. Soc. Chang. 2022, 174, 121301.

16. Verma, D.; Shukla, A.; Jain, P. COVID-19: Impact on Indian power sector. 2020. Available online: https://prsindia.org/covid-19/covid-blogs/impact-of-covid-19-on-the-power-sector (accessed on 19 August 2022).

17. Auerbach, A.J.; Gorodnichenko, Y.; Murphy, D. Inequality, fiscal policy and COVID-19 restrictions in a demand-determined economy. Eur. Econ. Rev. 2021, 137, 103810.

18. Rainisch, G.; Undurraga, E.A.; Chowell, G. A dynamic modeling tool for estimating healthcare demand from the COVID-19 epidemic and evaluating population-wide interventions. Int. J. Infect. Dis. 2020, 96, 376–383.

19. Sami, S.A.; Marma, K.K.S.; Chakraborty, A.; Singha, T.; Rakib, A.; Uddin, M.G.; Hossain, M.K.; Uddin, S.M. A comprehensive review on global contributions and recognition of pharmacy professionals amidst COVID-19 pandemic: Moving from present to future. Future J. Pharm. Sci. 2021, 7, 119.

20. Chtioui, A.; Bouhaddou, I.; Benghabrit, A.; Benabdellah, A.C. Impact of COVID-19 on the hospital supply chain. In Proceedings of the 2020 IEEE 13th International Colloquium of Logistics and Supply Chain Management (LOGISTIQUA), Fez, Morocco, 2–4 December 2020; pp. 1–7.

21. Cardi, V.; Albano, G.; Gentili, C.; Sudulich, L The impact of emotion regulation and mental health difficulties on health behaviors during COVID-19. J. Psychiatr. Res. 2021, 143, 409–415.

22. Sridevi, P.; Selvameena, M.; Priya, S.; Saleem, M.; Saran, R. A cross-sectional study on the psychological impact of COVID-19 on post-graduate doctors and compulsory rotatory residential interns in COVID isolation ward of a tertiary care center, Madurai. Clin. Epidemiol. Glob. Health. 2022, 13, 100928.

23. Guberina, T.; Wang, A.M. Entrepreneurial leadership and fear of COVID-19 pandemic impact on job security and psychological well-being: A conceptual model. In Proceedings of the 2021 7th International Conference on Information Management (ICIM), London, UK, 27–29 March 2021; pp. 144–148.

24. Agarwal, A. Moving beyond DSM5 and ICD11: Acoustic analysis for psychological stress on daily-wage workers in India during COVID-19. Comput. Hum. Behav. Rep. 2021, 3, 100075.

25. Kaye, A.D.; Okeagu, C.N.; Pham, A.D.; Silva, R.A.; Hurley, J.J.; Arron, B.L.; Sarfraz, N.; Lee, H.N.; Ghali, G.; Gamble, J.W.; et al. Economic impact of COVID-19 pandemic

on healthcare facilities and systems: International perspectives. Best Pract. Res. Clin. Anaesthesiol. 2021, 35, 293–306.

26. Kumar, V.; Klanidhi, K.B.K.; Chakrawarty, A.; Singh, J.; Chatterjee, P.; Dey, A.B. Assessment of mental health issues among geriatric population during COVID-19 pandemic, Indian perspective. Asian J. Psychiatry. 2021, 66, 102897.

27. Liashenko, O.; Kravets, T.; Prokopenko, M. Analysis of structural shifts in students' behavioral patterns during COVID-19. In Proceedings of the 2021 11th International Conference on Advanced Computer Information Technologies (ACIT), Deggendorf, Germany, 15–17 September 2021; pp. 368–371.

28. Kamal, M.; Aljohani, A.; Alanazi, E. IoT meets COVID-19: Status, challenges, and opportunities. arXiv 2020, arXiv:2007.12268.

29. Ndiaye, M.; Oyewobi, S.S.; Abu-Mahfouz, A.M.; Hancke, G.P.; Kurien, A.M.; Djouani, K. IoT in the wake of COVID-19: A survey on contributions, challenges and evolution. IEEE Access. 2022, 8, 186821–186839.

30. Tarek, D.; Benslimane, A.; Darwish, M.; Kotb, A.M. A new strategy for packets scheduling in cognitive radio internet of things. Comput. Netw. 2020, 178, 107292.

31. Kakkar, R.; Gupta, R.; Tanwar, S.; Rodrigues, J. Coalition game and blockchain-based optimal data pricing scheme for ride sharing beyond 5G. IEEE Syst. J. 2021, 1–10.

32. Marbouh, D.; Abbasi, T.; Maasmi, F.; Omar, I.A.; Debe, M.S.; Salah, K.; Jayaraman, R.; Ellahham, S. Blockchain for COVID-19: Review, opportunities, and a trusted tracking system. Arab. J. Sci. Eng. 2020, 45, 9895–9911.

33. Kalla, A.; Hewa, T.; Mishra, R.A.; Ylianttila, M.; Liyanage, M. The role of blockchain to fight against COVID-19. IEEE Eng. Manag. Rev. 2020, 48, 85–96.

34. Jourenko, M.; Kurazumi, K.; Larangeira, M.; Tanaka, K. SoK: A taxonomy for layer-2 scalability related protocols for cryptocurrencies. IACR Cryptol. ePrint Arch. 2019, 2019, 352.

35. van den Hooff, J.; Kaashoek, M.F.; Zeldovich, N. VerSum: Verifiable computations over large public logs. In Proceedings of the 2014 ACM SIGSAC Conference on Computer and Communications Security (CCS '14), Scottsdale, AZ, USA, 3–7 November 2014; Association for Computing Machinery: New York, NY, USA, 2014; pp. 1304–1316.

36. Yu, G.; Wang, X.; Yu, K.; Ni, W.; Zhang, J.A.; Liu, R.P. Survey: Sharding in blockchains. IEEE Access. 2022, 8, 14155–14181.

37. Naudé, W. Artificial intelligence vs COVID-19: Limitations, constraints and pitfalls. AI Soc. 2020, 35, 761–765.

38. Leslie, D. Tackling COVID-19 through responsible AI innovation: Five steps in the right direction. Harv. Data Sci. Rev., Special Is(no. 1), 1–11, Jun. 2020, doi: 10.1162/99608f92.4bb9d7a7.

39. Roberts, M.; Driggs, D.; Thorpe, M.; Gilbey, J.; Yeung, M.; Ursprung, S.; Aviles-Rivero, A.I.; Etmann, C.; McCague, C.; Beer, L.; et al. Common pitfalls and recommendations for using machine learning to detect and prognosticate for COVID-19 using chest radiographs and CT scans. Nat. Mach. Intell. 2021, 3, 199–217.

40. Naudé W. Artificial intelligence against COVID-19: An early review. Available online: https://towardsdatascience.com/artificialintelligence-against-covid-19-an-early-review-92a8360edaba (accessed on 2 July 2022).

41. Luccioni, A.; Bullock, J.; Pham, K.H.; Lam, C.S.N.; Luengo-Oroz, M.A. Considerations, good practices, risks and pitfalls in developing AI solutions against COVID-19. arXiv 2020, arXiv:2008.09043.

7 The Microcontroller-Based Technology for Developing Countries in the COVID-19 Pandemic Era

Dolly Indra, Fitriyani Umar, Farniwati Fattah, Huzain Azis, and Abdul Rachman Manga
Universitas Muslim Indonesia
Makassar, Indonesia

7.1 INTRODUCTION: BACKGROUND

The global spread of COVID-19 had changed behavior in human life. One example is the transformation of direct contact to less contact in interpersonal interactions. Maintaining relationships between humans at a safe distance or humans with an object that had to be in direct contact became impractical during the pandemic. This behavior followed the government health regulation to contain the spread of COVID-19. Technology aided humans in carrying out their activities in pandemic conditions.

The Internet-fueled fast spread of technology had resulted in favorable cultural shifts in developing countries. During the COVID-19 era, digital technology was unquestionably crucial for decreasing and eliminating social, physical, and psychological risk factors and managing the long-term implications of social isolation and lockdown loneliness. In reaction to the epidemic, several developing nations had embraced technology and adapted it to local conditions throughout the past decade, including developing countries.

Some researchers were working in the field of Internet of Things (IoT) technology. For example, a remote health monitoring system (Ngo Manh et al., 2015) for elderly patients (Mubin & Ahmed, 2017) and LoRa monitoring and support for senior people (Lousado & Antunes, 2020). Another instance was a daily living activity remote monitoring system for solitary older people (Maki et al., 2011). The system was supported by a smart embedded home monitoring system (Yu et al., 2013) with a Zigbee gateway (AlSharqi et al., 2014). The technologies are beneficial and could be developed for broader aspects.

In this chapter, we would like to elucidate the implementation of several technologies, such as automatic barier gate, a smart stick for the blind, and automatic

DOI: 10.1201/9781003331674-7

handwashing. These tools implemented microcontroller technology (Sheng, 2019), to minimize direct contact. We used Arduino Uno, an open-source microcontroller platform (Yang et al., 2019) with C/C++ language for communication (Vijaya Rajan et al., 2019), which has a single board for flexible project creation (Arasu, 2018).

7.2 AUTOMATIC BARRIER GATE FOR MOTORCYCLE

We created a microcontroller-based automatic parking gate control system using an ID card that functions as access to this prototype. The system is only for motorbikes or two-wheeled vehicles, in which the motorbike riders do not require direct contact with the parking attendants. The circuit of the automatic parking barrier gate using Arduino ATmega328 is shown in Figure 7.1.

The working principle of the system we created in this research is that the motorbike rider first attaches the ID card to the Radiofrequency Identification (RFID) as an entry access (Lousado & Antunes, 2020). RFID is often used as access to enter or sign in to a system (Kristyawan & Rizhaldi, 2020; Landaluce et al., 2020). The Arduino Uno will process the signal from this RFID as a controller (Hasibuan & Sartika, 2021). If the ID card is readable, the receipt will be printed through the printer, an audio

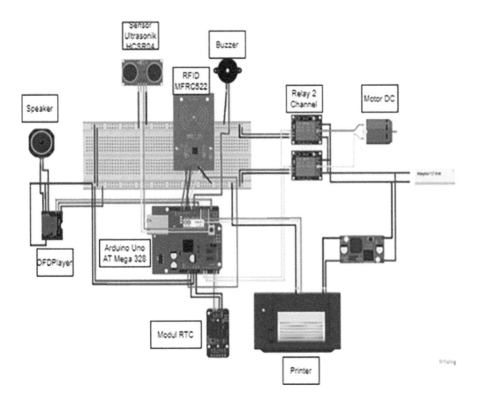

FIGURE 7.1   Arduino-based automatic parking barrier circuit.

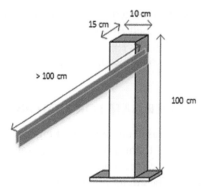

FIGURE 7.2   The design of the dimension of the parking barrier gate.

signal in the form of "Welcome" will be further forwarded via the DFPlayer module (Juhariansyah & Hendrawan, 2020), and the buzzer (Luque-Vega et al., 2020) will alarm. DFplayer is an audio decoder used to convert digital audio files into sound and store data in audio files (Jahangir et al., 2020; Subbiah, n.d..). The buzzer is an electronic component that produces sound vibrations through continuous sound waves for warning signals (Nooruddin et al., 2020). The ultrasonic sensor works as a tool to detect the presence of a vehicle for open and close parking gate purposes (Koval et al., 2016). If the ID card cannot be read, the audio information will notify, "Sorry, ID card is not detected, please try again," and the buzzer will not sound. Figure 7.2 is the design of the dimension of the parking barrier gate. The position of RFID and printer is shown in Figure 7.3. The design of an ID card as entry access is illustrated in Figure 7.4.

The implementation of the automatic barrier gate for motorcycle is depicted in Figure 7.5.

Figure 7.5 shows the initial step of implementation during which the motorcyclist registers to the system by attaching an ID card to the RFID. If the system detects the card, the buzzer will sound, the printer will further print the time of entry, and the barrier gate will open. Then the barrier gate is fully open, and the driver is ready to go to the parking area. Hence, the system is advantageous because it avoids direct human contact.

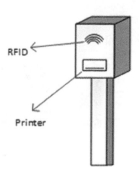

FIGURE 7.3   Design of position RFID and printer.

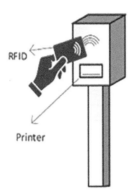

FIGURE 7.4 The design of the use of an ID card as entry access.

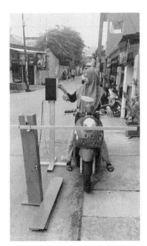 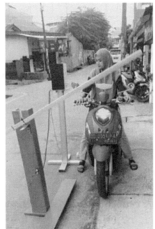

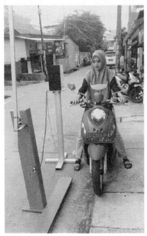

FIGURE 7.5 The implementation of automatic barrier gate.

TABLE 7.1

ID Card Reading Tests with Various RFID Distance

No	ID Card	Distance from ID Card to RFID (mm)				Barrier Gate Status
		0	5	10	20	
1	ID Card 1	Yes	Yes	Yes	Yes	Open
2	ID Card 2	Yes	Yes	Yes	Yes	Open
3	ID Card 3	Yes	Yes	Yes	Yes	Open
4	ID Card 4	Yes	Yes	Yes	Yes	Open
5	ID Card 5	Yes	Yes	Yes	Yes	Open
6	ID Card 6	Yes	Yes	Yes	Yes	Open
7	ID Card 7	Yes	Yes	Yes	Yes	Open
8	ID Card 8	Yes	Yes	Yes	Yes	Open
9	ID Card 9	No	No	No	No	Not Open
10	ID Card 10	No	No	No	No	Not Open

Several tests for using this automatic parking gate are carried out using several ID cards with various RFID distances, as shown in Table 7.1.

In this ID card reading test, 10 ID cards are used: ID card numbers 1–4 are in good condition, ID card numbers 5–8 are scuffed, and ID card numbers 9–10 are damaged. Each ID card is tested six times with the distance from the ID card to the RFID is 0–20 mm. The results show that the automatic barrier gate we made can work very well and achieve 100% results.

The automatic barrier gate is part of a comprehensive series of automated barriers that may be expanded into a high-speed, intense commercial-use model. Depending on the actual circumstances, a backup battery system is also required for low-voltage versions. It may be utilized as a security barrier gate in the future, which is the suggested option for protecting metropolitan areas, private properties, or public buildings from terrorists or unwanted guests. To achieve safe and verified access in entrance and exit gates, automatic barrier gate systems are now the need of the hour in residential areas and parking sites. The barriers are a contemporary and practical parking area management, and garage security solution.

7.3 SMART BLIND STICK

In this study, we also designed a microcontroller-based innovative stick prototype. This smart stick prototype can detect the distance of obstacles from the left, right, and front, as well as holes, and detect the presence of a moving object in front of the stick. This prototype aids blind people (or individuals with impaired vision) so they do not directly contact humans in their activities. The smart blind stick circuit is shown in Figure 7.6.

This system works by using four ultrasonic sensors where three ultrasonic sensors are used to detect the presence of obstructions placed in the front, left, and right positions while one is used to detect holes. The distance between the object and the

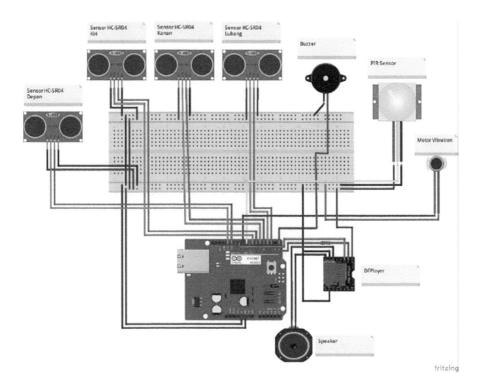

FIGURE 7.6 Arduino-based smart blind stick circuit.

barrier obtained from the ultrasonic sensor will be processed by Arduino as a micro-controller (Ma'arif, 2021; Syllignakis, 2016). Subsequently, the signal is forwarded to the user in the form of a sound alert through earphones or buzzers and vibrations in the stick grip through a vibrator. Furthermore, if an object moves in front of the stick, it will be detected by the PIR sensor (Andrews et al., 2020). The PIR sensor is used for object movement detection in a residential area or environment (Rueda et al., 2020). The prototype that we made can be used for blind people to maintain social distance and direct contact with humans.

The smart blind stick design is shown in Figure 7.7. Four ultrasonic sensors support this smart stick to detect the presence of obstructions or holes on the front, left, right, and bottom, and a PIR sensor is used to detect moving objects in the front area of the stick. The microcontroller used in this prototype is the Arduino Uno, which functions as a controlling component, and the power bank is used to supply electricity to the Arduino Uno. The output of Arduino Uno is in the form of helpful information stored in the SD card module and issued through earphones or a buzzer. The vibrations in the stick grip area through a vibrator motor are in response to the hand holding the stick. The movement of this smart stick is facilitated by three wheels for easy use.

The implementation of smart blind sticks is carried out for people with disabili-ties, especially blind people, as shown in Figure 7.8. The smart stick that we made

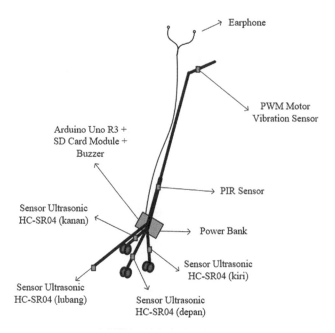

Earphone

PWM Motor
Vibration Sensor

Arduino Uno R3 +
SD Card Module +
Buzzer

PIR Sensor

Sensor Ultrasonic
HC-SR04 (kanan)

Power Bank

Sensor Ultrasonic
HC-SR04 (kiri)

Sensor Ultrasonic
HC-SR04 (lubang)

Sensor Ultrasonic
HC-SR04 (depan)

FIGURE 7.7   Design of Arduino-based smart blind stick.

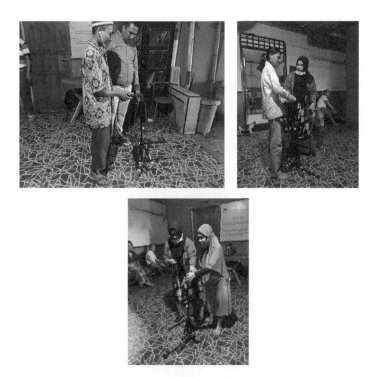

FIGURE 7.8   Implementation of smart sticks for blind people.

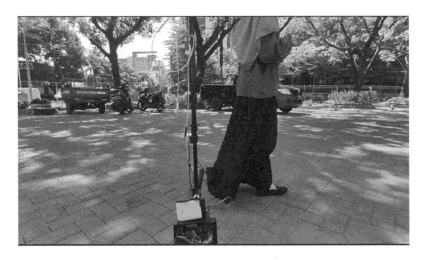

FIGURE 7.9   PIR sensor detects object movement in front of the stick.

is used by blind people. This stick is straightforward and helpful for blind people's activities during the COVID-19 pandemic.

This smart blind stick helps to detect object movement through the PIR sensor shown in Figure 7.9. If the object is moved, it will be detected by PIR sensor, and the buzzer will sound.

The ultrasonic sensor has experimented with different directions, and the results are shown in Tables 7.2–7.5. The tests' purpose is to investigate where distance detects the obstacles from the front, left, and right. In testing the front ultrasonic sensor, we conducted 10 tests with distances to the obstacle ranging from 10–100 cm. The results show that the average error difference is 0.42 cm. The overall test results of the front sensor on the smart stick are shown in Table 7.2.

TABLE 7.2
Test Results of the Front Ultrasonic Sensor on the Smart Blind Stick

No	Actual Distance from Front Sensor to Barrier Gate (cm)	Sensor Detected Results (cm)	Error Difference (cm)
1	10	10.4	0.4
2	20	19.5	0.5
3	30	29.5	0.5
4	40	40.5	0.5
5	50	50.1	0.1
6	60	60.1	0.1
7	70	70.5	0.5
8	80	80.8	0.8
9	90	90.2	0.2
10	100	99.4	0.6
	Average		0.42

TABLE 7.3

Test Results of the Left Ultrasonic Sensor on the Smart Blind Stick

No	Actual Distance from Left Sensor to Barrier Gate (cm)	Sensor Detected Results (cm)	Error Difference (cm)
1	10	10.5	0.5
2	20	20.1	0.1
3	30	29.6	0.4
4	40	39.7	0.3
5	50	49.5	0.5
6	60	60.4	0.4
	Average		0.37

The left ultrasonic sensor experiment used six tests with distances varying from 10–60 cm. The results show that the average error difference is 0.37 cm. The overall test results of the left sensor on the smart stick are shown in Table 7.3.

We tested the right ultrasonic sensor six times, and the sensor distance and the obstacle were 10–60 cm. The results show that the average error difference is 0.37 cm. The overall test results of the right sensor on the smart stick are shown in Table 7.4.

In testing the bottom ultrasonic sensor, which functions to detect holes, we tested the sensor 10 times with the sensor distance and the hole depth being 42–75 cm, where the average difference in system error is 1.31. The overall test results of the left sensor on the smart blind stick are shown in Table 7.5.

Based on ultrasonic sensor testing from the front, left, right, and bottom, the error difference in the system is relatively small, and the PIR sensor on the front can detect the presence of moving objects in front of it.

The smart stick for the blind, as the name implies, is a gadget for the visually impaired that guides the user to their goal while avoiding collisions with objects. Smart blind stick technology detects things and displays the information to the sight

TABLE 7.4

Test Results of the Right Ultrasonic Sensor on the Smart Blind Stick

No	Actual Distance from Right Sensor to Barrier Gate (cm)	Sensor Detected Results (cm)	Error Difference (cm)
1	10	10.5	0.5
2	20	20	0
3	30	30.1	0.1
4	40	40.4	0.4
5	50	50.6	0.6
6	60	60.6	0.6
	Average		0.37

TABLE 7.5

Test Results of the Bottom Ultrasonic Sensor on the Smart Blind Stick

No	Actual Distance from Bottom Sensor to Barrier Gate (cm)	Sensor Detected Results (cm)	Error Difference (cm)
1	42	37.3	4.7
2	44	39.7	4.3
3	48	47.2	0.8
4	50	49	1
5	55	54.7	0.3
6	58	57.5	0.5
7	60	60.4	0.4
8	64	64.1	0.1
9	70	69.2	0.8
10	75	75.2	0.2
	Average		1.31

impaired through voice. The benefit of our project is that it can identify any obstruction using ultrasonic sensors. As a result, it will assist blind persons while strolling outside their homes.

7.4 AUTOMATIC HAND WASH

The automatic hand wash we created in this study is a prototype that automatically dispenses soap and water for washing hands so the user will not need to touch devices. The automatic hand wash circuit is shown in Figure 7.10.

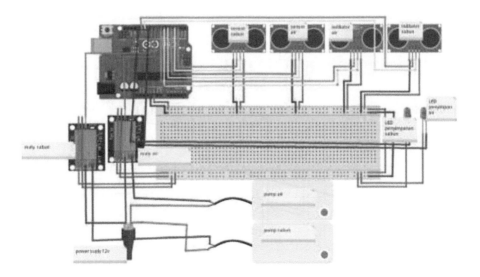

FIGURE 7.10 Automatic handwashing circuit.

The system uses four ultrasonic sensors. The first ultrasonic sensor is placed in a water reservoir to detect whether the water in the reservoir is available or not. The two ultrasonic sensors are placed in the soap dispenser to know the availability of the soap. The third ultrasonic sensor is placed near a pipe that functions as a water outlet. When the hand is brought under the water pipe, the water pump will automatically be turned on to transfer water from the water reservoir to the water pipe to be dispelled; when the hands are removed from the water pipe area, the water will automatically stop since the water pump is turned off. The fourth ultrasonic sensor is placed near the soap pipe, which functions as a soap outlet. When the hand is placed under the soap pipe, the water pump will automatically turn on to transfer soap from the dispenser to the soap pipe channel to be dispensed. When the hand is removed from the soap pipe proximity, the soap will automatically stop because the water pump is off. Hence, the prototype we made can be used as one of the ways to prevent the spread of COVID-19. This is in line with the government's recommendation to maintain the health protocol.

The design of the automatic hand wash is shown in Figure 7.11. The figure consists of a black box to store Arduino, relay, water pump, and soap. Four ultrasonic sensors support this automatic handwashing: ultrasonic sensor 1 is placed in water reservoir, ultrasonic sensor 2 is placed in a soap dispenser, ultrasonic sensor 3 is placed near the water pipe, and ultrasonic sensor 4 is placed near the soap line. The microcontroller used in this prototype is Arduino Uno, which functions as the controller component in this prototype. It uses two water pumps that function to transfer water and soap into the pipe as a water and soap outlet, two relays to control the water

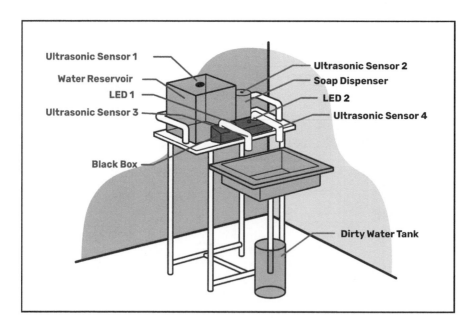

FIGURE 7.11   Automatic handwashing design.

and soap water pump, and two light emitting diodes (LEDs) as an indicator of the availability of water and soap.

The implementation of the automatic handwashing machine is shown in Figure 7.12. When the hands are placed under the water pipe, the water will automatically come out, and when the hands are placed under the soap pipe, the soap will automatically dispense. We made this handwashing tool to help one of the government programs maintained the COVID-19 protocol.

The ultrasonic sensor was placed near the water and soap dispenser for experimental purposes, as shown in Table 7.6.

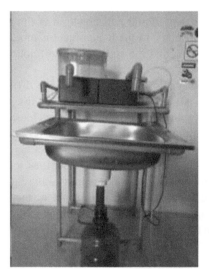
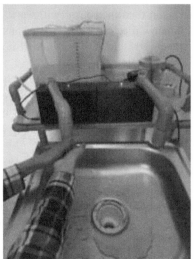
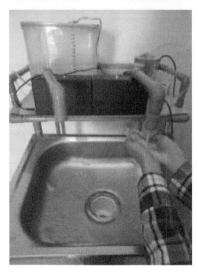

FIGURE 7.12   Implementation of automatic handwashing.

TABLE 7.6

Sensor Distance Test with Hand Object

No	Distance from Sensor to Hand	Sensor Condition	Water Flow
1	<15 cm	On	Flow
2	>15 cm	Off	Does not flow

In this experiment, if the ultrasonic sensor distance to the hand object is smaller than 15 cm, then the sensor will work, and soap liquid will flow (out of the pipeline). Meanwhile, if the ultrasonic sensor distance to the hand object is more significant than 15 cm, the sensor will not work, and the soap liquid will not come out of the pipeline.

Next, we tested the time duration for water flow. Here, we used five different amounts of water 50 mL, 60 mL, 70 mL, 80 mL, and 90 mL. The results show that it required 3.438 seconds on average to finish 50 mL of water, 4.447 seconds for 60 mL, 6.063 seconds for 70 mL of water, and 90 mL on average required 6.571 seconds, as shown in Table 7.7.

Automated handwashing was a crucial tool after completing activities to prevent the infections transferred through touch. Proper handwashing was required to eradicate the majority of germs on the hands. The automatic hand washer was an entirely automated process requiring no user interaction. Providing automated handwashing in a method that minimized touch and contamination were, therefore, an extra advantage.

TABLE 7.7

Time Duration for Water Flow

No	Water (mL)	Duration	Water (mL)	Duration	Water (mL)	Duration	Water (mL)	Duration	Water (mL)	Duration
1	50	3.26	60	4.69	70	5.32	80	5.98	90	6.44
2	50	3.30	60	4.50	70	5.30	80	5.99	90	6.50
3	50	3.32	60	4.49	70	5.43	80	6.24	90	6.48
4	50	3.68	60	4.52	70	5.40	80	6.22	90	6.54
5	50	3.13	60	4.46	70	5.38	80	6.12	90	6.52
6	50	3.48	60	4.21	70	4.83	80	5.99	90	6.60
7	50	3.76	60	4.30	70	5.17	80	5.97	90	6.70
8	50	3.50	60	4.40	70	5.42	80	6.00	90	6.69
9	50	3.49	60	4.42	70	5.49	80	6.10	90	6.56
10	50	3.46	60	4.48	70	5.46	80	6.02	90	6.68
Average		3.438		4.447		5.32		6.063		6.571

7.5   CONCLUSION

We created systems of automatic parking, smart blind sticks, and handwashing using microcontroller technology that enabled practice during the COVID-19 pandemic. The Arduino Uno-based auto parking barrier gate prototype using an ID card as an entry identity marker functioned well to avoid direct contact with humans. The Arduino Uno-based smart blind stick prototype was very easy to use and very suitable for blind people who did not want to contact humans directly in carrying out their activities. The Arduino Uno-based automatic hand wash prototype worked very well. It was easy to operate and supported the government's recommendation to maintain the COVID-19 protocol. These tools were helpful, yet needed further development in the future.

REFERENCES

AlSharqi, K., Abdelbari, A., Elnour, A. A., & Tarique, M. (2014). Zigbee Based Wearable Remote Healthcare Monitoring System for Elderly Patients. *International Journal of Wireless & Mobile Networks, 6*(3), 53–67. https://doi.org/10.5121/ijwmn.2014.6304

Andrews, J., Kowsika, M., Vakil, A., & Li, J. (2020). A Motion Induced Passive Infrared (PIR) Sensor for Stationary Human Occupancy Detection. *2020 IEEE/ION Position, Location and Navigation Symposium, PLANS 2020*, 1295–1304. https://doi.org/10.1109/PLANS46316.2020.9109909

Arasu, K. (2018). Automated experimental procedure using sensors and Arduino. *Proceedings of the International Conference on Inventive Computing and Informatics, ICICI 2017, ICICI*, 383–387. https://doi.org/10.1109/ICICI.2017.8365378

Hamim, M., Paul, S., Hoque, S. I. (2019, Jan.) Rahman, M. N., & Baqee, I.-A. IoT based remote health monitoring system for patients and elderly people. in *2019 International Conference on Robotics, Electrical and Signal Processing Techniques (ICREST)*, pp. 533–538, Dhaka, Bangladesh, doi: 10.1109/ICREST.2019.8644514.

Hasibuan, A., & Sartika Tambunan, D. (2021). Design and Development of An Automatic Door Gate Based on Internet of Things Using Arduino Uno Internet of Things IoT Arduino Automatic Door Gate Bluetooth. *Bulletin of Computer Science and Electrical Engineering, 2*(1), 17–27.

Jahangir, R., Teh, Y. W., Memon, N. A., Mujtaba, G., Zareei, M., Ishtiaq, U., Akhtar, M. Z., & Ali, I. (2020). Text-Independent Speaker Identification Through Feature Fusion and Deep Neural Network. *IEEE Access, 8*, 32187–32202. https://doi.org/10.1109/ACCESS.2020.2973541

Juhariansyah, R., & Hendrawan, A. H. (2020). Design of an Automatic Bell Warning System for Prayer Times in a Net-Centric Computing Lab. *Journal of Robotics and Control (JRC), 1*(3), 92–95. https://doi.org/10.18196/jrc.1320

Koval, L., Vaňuš, J., & Bilík, P. (2016). Distance Measuring by Ultrasonic Sensor. *IFAC-PapersOnLine, 49*(25), 153–158. https://doi.org/10.1016/j.ifacol.2016.12.026

Kristyawan, Y., & Rizhaldi, A. D. (2020). An Automatic Sliding Doors Using RFID and Arduino. *International Journal of Artificial Intelligence & Robotics (IJAIR), 2*(1), 13–21. https://doi.org/10.25139/ijair.v2i1.2706

Landaluce, H., Arjona, L., Perallos, A., Falcone, F., Angulo, I., & Muralter, F. (2020). A Review of IOT Sensing Applications and Challenges Using RFID and Wireless Sensor Networks. *Sensors (Switzerland), 20*(9), 1–18. https://doi.org/10.3390/s20092495

Lousado, J. P., & Antunes, S. (2020). Monitoring and Support for Elderly People Using Lora Communication Technologies: IOT Concepts and Applications. *Future Internet, 12*(11), 1–30. https://doi.org/10.3390/fi12110206

Luque-Vega, L. F., Michel-Torres, D. A., Lopez-Neri, E., Carlos-Mancilla, M. A., & González-Jiménez, L. E. (2020). IOT Smart Parking System Based on the Visual-Aided Smart Vehicle Presence Sensor: SPIN-V. *Sensors (Switzerland), 20*(5), 1–21. https://doi.org/10.3390/s20051476

Ma'arif, A. (2021). Embedded Control System of DC Motor Using Microcontroller Arduino and PID Algorithm. *IT Journal Research and Development, 6*(1), 30–42. https://doi.org/10.25299/itjrd.2021.vol6(1).6125

Maki, H., Ogawa, H., Matsuoka, S., Yonezawa, Y., & Caldwell, W. M. (2011). A daily living activity remote monitoring system for solitary elderly people. *Proceedings of the Annual International Conference of the IEEE Engineering in Medicine and Biology Society, EMBS*, 5608–5611. https://doi.org/10.1109/IEMBS.2011.6091357

Ngo Manh, K., Saguna, S., Mitra, K., & Ahlund, C. (2015). IReHMo: An efficient IoT-based remote health monitoring system for smart regions. *2015 17th International Conference on E-Health Networking, Application and Services, HealthCom 2015*, 563–568. https://doi.org/10.1109/HealthCom.2015.7454565

Nooruddin, S., Milon Islam, M., & Sharna, F. A. (2020). An IoT Based Device-Type Invariant Fall Detection System. *Internet of Things (Netherlands), 9*, 100130. https://doi.org/10.1016/j.iot.2019.100130

Rueda, L., Agbossou, K., Cardenas, A., Henao, N., & Kelouwani, S. (2020). A Comprehensive Review of Approaches to Building Occupancy Detection. *Building and Environment, 180*, 106966. https://doi.org/10.1016/j.buildenv.2020.106966

Sheng, J. (2019). Real Time DC Water Tank Level Control using Arduino Mega 2560. *IEEE International Symposium on Industrial Electronics, 2019-June*, 635–640. https://doi.org/10.1109/ISIE.2019.8781174

Subbiah, S. (n.d.). *Smart Room for kids*. 1–4.

Syllignakis, J., Panagiotakopoulos, P., & Karapidakis, E. (2016). *Automatic Speed Controller of a DC Motor Using Arduino, for Laboratory Applications. December*. https://doi.org/10.22618/tp.ei.20163.389029

Vijaya Rajan, P., Babu, T., Karthik Pandiyan, G., Venkatragavan, D., & Shanmugam, R. (2019). Auxillary Safety Locking System of Vehicle Doors Using Arduino. *International Journal of Innovative Technology and Exploring Engineering, 9*(1), 277–281. https://doi.org/10.35940/ijitee.A4022.119119

Yang, S., Liu, Y., Wu, N., Zhang, Y., Svoronos, S., & Pullammanappallil, P. (2019). Low-Cost, Arduino-Based, Portable Device for Measurement of Methane Composition in Biogas. *Renewable Energy, 138*, 224–229. https://doi.org/10.1016/j.renene.2019.01.083

Yu, S. F., Shi, X. P., & He, Z. Y. (2013). Design of Remote Monitoring System Based on Embedded System. *Applied Mechanics and Materials, 336–338*, 1474–1478. https://doi.org/10.4028/www.scientific.net/AMM.336-338.1474

8 A Wireless Infrastructure Prototype Based on a Cloud Networking Solution to Optimize Service Provision in a Health Provider Entity

Leonel Hernández
Corporación Universitaria Reformada
Barranquilla, Colombia

Fachrul Kurniawan
Universitas Islam Negeri Maulana Malik Ibrahim Malang
Malang, Indonesia

Rayner Alfred
Universiti Malaysia Sabah
Kinabalu, Malaysia

8.1 INTRODUCTION

The COVID-19 pandemic had dramatically altered our lives and our society which was being felt throughout the world. However, it had affected almost all aspects of life and the economy, also, it had seriously affected the health sector. The magnitude of the outbreak had overwhelmed health centers, which had caused it to be even more noticeable in places where there had always been a care deficiency in the different public hospital centers.

Cloud networking represents a significant change from the traditional way companies think about Information Technology (IT) resources. It is a vital enabler by providing a seamless connection of devices and storage and active agents such as doctors, patients, hospitals, analytics laboratories, and emergency services. A typical eHealth system consists of four layers: (1) a sensing layer, which integrates with all the different types of hardware that connect to the physical world and collect data; (2) a network layer, which provides network support and data transfer in wired and wireless networks; (3) a service layer, which creates and manages all kinds of services to meet user requirements; and (4) an interface layer,

DOI: 10.1201/9781003331674-8

which offers interaction methods to users and other applications (Gutierrez, 2019). This approach focuses on the second layer, or the network layer, which offers the network support and data transfers either/or through wireless connections. Many hospitals have corporate Wireless Local Area Networks (WLANs) with multiple Access Points (APs) covering a given area. In these networks, interference is mitigated by assigning different channels to neighboring APs. In addition, stations are allowed to associate with any AP in the network, by default selecting the one that receives the most power, even if it is not the best option in terms of network performance. Finding a suitable network configuration capable of maximizing the performance of enterprise WLANs is a challenging task, given the complex dependencies between APs and stations. Recently, in wireless networks, reinforcement learning techniques have emerged as an effective solution to efficiently explore the impact of different network configurations on system performance, identifying those that provide better performance.

Cloud networking can help improve network performance, plus cloud-based resource management. Implementing a highly efficient WLAN network offers many benefits, which require addressing many challenges, including data management, scalability, and efficient wireless network interaction (Hucaby, 2016). This is where cloud networking will be used because it has different advantages, including scalability, versatility, and ubiquity, which are the main characteristics of cloud computing services. They can adapt to the user's needs at a particular moment. They also allow the use of a wide range of resources according to their demands, have a large storage capacity, and allow access to information from any place or device (i.e., PC, smartphone, or any other mobile device).

This chapter consists of several sections explaining the research method, results, discussion, and conclusion.

8.2 METHODS

8.2.1 Literature Review

In Colombia, the COVID-19 pandemic had caused significant changes in the health sector; *Semana* magazine published a story called "The Pandemic Accelerated the Digital Transformation in the Health Sector," where it mentioned the following: "Telemedicine was just the tip of the iceberg" (Semana, 2020). For Alonso Verdugo, Microsoft's chief medical officer for Latin America, advances in virtual patient care opened the field for the sector to look deeper and apply new developments to improve its operation and efficiency. In this regard, he assured us that in the future medical institutions will bet more confidently on implementing technologies such as cloud networking, artificial intelligence, data analytics, and even blockchain to traceability in several of their processes. "For this to be achieved, there must be a proactive attitude from all the actors involved in the system: the government, institutions, doctors, and patients," he said. In the news, several experts pointed out the following: "The digital transformation in the health sector that could take place in about ten years was achieved in less than ten weeks, thanks to the fact that the technology was ready, it was only necessary to use it."

Cloud computing provides advanced infrastructure to facilitate digital transformation. Cloud computing facilitated collaboration, communication, and essential online services during the COVID-19 crisis (Fana et al., 2020; Garcia-Contreras et al., 2021). The COVID-19 pandemic had forced people to work from home, but they must communicate and collaborate online. Therefore, we saw an essential role of cloud computing in meeting this challenge of working from home and delivering efficiently (Riva et al., 2020; Hernandez et al., 2021). During the lockdown situation, cloud computing technology helped to provide commendable service in the field of healthcare. There had been a brief discussion about how the components of cloud computing were vital to overcoming that situation. This chapter also studied cloud computing remote work during the COVID-19 pandemic and finally identified significant cloud computing applications in the past-COVID-19 pandemic. All countries were focused on reducing the spread of this virus, so this technology helped minimize the reach of the virus by providing services online. It provided an innovative environment that enhanced the creativity and productivity of healthcare workers. This technology efficiently detected, tracked, and monitored newly infected patients at that moment (Ahmadi et al., 2019; Abdelmoneem et al., 2020).

In the future, this technology will help to know and control this infection to save millions of lives worldwide (Aski et al., 2022). This technology is also instrumental in forecasting the future impact of SARS-CoV-2. Implementing more robust networks with easy implementation and cloud networking and cloud computing opens the possibility of telemedicine and eHealth more decisively in hospital centers in the future. Therefore, proper utilization of physical resources to meet various traffic demands and improve system performance will be critical (Hernandez et al., 2018). Cloud networking solutions are made up of a complex architecture (Aguilar & Rodriguez, 2021), which allows them to be implemented in multiple fields (Gonnet et al., 2015) (Salkenov & Bagchi, 2019; Zamora, 2020).

8.2.2 RESEARCH METHODOLOGY

During exploratory and documentary study all the information is collected regarding the needs, problems that arise in wireless connectivity, expectations of IT personnel, medical staff, and patients, and the theory regarding cloud networking and cloud computing. The research methodology brought together the characteristics of exploratory and applied research. It is required to characterize the current WLAN network of the hospital center (Hernandez et al., 2019). The critical processes that exist within the facilities of the hospital centers and the different internal protocols must be considered in this compiled information to achieve an appropriate design/planning to meet all the requirements.

Applied research is done because the designed prototype will be implemented as a connectivity solution for the hospital center, meeting the technical and business goals initially set. A Wi-Fi site survey is performed to understand the site's Radiofrequency (RF) environment. Collect detailed data from your wireless network and view that data. Table 8.1 summarizes the most relevant aspects of the research.

TABLE 8.1

Research Methodology Aspects

Specific Objective	Activities	Method	Techniques Used	Result
Design a WLAN network based on a cloud networking solution for a hospital center in the city of Barranquilla	Collection of current WLAN network information Topology design Choose technology to use	Different software will be used for the execution of the activities	Software to use packet tracer, Acrylic Wi-Fi	Design of a WLAN network based on a cloud networking solution such as Meraki
Build the prototype of a WLAN network based on a cloud networking solution	Provisioning of Cisco Meraki equipment Wireless network settings in the dashboard	Configuration of the WLAN Hospital network with the respective specifications	The configuration will be done from the Cisco Meraki dashboard	Prototype of a WLAN network based on cloud networking
Present prototype functionality on the Cisco Meraki cloud platform	Run different functionality tests on the Cisco Meraki platform	Connect a device to the network created in Meraki dashboard	Connect a client to the Hospital 1 WLAN network and browse	Functional prototype of a cloud-based WLAN network networking
Show the different data provided by the Cisco Meraki cloud platform	Visualize the different functionalities and information provided by the Cisco Meraki dashboard platform	Within the Cisco Meraki platform, different data supplied by the network and forms of monitoring of this are displayed	View the different data provided by the Cisco Meraki dashboard	Learn more about the functionalities of the Cisco Meraki dashboard and its advantages

8.3   RESULTS AND DISCUSSION

The network design implies the evaluation, understanding, and scope of the network to be implemented, which are included in this document. The complete network design is usually represented as a network diagram that serves as the blueprint for physically implementing the network, as shown in Figure 8.1.

A site survey is performed to understand the hospital's RF environment. It will be executed with Acrylic Wi-Fi heatmaps, which is a Wi-Fi planning and site survey tool that allows you to design, analyze, and troubleshoot wireless networks quickly and generate reports. The design's equipment and topology must be identified for this cloud-based WLAN network. The appropriate technology for the solution is Cisco Meraki. Cisco Meraki improves the IT experience, simplifies deployment and management, and creates compelling digital experiences.

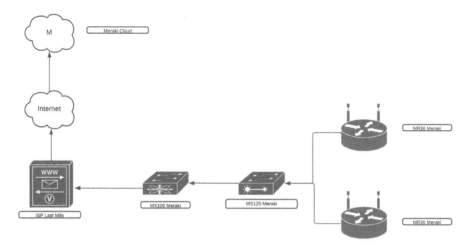

FIGURE 8.1 Physical network topology.

Figure 8.2 shows the simulated topology in the packet tracer tool. The design was implemented in a simulated environment and then prototyped with physical devices

The devices used for the prototype are Cisco Meraki MX100, Cisco Business CBS350-24T-4G, and Cisco Meraki MR36. The Cisco Meraki MX100 will act as a Dynamic Host Configuration Protocol (DHCP) server for the MR36s. In the APs, the Service Set Identifier (SSID) or wireless network called "Red WLAN Hospital 1" will be configured so that the wireless clients can access the services of the infrastructure.

Cisco Meraki's cloud-managed architecture enables plug-and-play deployments. It provides centralized visibility and control across locations, as Meraki MR Series APs are fully managed through the web-based control panel (Novák et al., 2019).

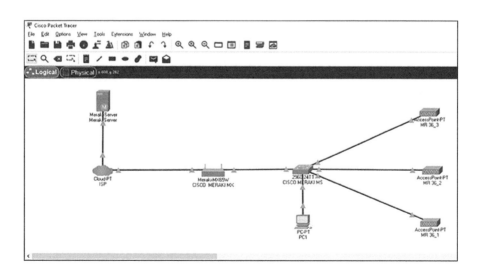

FIGURE 8.2 Design topology in Cisco packet tracer simulator.

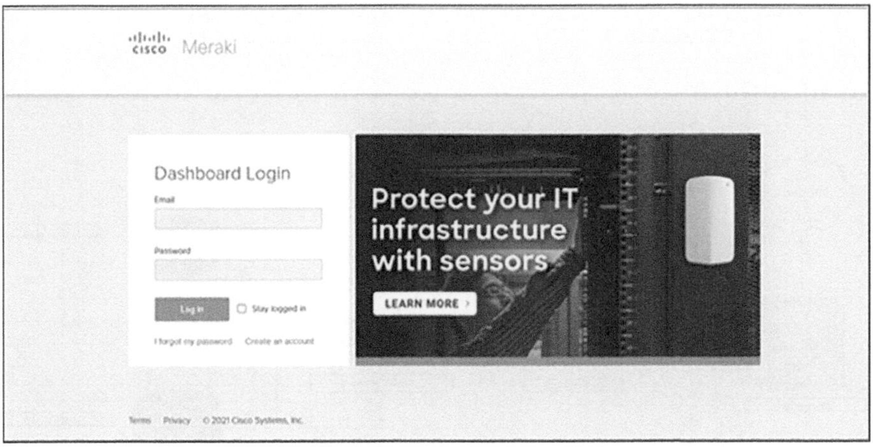

FIGURE 8.3   Cisco Meraki dashboard.

With Meraki, configuration and diagnostics can be done remotely as quickly as on-site (Cisco, 2019). A prototype was made based on the previously designed network and considering the limitations described in the scope and limitations section. Each device downloads its configuration through the Meraki cloud, applying its network and security policies automatically so that you do not have to provision them on-site. Therefore, the prototype focuses on providing the equipment from the dashboard; we enter the URL from any browser (see https://account.meraki.com/secure/login/dashboard_login) and join with the corresponding credentials. Figure 8.3 shows the Meraki dashboard.

The Meraki cloud is the backbone of the highly available, secure, and efficient Meraki solution, allowing instant access to all features within the Meraki dashboard (Cisco Systems, 2013). The Meraki dashboard is a centralized web browser-based tool to monitor and configure Meraki devices and services. It is made up of highly reliable servers in various data centers worldwide. A panel account is what you use to log in to a panel to manage and configure your organizations, networks, and devices. Once the Meraki devices to be used were identified, in this case, MX100 and MR36, an organization was created as follows (illustrated in Figure 8.4).

Dashboard networks provide a way to logically group and configure Cisco Meraki APs, security devices, switches, and systems managers. Devices on the same network can be configured and monitored simultaneously. Panel networks are also helpful for separating physically different sites within an organization. A network contains devices and information related to those devices. It can have any number of APs or switches, but only a single security appliance, hub Virtual Machine (VM), or systems manager instance (Santamaria, 2022). Figure 8.5 shows the creation of a new network, and Figure 8.6 shows the SSID configuration.

Although there are several ways in which devices can be added to a network (for the prototype, the MR36 APs and the MX100 switch are added), for this design, the simplest way that applies to all devices and network types was carried out, as shown in Figure 8.7 (Navigate to Network-wide > Configure > Add devices).

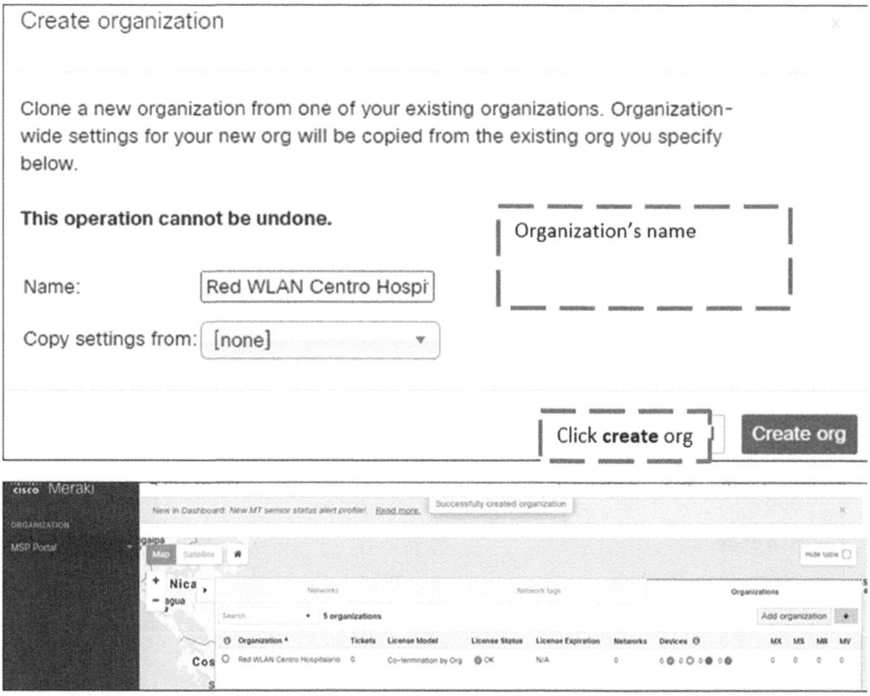

Create organization
Clone a new organization from one of your existing organizations. Organization-wide settings for your new org will be copied from the existing org you specify below.
This operation cannot be undone.
Organization's name
Name:
Red WLAN Centro Hospi
Copy settings from:
[none]
Click create org
Create org
Meraki
Successfully created organization
5 organizations
Add organization

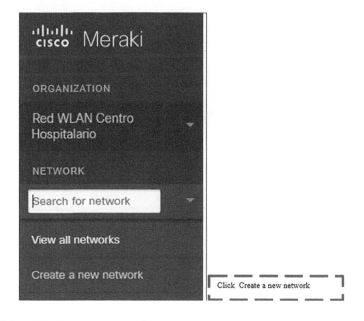

FIGURE 8.4 Creating an organization.

Meraki
ORGANIZATION
Red WLAN Centro Hospitalario
NETWORK
Search for network
View all networks
Create a new network
Click Create a new network

FIGURE 8.5 Creating a new network.

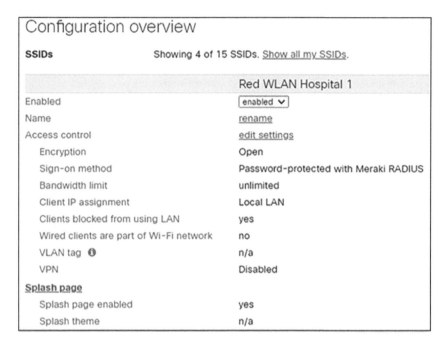

FIGURE 8.6   SSID configuration.

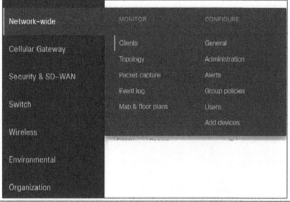

FIGURE 8.7   Adding devices to the network topology.

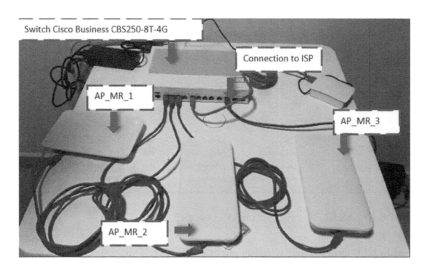

FIGURE 8.8 Meraki physical topology.

Once you have finished configuring the SSID, you turn on the APs added to the platform previously, which will be done through the POE+ ports of the Cisco Business CBS250-8T-4G Switch. Figure 8.8 shows the equipment.

Once the AP is connected to the switch, you must wait a few minutes while the APs are synchronized to the Meraki cloud and download the configuration previously made. When this physically happens, the AP Light Emitting Diode (LED) will be green, as shown in Figure 8.9.

Figure 8.10 shows the list of APs connected and synchronized in the Meraki dashboard.

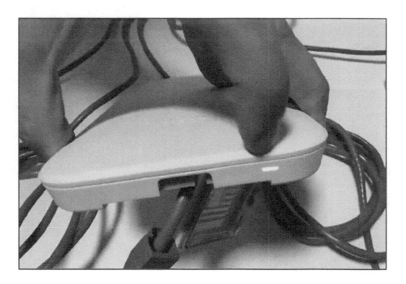

FIGURE 8.9 AP synchronized.

Access points

List   Health   Map   Connection log

APs for the last day ▾

	OFFLINE	ALERTING	ONLINE	REPEATERS
	•0	•0	•3	○0

Edit ▾   Search...   ▾   3 access points   Add APs   Download As ▾

#	Status ⊖	Name ▾	Serial number	MAC address	Model	Connectivity	🔧
☐1	●	AP_MR_36_2	▬▬▬▬▬	▬▬▬▬▬	▬▬	▬▬▬▬	
☐2	●	AP_MR_36_1	▬▬▬▬▬	▬▬▬▬▬	▬▬	▬▬▬▬	
☐3	●	AP_MR_36_1	▬▬▬▬▬	▬▬▬▬▬	▬▬	▬▬▬▬	

FIGURE 8.10   Meraki dashboard with AP connected.

Figure 8.11 shows that a wireless client is connected successfully to the network LAN Hospital 1 and it got an IP address.

A ping test is carried out toward the computer from the Meraki dashboard, executed by clicking (Figure 8.12). The result is thriving, with a latency of 26 ms and Received Signal Strength Indication (RSSI) signal strength of 32 db.

Once the WLAN network has been configured, the equipment has been installed, and users have started connecting and browsing the Wi-Fi network WLAN Hospital 1 Network, it is now possible to enter the different monitoring options and the data provided by the Cisco Meraki dashboard. Next, the monitoring options and relevant data provided by the dashboard will be named, as shown in Table 8.2.

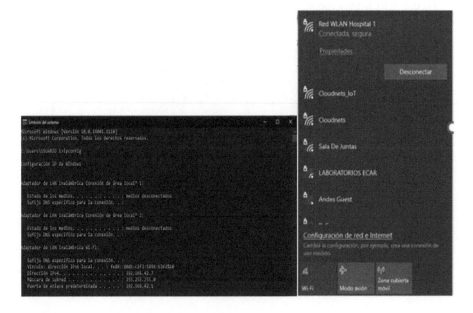

FIGURE 8.11   Wireless client successfully connected.

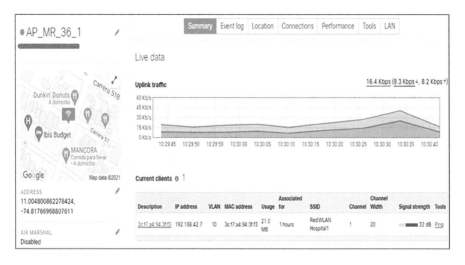

FIGURE 8.12 Network connectivity test.

TABLE 8.2
Dashboard Options

Monitoring Options	Relevant Data from the Meraki Dashboard
Real-time data	• Uplink Traffic • Current Customers: This count represents all associated customers. This includes customers who have not transferred data. • Radio and VLAN Request Status: Track the five most recent requests and corresponding responses, if received • Use in current channels • Mesh Neighbors: Shows nearby Meraki APs on the same channel that mesh neighbors
Device historical data	• Connectivity • Usage • Clients
Location	Real-time location of devices
Connections	• General connection statistics • Problems by SSID • The Connection Steps Chart quickly and easily shows each step of the process that clients go through each time they connect to an AP. This makes it easy to see where in the process customers may be experiencing issues • Customer Problems

(Continued)

TABLE 8.2 *(Continued)*
Dashboard Options

Monitoring Options	Relevant Data from the Meraki Dashboard
Performance	• Usage: This graph shows how much data the AP has transferred over time. If use is unusually high, it can contribute to latency • Clients: This graph shows how many clients connected to this AP over time. If an AP has an unusually high number of clients, it can reduce latency. • Signal Quality: This graph shows the average SNR for clients connected to the AP over time • Average wireless latency • Channel utilization • Data Transfer Rates: This graph shows the data rates used as a percentage of the maximum data rate supported by this Client
Tools	• Ping • Restart devices • Blink LEDs • Performance Panel
LAN	RADIUS and VLANs request status

8.4 CONCLUSIONS

All professionals in the area of networks always look for an objective in the company or projects in which they carry out their work; that is, to improve the network infrastructure and optimize the service provided to the different users. In this case, there is a focus on the WLAN network to strengthen its infrastructure and performance. This project worked on the design and prototyping of a WLAN network based on a cloud networking solution using Cisco Meraki technology for its robustness and simple administration.

Any project's fundamental goal is to anticipate inconsistencies when making a prototype or implementing a network. In this project, several achievable objectives were worked on. The first of them was the design of the network, which, thanks to the Packet Tracer simulator, was possible to simulate the design of the network. However, in Packet Tracer, it is impossible to carry out a series of configurations. Still, it does give an overview of the proposed design if it was viable.

Once the design has been tested in the simulator, the next stage continues, and a crucial step in this project is to make the prototype. Thanks to the experience with the management of the Meraki equipment and the dashboard, the elaboration of the prototyping did not have complications; in addition, it is the provisioning and configuration regarding Meraki that is straightforward and intuitive for rapid deployment, which helps an administrator of a network with little experience implement networks based on Meraki technology without any problems. Meraki has a broad-based proposed prototype, so a network administrator or related areas of hospital centers in Barranquilla will have visibility over the behavior of users, devices, and applications on the network, which allows data to be collected about usage trends and the number of visitors, and general or specific monitoring of a network computer to be carried out from anywhere. The simplicity and flexibility of implementing a WLAN network based on cloud networking using Cisco Meraki technology in hospitals in Barranquilla are evident. The future work that can be done with cloud architectures based on Meraki is far-reaching, as described by Noor et al. (2018) in their research. The solution proposed in this research must consider important aspects, such as security and traffic optimization, among others, focused on cloud networking.

REFERENCES

Abdelmoneem, R. M., Benslimane, A., & Shaaban, E. (2020). Mobility-Aware Task Scheduling in Cloud-Fog IoT-Based Healthcare Architectures. *Computer Networks*, *179*. https://doi.org/10.1016/j.comnet.2020.107348

Aguilar, C., & Rodriguez, J. (2021). Cloud Network Management: A Step Toward SDWAN. *Redes de Ingeniería*, *4*(1), 17.

Ahmadi, H., Arji, G., Shahmoradi, L., & Safdari, R. (2019). The Application of Internet of Things in Healthcare: A Systematic Literature Review and Classification. *Universal Access in the Information Society*, *18*(4), 837–869. https://doi.org/10.1007/s10209-018-0618-4

Aski, V. J., Kumar, S., Verma, S., & Rawat, D. B. (2022). Advances on Networked Ehealth Information Access and Sharing: Status, Challenges and Prospects. *Computer Networks*, *204*. https://doi.org/10.1016/j.comnet.2021.108687

Cisco. (2019). *Introducción a la tecnología de red en la nube Acerca de Meraki, parte de Cisco* (p. 28). Cisco Systems, https://www.youtube.com/watch?v=vIIO7KdwHTw [Accessed 18-09-2022].

Cisco Systems. (2013). *Deploying Apple IOS in Education. March.*

Fana, M., Milasi, S., Napierala, J., Fernandez-Macias, E., & Vazquez, I. G. (2020). Telework, Work Organization and Job Quality during the COVID-19 Crisis: A Qualitative Study. *JRC Working Papers on Labour, Education, and Technology*. https://ideas.repec.org/p/ipt/laedte/202012.html

Garcia-Contreras, R., Muñoz-Chavez, P., Valle-Cruz, D., Rubalcaba-Gomez, E., & Becerra-Santiago, J. (2021). Teleworking in times of COVID-19. Some lessons for the public sector from the emergent implementation during the pandemic period: Teleworking in times of COVID-19. *ACM International Conference Proceeding Series*, 376–385. https://doi.org/10.1145/3463677.3463700

Gonnet, S., Blas, M. J., Gonnet, S., & Leone, H. (2015). *Un Modelo para la Representación de Arquitecturas Cloud basadas en Capas por medio de la Utilización de ... November.*

Gutierrez, J. P. (2019). *Implementación de un Prototipo de una Red Inalámbrica de Sensores Biomédicos, para la Adquisición y Almacenamiento de Datos, Usando Cloud Computing, para Pacientes en Casa.* Universidad Nacional de San Agustín de Arequipa., https://www.youtube.com/watch?v=vIIO7KdwHTw [Accessed 18-09-2022]

Hernandez, L., Balmaceda, N., Guerra, J., Charris, A., Solano, L., Vargas, C., & Alcazar, D. (2021). *An Integrated Framework Based on Fuzzy AHP-TOPSIS and Multiple Correspondences Analysis (MCA) for Evaluate the Technological Conditions of the Teleworker in Times of Pandemic : A Case Study.* Springer International Publishing. https://doi.org/10.1007/978-3-030-90966-6

Hernandez, L., Balmaceda, N., Hernandez, H., Vargas, C., De La Hoz, E., Orellano, N., Vasquez, E., & Uc-Rios, C. E. (2019). Optimization of a WiFi Wireless Network that Maximizes the Level of Satisfaction of Users and Allows the use of New Technological Trends in Higher Education Institutions. *Lecture Notes in Computer Science (Including Subseries Lecture Notes in Artificial Intelligence and Lecture Notes in Bioinformatics)*. https://doi.org/10.1007/978-3-030-21935-2_12

Hernandez, L., Villanueva, H., & Estrada, S. (2018). Proposal for the Design of a New Technological Infrastructure for the Efficient Management of Network Services and Applications in a High Complexity Clinic in Colombia. *Advances in Intelligent Systems and Computing*. https://doi.org/10.1007/978-3-319-67621-0_7

Hucaby, D. (2016). *CCNA Wireless 200–355 Official Cert Guide*. Cisco Press. www.ciscopress.com

Noor, T. H., Zeadally, S., Alfazi, A., & Sheng, Q. Z. (2018). Mobile Cloud Computing: Challenges and Future Research Directions. *Journal of Network and Computer Applications*, *115*, 70–85. https://doi.org/10.1016/j.jnca.2018.04.018

Novák, V., Stočes, M., Kánská, E., Pavlík, J., & Jarolímek, J. (2019). Monitoring of Movement on the Farm Using WiFi Technology. *Agris On-Line Papers in Economics and Informatics*, *11*(4), 85–92. https://doi.org/10.7160/aol.2019.110408

Riva, G., Mantovani, F., & Wiederhold, B. K. (2020). Positive Technology and COVID-19. *Cyberpsychology, Behavior, and Social Networking*. https://doi.org/10.1089/cyber.2020.29194.gri

Salkenov, A., & Bagchi, S. (2019). Cloud Based Autonomous Monitoring and Administration of Heterogeneous Distributed Systems Using Mobile Agents. *Future Generation Computer Systems*, *99*, 527–557. https://doi.org/10.1016/j.future.2019.04.047

Santamaria, A. (2022). *Desarrollo de un Prototipo de Aplicación Web para el Control de Asistencia y de Movilidad del Personal de una Empresa Empleando Cisco Meraki*. Escuela Politécnica Nacional.

Semana (2020). *La pandemia aceleró la transformación digital en el sector de la salud*. Revista Semana. https://www.semana.com/pais/articulo/transformacion-digital-en-el-sector-de-la-salud-en-colombia/303539/

Zamora, J. (2020). *Diseño e implementación de una infraestructura inalámbrica basada en Alepo Meraki y Portal Cautivo para el control de acceso de empleados, proveedores y clientes en una entidad financiera*. Escuela Superior Politécnica del Litoral.

9 Virtual Reality as Social Interaction Medium Between COVID-19 Pandemic and Endemic Situations

Ong, Hansel Santoso, Hartarto Junaedi, and Joan Santoso
Institut Sains dan Teknologi Terpadu Surabaya
Surabaya, Indonesia

9.1 INTRODUCTION

The VR experience is immersive (Latoschik et al, 2019). Everyone used social media to communicate and maintain social needs during the COVID-19 pandemic. The impact of using social media for almost 3 years makes people change their behavior and attitude while communicating (Bautista et al., 2021; Reynolds, 1987). This impact was continued by using and developing social media Virtual Reality (VR). Companies in many fields try to give users a new experience while interacting in the virtual world up to now (Hürst & Geraerts, 2019).

Being immersed makes people feel, imagine, and interact with the virtual object. The key to a successful immersive experience often involves the presence of another character for social interaction (Kiourt et al., 2017). This can be done with a Non-Playable Character (NPC) with artificial intelligence to interact and communicate with the user. However, that is insufficient because one room or world needs more than one NPC (crowd) roaming the area. Another challenge is how to move the crowd (Stüvel et al, 2017) and not to attach with some pattern and make the user uncomfortable with their presence (Owaidah et al., 2021).

This chapter discusses a crowd simulation using Particle Swarm Optimization (PSO) (Clerc, 1999; Kennedy & Eberhart, 1995 for the education fair. The randomness of PSO makes each NPC walk to the destination without any pattern to create an immersive experience.

9.2 PROPOSED FRAMEWORK

The education fair is the simplest way to try NPC crowd intelligence. Some fairs have two leading roles: the booth is just staying and promoting, and the attendant

DOI: 10.1201/9781003331674-9

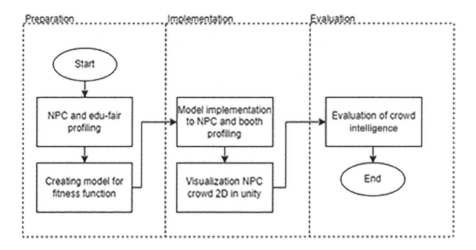

FIGURE 9.1   The fair education stages.

will roam and seek the best booth to attract them. The attendant represents the population, and the food or the objective by the PSO represents the booth.

Figure 9.1 shows the education fair's preparation, implementation, and evaluation.
The commencement of the preparation phase serves as the start of profiling the NPC,
the booth serves as the target, and each person moves randomly toward the target. The
implementation phase will implement the model into the profile in the scenario and
visualize it in 2D using the unity game engine. The last phase is to evaluate this
methodology from initialization and implementation.

Tables 9.1 and 9.2 show the profile of attendance and booth. With this profile, every
attendant has a target, which will be compatible with the booth. For this study case, there
will be 10 profiles of NPC and 10 profiles of the booth. Table 9.1 is the profile of NPC
using high school students with the type of different schools, ages, departments, and interests. Each of the profiles will have a random number with the rang as the initial value.

The content of Table 9.2 represents the booth as the target also will have a profile
like the NPC. The booth's three main requirements are department, school, and field
criteria. Each profile will start with a random numerical score. Every person in a population is profiled and initialized in the PSO algorithm (Shi & Eberhart, 1998). To represent the initial value as seen in Equation (9.1) and the velocity as seen in Equation (9.2):

$$X_i(t) = X_{i1}(t) + X_{i2}(t), \ldots, X_{iN}(t) \tag{9.1}$$

$$V_i(t) = V_{i1}(t) + V_{i2}(t), \ldots, V_{iN}(t) \tag{9.2}$$

where

X: Position of the particle,
V: Particle velocity
i: Particle index
t: Iteration-t
N: Size of the dimension

TABLE 9.1

NPC Profiles

NPC Profiles						
No.	Student	School	Age	Department	Interest	Score
1	Student A	Private	Random (17–19)	Science	Engineering	0.0–0.1
2	Student B	Public	Random (17–19)	Science	Information Technology	0.1–0.2
3	Student C	Private	Random (17–19)	Science	Natural Science	0.2–0.3
4	Student D	Public	Random (17–19)	Science	Architecture	0.3–0.4
5	Student E	Private	Random (17–19)	Social	History	0.4–0.5
6	Student F	Public	Random (17–19)	Social	Economics	0.5–0.6
7	Student G	Private	Random (17–19)	Social	Business	0.6–0.7
8	Student H	Public	Random (17–19)	Social	Law	0.7–0.8
9	Student I	Private	Random (17–19)	Language	Literature	0.8–0.9
10	Student J	Public	Random (17–19)	Language	Communication	0.9–1.0

This model represents the movement mechanism of each individual in one population (Kennedy & Eberhart, 1995).

$$V_i(t) = V_i(t-1) + c_1 r_1 (Pbest - X_i(t-1)) + c_2 r_2 (Gbest - X_i(t-1)) \qquad (9.3)$$

where

$V_i(t)$: Velocity of each individual in iteration
c_1, c_2: Learning factor
r_1, r_2: Random number with a range of 0-1
Pbest: Best position of each individual
Gbest: Best position of the swarm/crowd/population.

9.2.1 GAME SCENARIO

Simulating the algorithm and the model from the framework will be done using a game scenario to make it easier. Every game always has more than one NPC wandering or roaming a crowd. This case will use one scenario using 10 booths and 10 NPCs with random profiles to amplify this algorithm and increase the population's size according to time development.

TABLE 9.2
Education Fair Booth Profile

Education Fair Booth Profiles

No.	University	Major 1	Major 2	Major 3	Department Requirement	School Requirement	Field	Score
1	University A	Automotive	Civil Engineering	Industrial Production Technologies	Science	Mixed	Engineering	0.0–0.1
2	University B	Information System	Artificial Intelligent	Data Science	Science	Private	Information Technology	0.1–0.2
3	University C	Chemistry	Biology	Physics	Science	Public	Natural Science	0.2–0.3
4	University D	Landscape Architecture	Architecture, General	City/Urban/Regional Planning	Science	Mixed	Architect	0.3–0.4
5	University E	Archeology	Geography	Sociology	Social	Private	History	0.4–0.5
6	University F	Economy	Banking	Tourism	Social	Private	Economics	0.5–0.6
7	University G	Accountant	Finance	Management	Social	Mixed	Business	0.6–0.7
8	University H	Law	Criminology	Legal Studies	Social	Mixed	Law	0.7–0.8
9	University I	English Language and Literature, General	Linguistics	Creative Writing	Language	Mixed	Literature	0.8–0.9
10	University J	Public Relations	Advertising	Communications Technology	Language	Mixed	International Relation	0.9–1.0

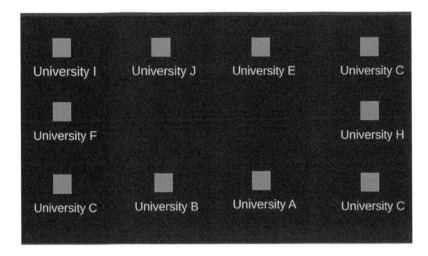

FIGURE 9.2   Ten booths with random profiles.

As seen in Figure 9.2, 10 types of universities have random values to make their profile. The color of the booth is magenta with the label of their type. This example is trying to mimic the real world, where more than one university will have the same field but a different facility.

As seen in Figure 9.3, there are five individuals to represent the attendants in the education fair with a red block. In the first iteration, all individuals will be spawned on the middle of the education fair calculating the fitness function for every individual. The best fitness function value will be this iteration's global solution. For others, individuals will be following the best solution. Each iteration will have the same steps, determining the best individual and others following the best individual until convergent or the maximum iteration has been reached.

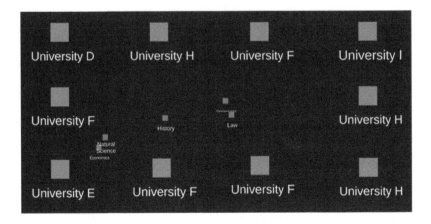

FIGURE 9.3   First trial using five individuals.

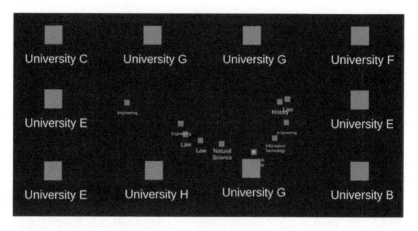

FIGURE 9.4   The second trial using 10 individuals.

9.2.2   CROWD SIMULATION PROFILE USING PSO

The NPC crowd will simulate in Figure 9.4 as the initial condition where the attendants are in the environment and try to visit the best booth from the global best.

Use the ideal parameter, as shown in Figure 9.4, to mimic the NPC population where c1 is the cognitive coefficient, and c2 is the social coefficient, which has values of 2. The start inertia is 0.9, the end inertia is 0.4, the max velocity is 9, the population size is ten, and the max iteration is 100.

9.3   EXPERIMENT AND SIMULATION

The scenario trial uses different parameters to compare the result, which is needed for a better experience. First, the fitness function will use the Euclidian distance and Manhattan distance. The Euclidian distance is used to measure the closest booth, and the Manhattan distance is used to measure the similarity of the NPC profile.

$$d = \sqrt{(x_2 - x_1)^2 - (y_2 - y_1)^2} \tag{9.4}$$

$$p = |x_2 - x_1| \tag{9.5}$$

$$f(x) = d + p \tag{9.6}$$

As can be observed in Equations (9.4) and (9.5), d is the value of the Euclidian distance between the NPC and the nearest booth, and p is the Manhattan distance between the NPC's profile and the closest booth's profile. The fitness function is on Equation (9.6) to sum the distance and the profile.

This trial will decrease the max velocity from the ideal parameter because it moves too fast, and it is unrealistic if the attendants walk too fast or look like they are running toward the booth. So, the max velocity decreases from 9 to 2 to maintain the movement speed and become convergent.

TABLE 9.3

Experiment's Average Result Using Different Populations

Population	Trial	Time for All Agents to Reach the Target (s)	Average Time (s)
10	1	29	
10	2	44.35	40.3133333
10	3	47.59	
20	1	63	
20	2	47	58.6666667
20	3	66	
40	1	47	
40	2	73	57.3333333
40	3	52	
80	1	50.2	
80	2	46.31	57.8366667
80	3	77	
100	1	51	
100	2	63	59.6666667
100	3	65	

Table 9.3 shows the experiment's average result using different populations, and each trial is conducted three times. The time difference occurs because a random factor gives different ways and velocities. Figure 9.5 shows another visualization of the inertia from start to end.

As seen in Figure 9.5, for 100 iterations, there is a best solution fitness function value, which is the smallest fitness value among the other individuals. As the iteration

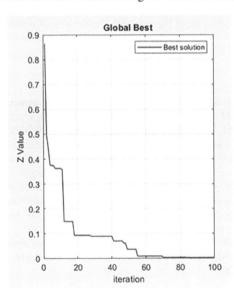

FIGURE 9.5 Fitness value in every iteration.

goes from 0 to 100, the fitness value for the best solution is more minor. In this trial, the best solution touches the zero value in approximately 70 iterations on average. A value of 0 in this experiment means the same as convergent, and this result can be considered satisfactory through a process that does not take long enough to reach convergence with several populations that have been tested.

To test the success of this algorithm, it was been carried out repeatedly and had more or less the same results. Therefore, future research will continue by incorporating this algorithm into VR to test the effect of NPC movement on users. The movement of the NPC in VR is still the same, using 2D and 3D characters for the NPC and 3D objects to create the virtual environment.

9.4   CONCLUSION

PSO is a metaheuristic optimization technique that can be applied to optimize the behavior of NPCs in a metaverse environment. By using PSO to optimize the behavior of NPCs, it is possible to create a more realistic and engaging experience for players in the metaverse. For example, PSO can be used to optimize NPCs' movement patterns and decision-making processes, which can improve the overall gameplay experience.

However, some challenges are associated with using PSO for a crowd of NPC intelligence in a metaverse environment. One of the main challenges is the complexity of the environment and the large number of parameters that need to be optimized. Additionally, the effectiveness of PSO can be sensitive to the fitness function used, and the initial conditions and algorithm parameters can affect the results.

In conclusion, while PSO is a promising approach for optimizing the behavior of NPCs in a metaverse environment, it requires careful consideration and evaluation to ensure its effectiveness. Further research is needed to explore how PSO can be adapted and improved to meet the specific challenges of optimizing NPC behavior in a metaverse.

REFERENCES

Bautista, Y. J. P., Liu, J., & Aló, R. (2021). Behavior analysis of pandemic source media communications. *2021 IEEE International Conference on Big Data and Smart Computing (BigComp)*, 48–51. https://doi.org/10.1109/BigComp51126.2021.00018

Clerc, M. (1999). The swarm and the queen: Towards a deterministic and adaptive particle swarm optimization. *Proceedings of the 1999 Congress on Evolutionary Computation-CEC99 (Cat. No. 99TH8406)*, 3, 1951–1957. https://doi.org/10.1109/CEC.1999.785513

Hürst, W., & Geraerts, R. (2019). Augmented and Virtual Reality Interfaces for Crowd Simulation Software-A Position Statement for Research on Use-Case-Dependent Interaction. *2019 IEEE Virtual Humans and Crowds for Immersive Environments (VHCIE)*, 1–3. https://doi.org/10.1109/VHCIE.2019.8714733

Kennedy, J., & Eberhart, R. (1995). Particle swarm optimization. *Proceedings of ICNN'95 – International Conference on Neural Networks*, 4, 1942–1948. https://doi.org/10.1109/ICNN.1995.488968

Kiourt, C., Pavlidis, G., Koutsoudis, A., & Kalles, D. (2017). Multi-agents based virtual environments for cultural heritage. *2017 XXVI International Conference on Information, Communication and Automation Technologies (ICAT)*, 1–6. https://doi.org/10.1109/ICAT.2017.8171602

Latoschik, M. E., Kern, F., Stauffert, J.-P., Bartl, A., Botsch, M., & Lugrin, J.-L. (2019). Not Alone Here?! Scalability and User Experience of Embodied Ambient Crowds in Distributed Social Virtual Reality. *IEEE Transactions on Visualization and Computer Graphics*, 25(5), 2134–2144. https://doi.org/10.1109/TVCG.2019.2899250

Owaidah, A. A., Olaru, D., Bennamoun, M., Sohel, F., & Khan, R. N. (2021). Modelling Mass Crowd Using Discrete Event Simulation: A Case Study of Integrated Tawaf and Sayee Rituals During Hajj. *IEEE Access*, 9, 79424–79448. https://doi.org/10.1109/ACCESS.2021.3083265

Reynolds, C. W. (1987). Flocks, herds and schools: A distributed behavioral model. *Proceedings of the 14th Annual Conference on Computer Graphics and Interactive Techniques*, 25–34. https://doi.org/10.1145/37401.37406

Shi, Y., & Eberhart, R. (1998). A modified particle swarm optimizer. *1998 IEEE International Conference on Evolutionary Computation Proceedings. IEEE World Congress on Computational Intelligence (Cat. No.98TH8360)*, 69–73. https://doi.org/10.1109/ICEC.1998.699146

Stüvel, S. A., Magnenat-Thalmann, N., Thalmann, D., Stappen, A. F., & Egges, A. (2017). Torso Crowds. *IEEE Transactions on Visualization and Computer Graphics*, 23(7), 1823–1837. https://doi.org/10.1109/TVCG.2016.2545670

10 The Integration of Ambient Intelligence with Serious Game for Recommendation System of Tourist Destinations Post-COVID-19 Pandemic

Yunifa Miftachul Arif, Fachrul Kurniawan,
Hani Nurhayati, Fresy Nugroho, Muhamad Faisal,
Ahmad Fahmi Karami, and Ashri Shabrina Afrah
Universitas Islam Negeri Maulana Malik Ibrahim Malang
Malang, Indonesia

Roman Voliansky
Dniprovsky State Technical University
Kamianske, Ukraine

10.1 INTRODUCTION

The COVID-19 pandemic had hit the world and hampered the development of Indonesia's tourism sector. In the wake of the COVID-19 pandemic, tourists will be more careful in choosing Tourist Destinations (TDs). More detailed knowledge and information must be available about TDs. The information is expected to be used to select and plan destinations and determine the schedule of TDs being visited [1]. The developing digital technology makes information about the characteristics of TDs available and can be obtained easily through the Web and social media. However, tourists still have to make more effort in the decision-making process to choose destinations that suit their characteristics and desires. In other words, tourists need recommendations to help determine the TDs to be visited [2]. Furthermore, to maximize understanding of the content being taught, the tourism learning media should be fun for the user through games.

A serious game is a fun multimedia pedagogic that helps players develop knowledge and expertise [3]. Furthermore, serious games require technical support to provide responses and knowledge following the conditions and characteristics of the player to improve interaction, efficiency, and learning accuracy [4]. In the serious game of TDs, multimedia feedback can be visualized in the form of changes in the

DOI: 10.1201/9781003331674-10

choice of travel scenarios set automatically in the game. The scenario represents the choice of tourist TDs recommended by the serious game. Therefore, an integrated recommendation engine is needed in the serious game to determine recommendations for selecting TDs according to the characteristics and wishes of the player.

A potential component for the integrated recommendation engine is the Ambient Intelligence (AML), virtual environment development technology that can respond adaptively to users. A virtual environment with AML has several characteristics: it is sensitive, responsive, adaptive, transparent, ubiquitous, and intelligent [5]. The presence of AML in the game is expected to increase interest and understanding through the suitability of visualization of knowledge based on the awareness of players' presence, needs, and characteristics/preferences [6]. Systems in the AML environment can detect and interpret human activities and provide multimedia feedback to provide guidance, recommendations, and learning [7].

A recommender system uses algorithms to analyze vast volumes of data, especially product and user information, and then provides relevant suggestions or recommendations based on a data mining approach [8]. The reference for generating recommendations for selecting TDs is based on the factors that influence tourists in choosing TDs. In general, two things influence tourists in determining their TDs, namely Personal Characteristics (PCs) and Destination Attributes (DAs), each of which has several attributes that vary. All attributes possessed by PCs describe the inherent characteristics of each traveler. In comparison, the attributes of DAs describe the characteristics inherent in each TD [9, 10]. Furthermore, using more detailed rating criteria can improve the prediction and accuracy of the recommendations [11]. The development of the recommendation system should consider all tourist characteristics and attributes of TD assessments.

10.2   SERIOUS GAME

A serious game is a game genre that contains interactive technology applications that have more comprehensive functions than ordinary games. It can contain training, policy exploration, analytics, visualization, simulation, education, military, and health. Serious games can also be defined as applications that combine educational content with gameplay by integrating learning objectives into the game environment. This genre aims to educate or train players but is wrapped in a fun game [12]. The application areas of serious games include simulators, education, health, advertising and services, archaeology, politics, and project management. Serious games are a new, practical approach to training and exploration with low cost and risk possibilities. Games can be an adequate substitute for direct experience in the real world or actual infrastructure because games can produce learning experiences relatively quickly and safely [13].

One of the studies on incorporating tourism content into games explained that tourism games contribute to more valuable interactions with higher satisfaction levels and increase awareness and loyalty to the destination [14]. The research object is several online tourism games in Canada, Thailand, and Brazil. An example of a game scenario used in this research is about treasure hunting in a TD, which aims to help visitors explore various areas and collect points, photos, memories, and experiences. Another study stated that the focus on tourism in a game is sometimes not well developed and can even damage the game's purpose [15]. Therefore, an appropriate scenario is needed to adopt tourism elements in a game.

10.3 AMBIENT INTELLIGENCE (AML)

AML is a technology that originates from a broad computing application and aims to respond appropriately to humans' presence and characteristics in a virtual or real environment. AML provides services that work automatically, which are useful for facilitating human work. AML technology features include being sensitive, responsive, adaptive, transparent, ubiquitous, and intelligent. The presence of AML can increase the interaction between users and the technology using computer equipment that can be accessed from different places through ubiquitous computing [5]. The application of AML in game technology supports adjusting the virtual environment's behavior to the players' needs and preferences.

Game technology provides an interface for the user and seeks to maintain their existence and interaction through attractive interactions with features and tools [6]. Characteristics of games and entertainment can be combined with AML technology to give rise to new entertainment applications described by ambient entertainment. One example of ambient entertainment is an ambient entertainment application about virtual conductors that provide direction to musicians through animated hand movements that can change adaptively in response to sound analysis data produced by musical instruments [7]. Hence, ambient technology creates an adaptive game environment.

10.4 AMBIENT INTELLIGENCE FOR TOURISM
DESTINATIONS SERIOUS GAME

In this chapter, AML technology supports interaction between players and serious games. The AML responds to the knowledge of TDs through a choice of scenarios recommended by the serious game system. The recommendation response is adjusted to the player's preference. The TD selection features are PCs, Rating Destinations Attribute (RDA), and Player Expectations (EPs). Figure 10.1 shows the AML system's serious game design for selecting TDs.

Three main parts of the AML serious game are decentralized data sharing, a recommendation system for selecting TDs, and scenario control serious games. In general, the system works based on three types of input as a feature of selecting TDs. The three features include PC, RDA, and player EPs. A decentralized data filter is one part of this research that is responsible for the circulation, availability, and security of data needed by the system. Among the three datasets for selecting TDs, PC and RDA are data circulated through a decentralized data-sharing system. The two data types are a reference for the recommendation system to produce recommendations for TDs. The recommendations produced with the EP data become input for the serious game scenario control system to determine scenario choices for players in which every change in scenario choice will affect changes in the virtual environment faced by players in the game.

Two method approaches are used in this chapter: known and unknown. The known rating approach is used for calculations when the user already has a rating of

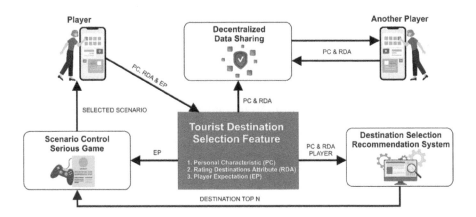

FIGURE 10.1 Ambient intelligence in the serious game of tourism destinations selection.

at least two items. The recommendation calculation is carried out using the known rating approach when the player, as a potential tourist, already has an assessment or rating (RDA) of at least two TD items. The method in the known rating approach used in this study is the Multi-Criteria Recommender System (MCRS). In contrast, the unknown rating is the approach used if the player, as a potential tourist, does not yet have an overview of the rating for the tourism destinations that are the recommendation system items. So that the ranking of Top N recommendations is generated based on PC data reference, we used the Artificial Neural Network (ANN) method to classify the Top N items of TDs based on the player's PC data input.

10.5 MCRS-BASED KNOWN RATING APPROACH

In the known rating approach, the system assumes that the player has visited at least two TDs. This condition allows them to provide an assessment rating for each of the criteria for the TDs they visit. This study uses data RDA as a reference in generating recommendations using the MCRS method. RDA data are defined based on the criteria in the 6AsTD framework consisting of R1, R2, R3, R4, R5, R6, and R0. Each criterion becomes a reference in rating the value of halal TDs by tourists who collect rating data. The MCRS, in this study, uses RDA data from players as a reference to predict the rating criteria for TDs that are not yet known based on their resemblance to the RDA reference data in the database.

The MCRS is a method for generating recommendations that work by extending the traditional approach [16, 17]. The MCRS uses a heuristic-based approach to generate recommendation ranking predictions. This method expands by increasing the ratings to cover various item attributes and combining their ranks to improve prediction accuracy. To carry out its function, MCRS works in two phases: prediction and recommendation. Prediction is the phase in which the system performs the process of calculating predictions from user preferences, whereas the recommendation is the phase in which users get item recommendations [18]. This study defines a player as a user who wants to get recommendations for halal tourist attractions through games.

We use the MCRS to produce these recommendations using a heuristic approach. This neighborhood-based collaborative filtering approach has several steps to determine criteria for user u. The first step is to calculate the similarity rating on each user criterion to the previous tourist data as u'. To find $sim(u,u')$ similarity ratings, there are two methods: cosine-based similarity [Equation (10.1)] and Pearson correlation-based similarity [Equation (10.2)] [18, 19], where $I(u,u')$ is the item that gets the rating from the user u, u', and $R(u,i)$ is the rating from the user for the item.

$$sim(u,u') = \frac{\sum_{i \in I(u,u')} R(u,i)R(u',i)}{\sqrt{\sum_{i \in I(u,u')} R(u,i)^2} \sqrt{\sum_{i \in I(u,u')} R(u,i)^2}} \tag{10.1}$$

$$sim(u,u') = \frac{\sum_{i \in I(u,u')} \left(R(u,i) - \overline{R(u)}\right)\left(R(u',i) - \overline{R(u')}\right)}{\sqrt{\sum_{i \in I(u,u')} \left(R(u,i) - \overline{R(u)}\right)^2} \sqrt{\sum_{i \in I(u,u')} R(u',i) - \overline{R(u')}^2}} \tag{10.2}$$

The second step in the heuristic approach is finding a similarity ranking. Several methods that can be used to find the similarity ranking include average similarity $sim_{avg}(u,u')$, worst-case (smallest) similarity $sim_{min}(u,u')$, and aggregate similarity $sim_{agregate}(u,u')$, as shown by Equations (10.3–10.5) [18], where $sim_{avg}(u,u')$ is the average similarity criteria between user u and user u'. Meanwhile $sim_{min}(u,u')$ is the formula to get the worst-case (smallest) similarity between user u and user u'. In the three equations, the value of c is the criteria for TD items, whereas the value of n represents the number of criteria that get a rating from the user. Furthermore, in the calculation of aggregate similarity $sim_{agregate}(u,u')$, the value of w_c is the weight of the c criterion, owned by each TD item. In this study, the weight of each TD item criteria is assumed to have the same value.

$$sim_{avg}(u,u') = \frac{1}{n+1} \sum_{c=0}^{n} sim_c(u,u') \tag{10.3}$$

$$sim_{min}(u,u') = \frac{min}{c = 0,\ldots,n} sim_c(u,u') \tag{10.4}$$

$$sim_{agregate}(u,u') = \sum_{c=0}^{n} w_c sim_c(u,u') \tag{10.5}$$

Where:

$$u' = (u'_1, u'_2, \ldots, u'_m) \tag{10.6}$$

In Equation (10.6), m is the number of users u', which is used as a reference in finding the similarity of each user u. Furthermore, to find user u' who has the highest similarity to user u, it is necessary to rank the calculation results of average similarity, worst-case (smallest) similarity, or aggregate similarity.

10.6 ARTIFICIAL NEURAL NETWORK-BASED UNKNOWN RATING APPROACH

In producing system recommendations, it is possible to be faced with a condition where the player is a potential tourist who has never come to one of the destinations in the tourist area. So an unknown rating approach is needed in producing recommendations for selecting TDs. One part of MCRS works based on tourist PC data, using ANN to classify the selection of TD on PC_1 to PC_n data. With the recommendation system using tourist PC data, it is hoped that it can produce recommendation predictions in the early stages of using the system before the user assessment data are known against the DA criteria. The 10 PC criteria proposed in this study are gender (Gdr), age (Age), job (Job), hobby (Hob), motivations (Mot), marital status (Mrt), Origin (Org), people in a group (PIG), educations (Edu), and repetition (Rep). The dataset for each criterion is training data obtained from previous tourists. After training and obtaining the preferred TD classification model based on PC1 to PC9 data, the PC User data input is matched with the classification results to estimate the TD choice recommendation according to the User PC. The design of a machine learning-based MCRS system using PC data is shown in Figure 10.2.

In the learning process phase, training data containing PC data and five tourist options are trained using one of the ANN methods, Multi-Layer Perceptron (MLP). At this stage, we tested several MLP architectural models to find the architecture with the best accuracy. In this study, the weight and bias values generated from data training are used in the data testing process to produce recommendations for the choice of TDs for players as new tourists. This process is the same as the system can overcome the cold-start problem in the recommendation system based on the

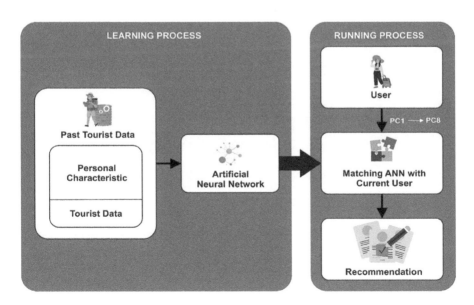

FIGURE 10.2 ANN-based unknown rating recommender system using PC data.

known rating approach. The system can still recommend items even to new users whose rating models are unknown.

In the training process, the data are trained using a backpropagation learning algorithm to form the best network and produce the appropriate weight and bias values. This process is done to produce the best output in the testing process.

10.7 AMBIENT INTELLIGENCE-BASED SERIOUS GAME FOR TOURISM RECOMMENDATION SYSTEM

The recommendation system uses two types of datasets. The first contains rating data on tourist ratings of TDs (RDA). These data are used as the MCRS reference data in the known rating approach. The second dataset contains a collection of PC data for tourists and their five choices of TDs. The data are used as training data in the ANN classification to generate recommendations based on the unknown rating approach. This study's two datasets were taken in Batu, a tourism area in Indonesia.

10.7.1 KNOWN RATING RESULT

The recommender system testing phase aims to analyze the MCRS performance in creating recommendations. One crucial part of the MCRS method is to look for similarities in the user assessment model. Each criterion for halal tourism destinations is based on other tourist RDA datasets. We used 158 RDA data obtained by filling out questionnaires.

Furthermore, Figure 10.3 compares the accuracy performance of MCRS with a conventional recommender system that only uses single criteria. The results of this comparison indicate that MCRS generally has a higher accuracy level than the single-criteria recommendation system.

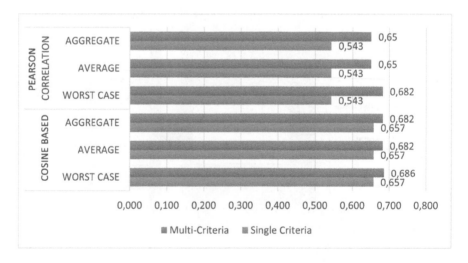

FIGURE 10.3 Comparison of accuracy for cosine-based similarity and Pearson correlation-based similarity.

TABLE 10.1

Comparison of Known and Unknown Rating Recommender Systems

Recommender Approach	Accuracy	Precision	Recall	F1 Score
Known rating using MCRS	0.743	0.640	0.640	0.640
Unknown rating using ANN	0.660	0.590	0.675	0.630

10.7.2 Unknown Rating Result

The unknown rating-based recommendation system in this study uses PC data and choice of TDs obtained through a questionnaire, which is then processed and used in determining TD recommendations in Batu. This research uses an MLP ANN method with a backpropagation learning algorithm. In the experiment process, the error/loss value that does not match the target error will be weighted to produce an error value that matches the target error. A neural network-based recommendation system is used to model the interaction of user features and items through an MLP architecture. The architecture will add a hidden layer to the item and user vectors in the MLP framework to learn about the interaction between items and users. It provides a great deal of flexibility and nonlinearity to learning about interactions between users and items [20].

The testing process was carried out to compare the results of testing data using the ANN method with the actual testing data from the tourist data collection. The data consist of 227 actual data, with 80% training data and 20% testing data. Table 10.1 shows the differences in the results of the recommendations using the known rating approach with the unknown rating. The accuracy of the recommender system based on the known rating is 0.743, whereas the recommender system based on the unknown rating produces an accuracy of 0.660. Figure 10.4 is an example of a virtual environment visualization of the scenario options determined based on the recommendations. These recommendations are adaptively generated based on PC data and DA player ratings.

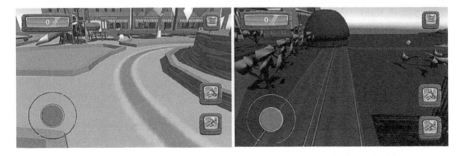

FIGURE 10.4 Visualization of the selected scenario of the virtual environment in the tourism promotions serious game.

10.8   CONCLUSION

This study discusses the development of serious game-based tourism promotion media in the post-COVID-19 pandemic. Serious games that are built are equipped with AML technology based on a recommender system using a known and unknown rating approach. We use MCRS to generate recommendations based on a known rating approach. As for the unknown rating approach, we use the ANN method based on user PC data. The experimental results show that the recommender system can provide an adaptive response to players through recommendations for the choice of TDs, which are visualized in a virtual environment scenario of a serious game. These results indicate that the known rating approach has a higher level of accuracy than the unknown rating approach.

REFERENCES

1. F. Peyghambari, M. Salehnia, M. F. Moghadam, M. R. Valujerdi, and E. Hajizadeh, "The correlation between the endometrial integrins and osteopontin expression with pinopodes development in ovariectomized mice in response to exogenous steroids hormones," *Iran Biomed J*, vol. 14, no. 3, pp. 109–119, 2010, doi: 10.1007/978-3-319-14343-9.
2. L. Etaati, and D. Sundaram, "Adaptive tourist recommendation system: Conceptual frameworks and implementations," *Vietnam Comput Sci*, vol. 2, no. 2, pp. 95–107, 2015, doi: 10.1007/s40595-014-0034-5.
3. I. Marfisi-Schottman, S. George, and F. Tarpin-Bernard, "Tools and Methods for Efficiently Designing Serious Games," in *4th European Conference on Game-Based Learning*, 2010, no. October, Copenhagen, Denmark, pp. 226–234.
4. Y. M. Arif, S. Harini, S. M. S. Nugroho, and M. Hariadi, "An automatic scenario control in serious game to visualize tourism destinations recommendation," *IEEE Access*, vol. 9, 2021, doi: 10.1109/ACCESS.2021.3091425.
5. D. J. Cook, J. C. Augusto, and V. R. Jakkula, "Ambient intelligence: Technologies, applications, and opportunities," *Pervasive Mob Comput*, vol. 5, no. 4, pp. 277–298, 2009, doi: 10.1016/j.pmcj.2009.04.001.
6. F. Benzi, F. Cabitza, and D. Fogli, "Gamification Techniques for Rule Management in Ambient Intelligence," in *European Conference on Ambient Intelligence*, 2015, pp. 353–356. doi: 10.1145/2909132.2926083.
7. A. Nijholt, D. Reidsma, and R. Poppe, *Games and Entertainment in Ambient Intelligence Environments*, 1st ed. Elsevier Inc., 2010. doi: 10.1016/B978-0-12-374708-2.00016-4.
8. Suresh Kumar Gorakala, *Building Recommendation Engine*, vol. 1, no. 1. Packt Publishing, 2016. doi: 10.1017/CBO9781107415324.004.
9. J. L. Nicolau, and F. J. Mas, "The influence of distance and prices on the choice of tourist destinations: The moderating role of motivations," *Tour Manag*, vol. 27, no. 5, pp. 982–996, 2006, doi: 10.1016/j.tourman.2005.09.009.
10. Y. M. Arif, S. M. S. Nugroho, and M. Hariadi, "Selection of Tourism Destinations Priority using 6AsTD Framework and TOPSIS," 2019. doi: 10.1109/ISRITI48646.2019.9034671.
11. M. Hassan, "Performance Analysis of Neural Networks-based Multi-criteria Recommender Systems," in *2017 2nd International Conferences on Information Technology, Information Systems and Electrical Engineering (ICITISEE)*, 2017, pp. 490–494, doi: 10.1109/ICITISEE.2017.8285556.

12. N. Thillainathan, and J. M Leimeister, "Serious Game Development for Educators – A Serious Game Logic and Structure Modeling Language," in *EDULEARN14 Proceedings*, 2014, no. 2014, pp. 1196–1206.
13. E. Vasconcelos *et al.*, "A serious game for exploring and training in participatory management of national parks for biodiversity conservation: Design and experience," *SBGAMES2009 - 8th Brazilian Symposium on Games and Digital Entertainment*, pp. 93–100, 2009, doi: 10.1109/SBGAMES.2009.19.
14. F. Xu, D. Buhalis, and J. Weber, "Serious games and the gamification of tourism," *Tour Manag*, vol. 60, pp. 244–256, 2017, doi: 10.1016/j.tourman.2016.11.020.
15. C. Corrêa, and C. Kitano, "Gamification in tourism: Analysis of Brazil quest game 1 introduction and theoretical background," *ENTER 2015 Conference on Information and Communication Technologies in Tourism*, vol. 8, no. 3, pp. 1–2, 2015, doi: 10.19080/PBSIJ.2018.08.555740.
16. Y. M. Arif, and H. Nurhayati, "Learning material selection for metaverse-based mathematics pedagogy media using multi-criteria recommender system," *Int Intell Eng Syst*, vol. 15, no. 6, pp. 541–551, 2022, doi: 10.22266/ijies2022.1231.48.
17. R. P. Pradana, M. Hariadi, Y. M. Arif, and R. F. Rachmadi, "A multi-criteria recommender system for NFT based IAP in RPG game," in *International Seminar on Intelligent Technology and Its Applications (ISITIA)*, 2022, pp. 214–219. doi: 10.1109/ISITIA56226.2022.9855272.
18. G. Adomavicius, and Y. Kwon, *Multi-Criteria Recommender Systems*, New York, NY: Springer Science+Business Media, 2015. doi: 10.1007/978-1-4899-7637-6.
19. Y. M. Arif, H. Nurhayati, S. Nugroho, and M. Hariadi, "Destinations ratings based multi-criteria recommender system for Indonesian halal tourism game," *Int Intell Eng Syst*, vol. 15, no. 1, 2022, doi: 10.22266/IJIES2022.0228.26.
20. I. Huseyinov, and T. Hamitovali, "Developing restaurant recommendation system with neural collaborative filtering method," *Emerg Technol Innov Res (JETIR)*, vol. 8, no. 8, pp. 103–108, 2021.

11 Designing A Virtual Expo Area Amidst the Pandemic

Herman Thuan To Saurik and Harits Ar Rosyid
Universitas Negeri Malang
Malang, Indonesia

Andreas Adi Purwanto, Hartarto Junaedi,
and Esther Irawati Setiawan
Institut Sains dan Teknologi Terpadu Surabaya
Surabaya, Indonesia

11.1 INTRODUCTION

The COVID-19 pandemic hit various countries worldwide, including Indonesia, and impacted various sectors. With the COVID-19 restrictions, the business sectors must find new ways to operate, participating in some events such as exhibitions and conferences [1]. Virtual exhibitions are cyberspace designed with concepts, topics, or ideas and utilize advanced technology and architecture to present an interesting experience for users. In this definition, the technology combines augmented reality and Virtual Reality (VR) technologies to improve the course of presentations [2]. Studying the transfer of the exhibition form, which was previously a virtual vehicle during this pandemic, can be an innovation that can be developed in the future. The use of virtual exhibitions indirectly will also provide a wide and unlimited space because every visual form of objects and spaces is designed through the reality of digital illusions [3].

In the innovation of an exhibition platform [4], there are several application development features for virtual exhibitions, such as chat text, snapshots, multimedia presentation systems, share screens, live audio, and virtual character interactions such as inventory systems and the use of teleportation system modes. The research that presents the invisible Museum [5] results in a platform designed following the Human-Centered Design (HCD) approach with the collaboration of end users, curators, and museum personnel. The platform is user centered, allowing users to collaboratively create interactive and unique virtual exhibitions where the platform is built on Web-based 3D/VR technology.

The development of virtual applications has been widely applied. It is also supported by the existence of several purposes for VR devices, such as art exhibitions equipped with interactive use in presenting digital artworks [6], virtual tour design of museums by Alin Moldoveanu [7], workplace design by bringing it into

DOI: 10.1201/9781003331674-11

the world of games [8], and VR lab application design by utilizing panoramic shooting technology to produce a different experience with student learning [9]. Furthermore, producing a virtual world is also inseparable from group navigation settings [10] and how to build a multiplayer application that can bring each user later to interact with other users and feel that they are in a virtual world that is built [11]. The application of virtual technology and the development of several methodologies, both in the application of virtual environment design, navigation settings, and building multiplayer applications, encourage the application of VR in educational promotion activities. Promotional activities or campus expos are one source of educational information for students and prospective new students about various campuses and departments.

The utilization of VR technology has been developed with a case study on the Institut Sains dan Teknologi Terpadu Surabaya (ISTTS). However, the technology is still in single-player mode [12], and the resulting 3D modeling is too broad. Thus, in this study, a case study of the ISTTS expo is used by focusing on the space area, which consists of three main points: the department promotion booth area, the laboratory area for workshop activities, and the stage area for performance and activity gathering points. The main contributions of this chapter are in designing a system flow that focuses on character interaction to facilitate various virtual activities, especially in virtual campus expos. In addition, we also aim for the virtual campus expo to help users understand information supported by visual and communication design.

This work is divided into five parts and organized as follows. The first section is the Introduction. Section 11.2 explains supporting libraries and tools. Section 11.3 describes the proposed framework. Section 11.4 explains the experiments and analysis in this study. Finally, Section 11.5 outlines the conclusion and future works.

11.2 SUPPORTING TOOLS AND LIBRARIES

This section will discuss some of the supporting tools and libraries for developing our proposed framework: Unity 3D, Mirror Networking, Firebase, and Agora.

11.2.1 UNITY 3D

Unity is a cross-platform game engine developed by Unity Technologies and used to create 2D or 3D games for PCs, consoles, mobile devices, and Web browsers [13]. Assets in Unity 3D can come from files created outside of Unity, such as 3D models, audio files, images, or any other file type that Unity supports. Several types of assets can be created within Unity, such as an animator controller, audio mixer, or render texture. The Unity license is ideal for research projects due to its low cost and support for cross-platform deployment, VR, and external assets and plugins [14]. In animation settings, Unity has tools to help create and organize animations, namely animation clips and animator controllers. The animation clip window represent in Figure 11.1.

Scripts are behavior components in Unity. They can be attached to the game object to set the behavior of the game object, and use C# as a programming language.

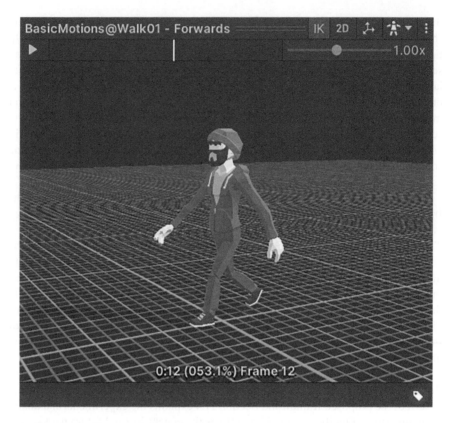

FIGURE 11.1   Animation clip window.

11.2.2   Mirror Networking

The mirror is a system for building multiplayer features in games made in Unity. The mirror is built on top of the lower-level transport real-time communication layer and handles various everyday tasks required by multiplayer games [15]. This section will discuss networking components, network behavior, and servers. The system overview of mirror networking can be seen in Figure 11.2.

Mirror provides two types of Remote Procedure Call (RPC) to perform remote actions in the network, such as running functions remotely. The first RPC is Command called from the client and executed on the server. Then, ClientRPC is called on the server and executed on the client.

11.2.3   Firebase

Firebase is a service from Google to make it easy and even more accessible for developers to develop applications [16]. Firebase, aka BaaS (backend as a service), is a solution offered by Google to speed up developer work. In this research, the Firebase services used are Realtime and Database and Authentication.

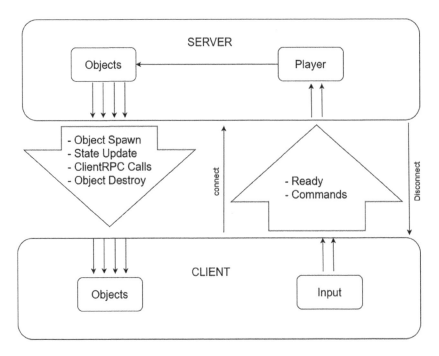

FIGURE 11.2   Diagram of remote action on mirror networking.

Here are some of the services offered by Firebase:

- Real-time database: It is a NoSQL database that can store and synchronize data in real time between applications and servers.
- Storage: It provides cloud file storage services for mobile and Web applications.
- Authentication: provides user authentication services for mobile and Web applications.
- Analytic: provides analytics services that can help app developers to know how users are using their apps.
- Hosting: provides deployment services that make it easy for application developers to deploy and manage their applications on the server.

Firebase is very useful for developers who want to build apps quickly because they can use the services available on the platform to eliminate the need for complex infrastructure management. In addition, Firebase also provides detailed documentation and many code examples that can help developers build an app.

11.2.4   AGORA

Agora is a real-time engagement platform that provides cross-platform Software Development Kit (SDKs) to implement voice calls, video calls, interactive live streaming, and real-time messaging features [17]. Agora SDKs available for Unity

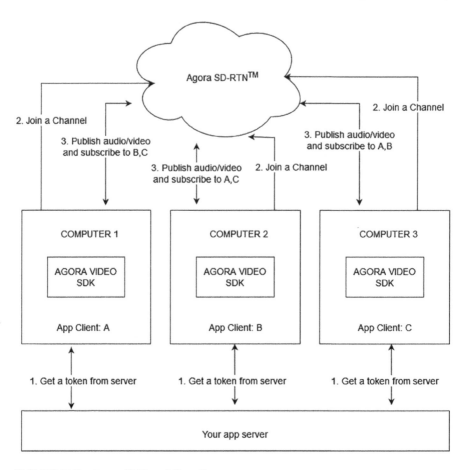

FIGURE 11.3 Agora SDK workflow diagram.

are Voice SDK, Video SDK, and Realtime Messaging SDK. The overview of the Agora computer system can be seen in Figure 11.3.

The SDK provides a set of APIs that allow developers to integrate communication services such as voice and video calls, video conferencing, and more into Unity applications created using the C# programming language. Unity's Agora SDK also allows developers to add features such as voice recognition, voice processing, and more into their applications. This SDK is available for the following platforms Windows, macOS, iOS, and Android

Using Unity's Agora SDK, developers can easily add real-time communication features to their Unity applications, making it easier for users to communicate with each other through the application.

11.3   RESEARCH FRAMEWORK

This section will discuss the details of the proposed framework for the virtual exhibition. The overall flow of the proposed architecture is displayed in Figure 11.4.

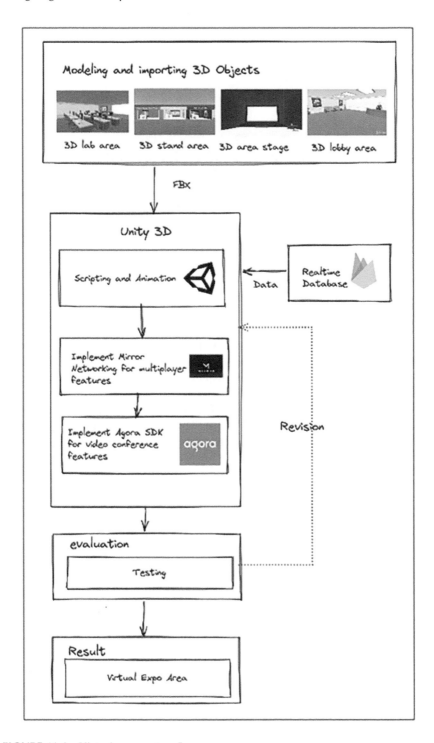

FIGURE 11.4 Virtual expo system flow.

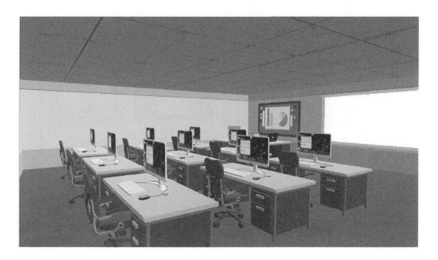

FIGURE 11.5   3D model of laboratory area.

The research flow begins with prototype modeling by designing 3D modeling of virtual expo requirement areas with three main points of the event: department promotion, workshop activities, and performances. Four main areas were produced from the three main points: the waiting room area, stage area, laboratory area, and stand area. Figure 11.5 displays one of the 3D model design areas in the laboratory.

Appealing to users about the dangers of COVID-19, this application is equipped with a poster and videos in several rooms. This interest can inform future users about the importance of understanding and preventing COVID-19. Figure 11.6 is an example of a display of a COVID-19 warning poster in the application.

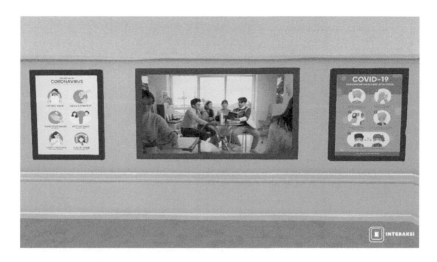

FIGURE 11.6   COVID-19 present in the form of a poster.

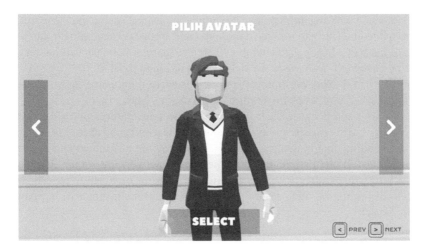

FIGURE 11.7   Avatar selection screen.

In the next stage, 3D models are created by providing several navigation controls in each area formed. Some 3D models are also equipped with features to display media in the form of images and videos that can be changed through the data management system provided. Finally, players will create an avatar used in the virtual expo area. The use of avatars, seen in Figure 11.7, is designed in multiplayer for each player who enters the virtual expo area to produce variants of avatar users. Each avatar comes with a nametag and photo to identify the avatar user.

Some areas are equipped with Non-Playable Characters (NPCs) and features designed per the event's three main points: department promotion, workshop activities, and performance. Each NPC is equipped with a dialog to provide information about the virtual campus expo and animation to give a livelier impression. For example, in Figure 11.8, the animations in the waiting room are divided into idle

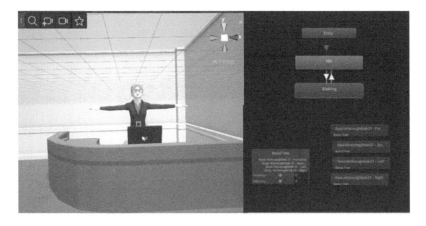

FIGURE 11.8   3D models of waiting room NPC.

animation and walking animations. The animation is made using the blend tree feature provided by Unity to provide a more flexible animation according to the movement of the NPC. Inside the blend tree, there are four animations: walking forward, walking backward, walking to the right, and walking to the left.

In the virtual expo, multiplayer testing was carried out using mirror networking and server and webcam features with Agora SDK. In this research, two libraries are used because each library has different features and roles. Mirror networking in this research plays a role in creating multiplayer rooms, spawning avatars, sending chat messages, and synchronizing the movement and animation of avatars to all clients connected to the mirror networking server. The mirror networking stage starts with the creation of a room or host. After which the process of joining by other users. After that, each user's avatar will be spawned on the server.

Algorithm 11.1. The Flow of Video Conference in the Lab Area

```
Initialize request_url, channel_name, token, app_id ="1234"
If RtcEngine Not null
   RtcEngine = IRtcEngine.GetEngine(app_id)
   RtcEngine.OnUserJoined = OnUserJoined
   RtcEngine.OnUserJoined = OnuserLeave
   Call RtcEngine.EnableVideo
   Call EnableVideoObserver
   token = Get(request_url+?channel=+"channel_name")
Endif
Function OnUserJoined(uint uid)
   surface = new RawImage
   surface.setForUser(uid)
endfunction
Function OnuserLeave(uint uid)
   surface = find_surface(uid)
   surface.destroy
endfunction
```

Agora SDK plays a role in conducting peer-to-peer connections for video conferencing features to conduct workshop activities in campus virtual expos. The Agora stage starts by connecting to the server to request an access token to enter the room. After getting access, the user will enter the room provided, and then the webcam from the user will be activated and displayed in the raw image object in Unity. To display all users who join the video conference, we can utilize the callback provided by Agora. In the callback function, we can create a new raw image object when a user enters and destroy the raw image object when a user leaves the video conference, as shown in Algorithm 11.1.

In Algorithm 11.1, the join function will be called to join the video call. Furthermore, the join function will check whether the RtcEngine has been loaded. Otherwise, the join will be rejected. If the RtcEngine has been loaded, it will bind

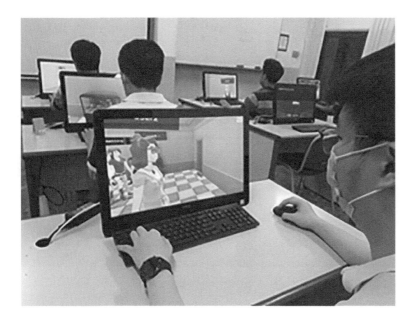

FIGURE 11.9   Application testing.

to several callback functions from Agora, namely OnUserJoined and OnUserLeave. In the OnUserJoined function, a RawImage will be created to display the video, and in OnUserLeave, the RawImage of the leaving user will be destroyed. Then the EnableVideo function and the EnableVideoObserver function of RtcEngine will be called, and the access token from the server will be obtained. Application testing can be seen in Figure 11.9.

The final step is testing to determine whether the existing features have appropriately functioned. One of the scenarios also evaluates users who fill out the guest book. The guest book data are stored in Firebase, which can later become evaluation material for the committee to screen students interested in the department. The appearance of the three main points and the four main areas produced. After testing, the application will be improved and developed into a virtual expo area application product.

11.4   RESULT AND EVALUATION

The results achieved in creating a virtual expo area are as follows.

11.4.1   PROMOTION OF CAMPUS DEPARTMENTS

At the point of department promotion, a booth area was created. Information about the department is in the form of videos and photos. The created booth has three templates with different images and video positions and filling out guest books by virtual expo participants. The display of the Bot area can be seen in Figure 11.10.

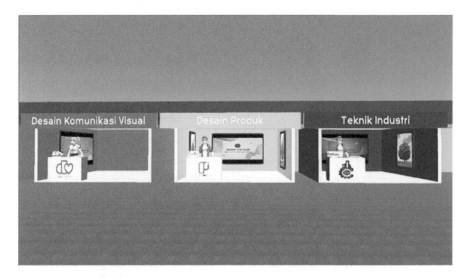

FIGURE 11.10   Booth area.

Presentation of information for departments using the image and video media can be arranged according to the data source created. Figure 11.11 is a display of information in the video.

There is also information in the form of images. For example, information on department brochures on the User Interface (UI) display is also attached to the brochure pdf download feature, a link to the website, and navigation to read the brochure as in Figure 11.12.

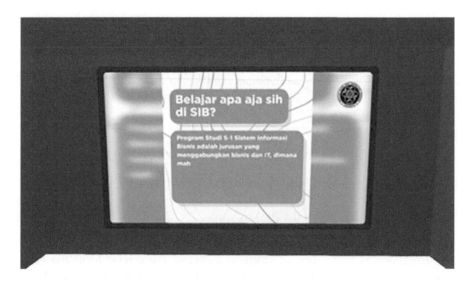

FIGURE 11.11   Information media in the form of video.

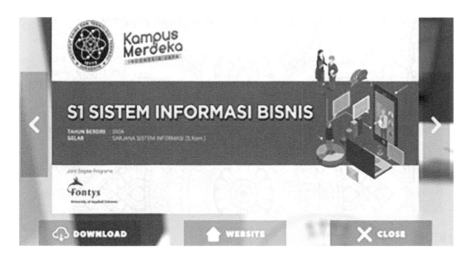

FIGURE 11.12 Brochure information in picture form.

In promoting departments, a feature is also added to fill out a guest book. Filling in this guest book is done so that later expo participants can provide data for a more detailed understanding of the department that interests participants. Filling in the guest book is designed efficiently by adding the contact number and email of the participant. Figure 11.13 is a user interface for using the guest book feature.

11.4.2 WORKSHOP ACTIVITIES

The results of the workshop activities are realized in the laboratory area, which is equipped with a design of 10 computers used to enter the video conference to conduct workshop activities in the virtual expo. The video conference feature is limited

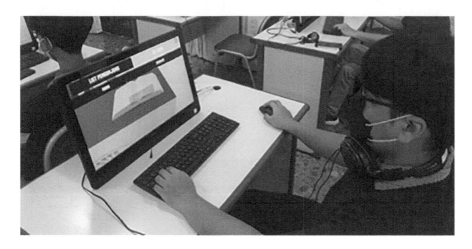

FIGURE 11.13 Filling in the guest book.

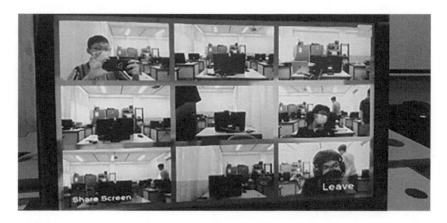

FIGURE 11.14   Video call feature.

to 10 users per session to provide a seamless experience. Figure 11.14 shows a display where the user activates the video call feature in the laboratory room.

11.4.3   PERFORMANCES AREA

The result that meets the goal of producing a performance area is a staging area, which will be used to display performances or as a gathering point area. In the design of this area, there is a large screen, mic, theater chairs, and laptop. A feature for the admin is available to display images and videos in the screen object by accessing the menu on the laptop object. Admin can also use the mic feature by standing in the stage area and interacting with mic objects. Figure 11.15 shows the stage area.

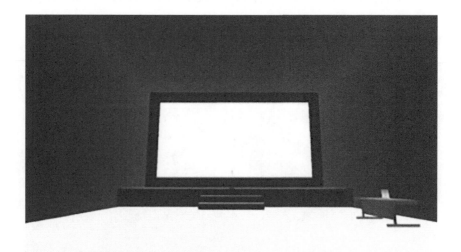

FIGURE 11.15   Stage area.

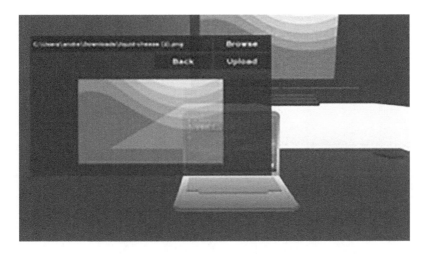

FIGURE 11.16   Stage screen media setting.

This mic feature is used to interact with expo participants, for example, by giving announcements. In addition, a feature to set the display into the stage screen based on data sources has been created in this area.

Figure 11.16 shows the stage display for the media settings screen, both photos and videos, to be displayed on the layer in the stage area. The admin displays images and videos in the screen object in this area. To access this feature, the admin must go to the laptop object provided and select the menu to load the image. There are three options for selecting media displayed: load images from local files, videos from local files, and videos and playlists from YouTube.

11.4.4   APPEAL FOR COVID-19 PREVENTION

In addition to providing user convenience through virtual applications, this application can also be used to encourage users regarding the prevention of COVID-19. Some areas in each room have posters that visitors can access. Providing posters and videos related to COVID-19, be it for prevention, appeals, or other information about COVID-19, can help explain to users the dangers of COVID-19 using interesting social campaigns in the application. It provides easy information about vaccines that can encourage users to vaccinate and information about COVID-19 tests, which makes it easier to inform users about COVID-19. Figure 11.17 is an example of a COVID-19 poster.

11.4.5   APPLICATION FEASIBILITY TEST

The feasibility test of the application was carried out by researchers using the following devices to run the program:

PC 1 Processor: i5 8250u I Nvidia MX 150, RAM: 8GB, Windows 11
PC 2 Processor: Ryzen 5 4600 I Nvidia GTX 1650, RAM: 16GB, Windows 10
PC 3 Processor: AMD A9 9425 I Radeon R5, RAM: 4GB, Windows 10

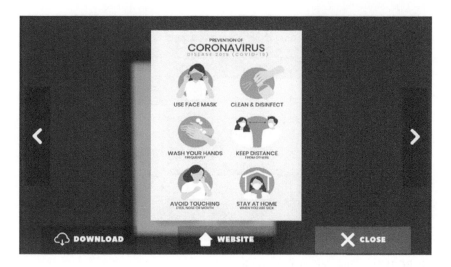

FIGURE 11.17   COVID-19 prevention poster.

Virtual expo application testing is conducted to determine the application's performance using devices with the previously listed specifications. The results show that the application can run smoothly on PC 1 and PC 2 devices, with better results on PC 2. However, on PC 3, the application runs with a little lag when entering the stand area, and the camera frame per second (fps) drops quite a lot when entering the video conference. Based on the Survey, the testing result is shown in Table 11.1.

TABLE 11.1

Testing Result Based on the Survey

No.	Engineering Aspect Software	5	4	3	2	1
1	Ease use of navigation in-app	90	4	6	0	0
2	Virtual expo navigation avatar control in the virtual expo	85	12	3	0	0
3	The visual display in the lab area	86	11	3	0	0
4	The visual display in the stage area	88	7	5	0	0
5	Visual display on stand area	84	10	6	0	0
6	Visual display of the area waiting room	86	10	4	0	0
	Lab Area Feature	5	4	3	2	1
7	Ease of use of video conference provided	97	3	0	0	0
	Area feature stage	5	4	3	2	1
8	Then choose videos and images on the stage area	97	3	0	0	0
	Feature of the space area wait	5	4	3	2	1
9	Explanation of information given by the NPC	96	3	0	0	0
	Global Feature	5	4	3	2	1
10	Ease of chat feature that exists in each area	96	4	0	0	0
11	Ease of providing information about COVID-19	88	5	7	0	0

11.5 CONCLUSION AND FUTURE WORKS

This research generated a virtual expo application that can be an alternative during a pandemic. We developed three main events: the promotion of departments, workshops, and performances. Using concise information and data management in the application is beneficial in handling the information content that is dynamically provided. However, this research is limited to images and videos. Appeals regarding COVID-19 can be easily presented in the form of posters and videos, and it can undoubtedly further influence users to present good information about the dangers of COVID-19 and countermeasures regarding the prevention of the spread of the virus. From our survey result, we concluded that our application carried out virtual expo activities and conveyed information about the department very well based on software engineering aspects of 86.5% and visual communication aspects of 96.5%, which is evident from interpreting the total evaluation score of 100 respondents from the ten questions asked.

For future works, we would like to utilize VR technology for users so that the perceived results can be in a virtual expo. Furthermore, in addition to adding some space areas, interactions are added to several objects, such as carrying books and moving objects.

REFERENCES

1. Stavrev, Stefan. "Virtual Exhibitions During a Pandemic–a Real-Time Online Expo With a Fictional Interior." Anniversary International Scientific Conference REMIA (2021): 113–120.
2. Kadam, P. "Virtual Exhibitions-Digitized World in Pre and Post-Covid." International Journal of Advance and Innovative Research, vol. 8, no. 3, pp. 93–95, 2021.
3. Arsita, P. "Virtual Exhibition Room in the Pandemic Era," Budapest International Research and Critics Institute-Journal (BIRCI-Journal), vol. 4, no. 3, pp. 5331–5338, 2021.
4. Deac, Gicu Calin, et al. "Virtual reality exhibition platform." Proceedings of the 29th DAAAM International Symposium. Vienna, Austria: DAAAM International, 2018.
5. Zidianakis, E., Partarakis, N., Ntoa, S., Dimopoulos, A., Kopidaki, S., Ntagianta, A., Ntafotis, E., Xhako, A., Pervolarakis, Z., Kontaki, E., Zidianaki, I., Michelakis, A., Foukarakis, M., & Stephanidis, C. "The Invisible Museum: A User-Centric Platform for Creating Virtual 3D Exhibitions with VR Support." Electronics, vol. 10, p. 363, 2021. https://doi.org/10.3390/electronics10030363
6. Donna, Carollina. "Graffiti Virtual Exhibition "Pandemic Youth." International Journal of Creative and Arts Studies, vol. 7, no. 2, p. 129, 2020.
7. Moldoveanu, A., Moldoveanu, F., Soceanu, A., & Victor, A. "A 3D Virtual Museum." UPB Scientific Bulletin, Series C: Electrical Engineering, vol. 70, no. 3, pp. 47–58, 2008.
8. Gabajová, Gabriela, Krajčovič, Martin, Matys, Marián, Furmannová, Beáta, & Burganova, Natalia. "Designing Virtual Workplace Using Unity 3D Game Engine." Acta Tecnología, vol. 7, pp. 35–39, 2021. doi: 10.22306/atec.v7i1.101.
9. Fang, H., Xiru, Y., Kun, H., Wenxin, L., & Haodong, T. "Design and Application of VR Lab Based on Unity." Journal of Physics: Conference Series, vol. 1982, no. 1, p. 012167, July 2021.
10. T. Weissker, & B. Froehlich, "Group Navigation for Guided Tours in Distributed Virtual Environments." IEEE Transactions on Visualization and Computer Graphics, vol. 27, no. 5, pp. 2524–2534, May 2021. doi: 10.1109/TVCG.2021.3067756.

11. Häkkinen, P., Bluemink, J., Juntunen, M. & Laakkonen, I. "Multiplayer 3D Game in Supporting Team-Building Activities in a Work Organization." 2012 IEEE 12th International Conference on Advanced Learning Technologies, 2012, pp. 430–432, doi: 10.1109/ICALT.2012.242.
12. Saurik, "Teknologi Virtual Reality Untuk Media Informasi Kampus," Junal Teknologi Informasi Dan Ilmu Komputer, vol. 6, no. 1, 2019.
13. Unity, User Manual 2021.3 (LTS) Documentation [online]. Available: https://docs.unity3d.com/Manual/index.html
14. T. Nieminen, "Unity game engine in visualization, simulation and modelling," Tampere University, 2021.
15. Mirror Networking [online]. Available: https://assetstore.unity.com/packages/tools/network/mirror-129321
16. Google Developer, Firebase for Unity [online]. Available: https://firebase.google.com/docs/unity/setup
17. Agora.io, Agora Unity SDK API Reference v3.7.0.1 [online]. Available: https//docs.agora.io/en/Video/API%20Reference/unity/index.html

12 Continuance Intention in Massive Open Online Courses Using Extended Expectation-Confirmation Model

Chow Shean Shyong and Edwin Pramana
Institut Sains dan Teknologi Terpadu Surabaya
Surabaya, Indonesia

12.1 INTRODUCTION

Since its rise in 2012, millions of individuals have enrolled in Massive Open Online Courses (MOOCs) over a relatively short period (Alraimi et al., 2015; Nong et al., 2022; Ouyang et al., 2017; Zhou, 2017). Hundreds of thousands of university students have been studying on MOOC platforms, mainly in North America and Europe (Ouyang et al., 2017). In recent years, the number of MOOCs offered and the number of participants has greatly increased, estimating over 11,400 active MOOCs have been launched by over 900 universities worldwide, and the cumulative number of enrolled learners has reached 101 million (Zhao et al., 2020).

The COVID-19 pandemic lockdown had impelled an unprecedented surge in the enrollment of MOOCs starting from early 2020. Udemy, a popular MOOC platform, had seen 425% enrollment growth from individuals, an 80% increased in use by businesses and governments, and 55% growth in new course creation (Impey & Formanek, 2021). Coursera, another popular MOOC platform, had 10 million enrollments in 30 days starting in March 2020, up by 640% from the previous year (Impey & Formanek, 2021).

Despite such popularity, on average, less than 10% of MOOC students completed the enrolled courses (Alraimi et al., 2015; Dai et al., 2020; Daneji et al., 2019; Jo, 2018; Joo et al., 2018; Lu et al., 2019; Nong et al., 2022; Ouyang et al., 2017; Tsai et al., 2018; Xiong et al., 2015; Zhao et al., 2020; Zhou, 2017). Such a low completion rate has raised questions about real learning effectiveness and sustainability for the future (Zhou, 2017). However, recent researchers have pointed out that, instead of completion rate, continuance intention in using MOOCs should be the right indicator for measuring the success of MOOCs (Alraimi et al., 2015; Dai et al., 2020;

DOI: 10.1201/9781003331674-12

Daneji et al., 2019; Joo et al., 2018; Lu et al., 2019; Ouyang et al., 2017; Zhou, 2017). Therefore, the following questions led to this study:

- What are the factors influencing the intention to continue the use of MOOCs?
- What are the relationships among the factors that influence the continuance intention in MOOCs?

According to Meet and Kala (2021), from 2013 through 2020, only 17 published papers studied MOOC engagement and continuance (Meet & Kala, 2021). Along with that, similar research focusing on Indonesia is rarely found. Of the 102 published papers reviewed by Meet & Kala (2021), 21 papers were published by institutions belonging to 16 countries, including Indonesia (Meet & Kala, 2021). In addition, while researching the role of motivation in MOOC retention rates, Badali et al., (2022) did not find any paper produced in Indonesia. Therefore, the main objective of this study is to fill in the research gap by examining the factors that enhance an individual's intention to continue using MOOCs, particularly in Indonesia.

This chapter is organized into multiple sections. The literature review section presents the literature review based on prior research on continuance intention in using MOOCs. The hypotheses development and the theoretical model section develops the hypotheses and the theoretical model for this study. The research methodology section describes the questionnaire development and sampling procedure. The results and discussions section discusses data preparation, structural equation modeling (SEM) analysis, and final results. The conclusion, limitations, and future studies section concludes the entire study, discusses the limitations, and provides suggestions for future studies.

12.2   MASSIVE OPEN ONLINE COURSES (MOOCs)

MOOCs are courses delivered in an online environment that are free and open to all (Alraimi et al., 2015). Coursera, EdX, Udacity, and Udemy are some of the major MOOC platforms. The courses in MOOCs are offered by renowned universities such as the Massachusetts Institute of Technology (MIT), Stanford University, Harvard University, and the University of Michigan (Voss, 2013). Typically MOOCs do not impose preconditions for course participants; there is no formal expectation or requirement on the participants' previous educational level or technical knowledge. Furthermore, it is primarily free and open for unlimited participation (Jo, 2018).

12.3   EXPECTATION-CONFIRMATION MODEL (ECM)

The expectation-confirmation model (ECM) was improved by Bhattacherjee (2001) from expectation-confirmation theory developed by Oliver (1980). ECM was used to study the continuance usage of information systems (IS), which was then proven to be a better measure of IS success than examining the initial adoption of IS (Bhattacherjee, 2001). Figure 12.1 shows the association among the constructs of ECM.

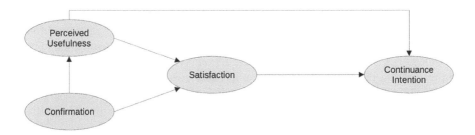

FIGURE 12.1 Expectation-confirmation model (ECM).

ECM posits that users' intention to continue using IS is primarily determined by the satisfaction with prior use of IS and is supported by the perceived usefulness following the use of the IS. In turn, satisfaction is significantly influenced by users' confirmation of their initial expectations and perceived usefulness of the IS (Bhattacherjee, 2001).

12.4 PRIOR RESEARCHES

Recent research has been focusing on continuance intention as the appropriate indicator for measuring the success of MOOCs (Alraimi et al., 2015; Dai et al., 2020; Daneji et al., 2019; Guo et al., 2016; Jo, 2018; Joo et al., 2018; Lu et al., 2019; Nong et al., 2022; Ouyang et al., 2017; Shanshan & Wenfei, 2022; Tsai et al., 2018; Zhao et al., 2020; Zhou, 2017). Alraimi et al. (2015) focused on openness and reputation, and concluded that perceived reputation was the strongest predictor of learners' intentions to continue using MOOCs, followed by perceived openness, perceived usefulness, and perceived enjoyment (Alraimi et al., 2015). Dai et al. (2020) studied the influence of attitude and curiosity on Chinese university students' intentions to use MOOCs, and found that both factors played a considerably dominant role in predicting subsequent continuance intention (Dai et al., 2020).

Another similar research on Chinese students focused on flow and interest and found that both factors were significant (Lu et al., 2019). A conducted similar research focused on employees rather than students, concluding that all ECM constructs were significant (Nong et al., 2022). Another study focused mainly on flow experience and concluded that telepresence and perceived hedonic value were the most significant factors transmitting the effects of flow onto online learners' continuance intentions (Guo et al., 2016). Along with the flow experience, Shanshan and Wenfei (2022), integrated more dimensions with quality elements and task-technology-fit, and concluded that teaching-based quality, platform-based quality, and task-technology-fit all had a positive and significant impact on continuance intention (Shanshan & Wenfei, 2022).

Research on Malaysian MOOC users concluded that users were willing to continue using MOOCs based on the significant positive influence of perceived usefulness and satisfaction (Daneji et al., 2019). Korean research concluded that continuance intention was influenced more by perceived ease of use than perceived usefulness for Korean K-MOOC users (Joo et al., 2018). Tsai et al. (2018) studied the effects of metacognition on online learning interest and concluded that metacognition was positively influencing the three levels of learning interest (liking, enjoyment, and engagement), which in turn were positively influencing continuance intention to use MOOCs (Tsai et al., 2018). Ouyang et al. (2017) added another aspect to the research by integrating the task-technology-fit model and concluded the role of task-technology-fit in improving students' continuance intention on MOOCs (Ouyang et al., 2017). Jo (2018) explored the determinants of MOOC continuance intention with a similar model and concluded positively influence on utilization and perceived usefulness in the MOOC usage environment (Jo, 2018). The additional integrated factors of social influence, knowledge outcome, and performance proficiency concluded that confirmation, perceived usefulness, satisfaction, social influence, knowledge outcome, and performance proficiency were all significant (Zhou, 2017).

12.5   HYPOTHESES DEVELOPMENT AND THE THEORETICAL MODEL

Confirmation refers to the users' perceptions of the congruence between the expectation of MOOC use and its actual performance (Bhattacherjee, 2001). ECM theorized that the extent of users' confirmations led to a positive effect on their perceived usefulness and satisfaction with MOOCs (Alraimi et al., 2015; Dai et al., 2020; Daneji et al., 2019; Lu et al., 2019; Nong et al., 2022; Ouyang et al., 2017; Shanshan & Wenfei, 2022; Zhou, 2017). When MOOC performance confirmed or overcame users' expectations, users would find satisfaction. When users' expectations were confirmed, they would feel the system was worth using and expect more in their future use (Zhou, 2017). Thus, this study hypothesizes that:

H1: Confirmation has a positive direct effect on the perceived usefulness of using MOOCs.

H2: Confirmation has a positive direct effect on satisfaction using MOOCs.

Perceived usefulness refers to the users' perceptions of the expected benefits of MOOC use (Bhattacherjee, 2001). Perceived usefulness has been found to have a strong positive impact on satisfaction in previous studies (Jo, 2018; Joo et al., 2018; Lu et al., 2019; Nong et al., 2022; Ouyang et al., 2017). If MOOCs were perceived to be helpful, the learner would be satisfied. Thus, perceived usefulness was significantly related to satisfaction (Lu et al., 2019). Perceived usefulness has also been found to positively influence continuance intention (Alraimi et al., 2015; Daneji et al., 2019; Jo, 2018; Nong et al., 2022; Ouyang et al., 2017). Ouyang et al. (2017) concluded that when users believed studying on MOOC platforms was beneficial in improving their capability or helpful for them to find new jobs, they tended to continue using MOOCs (Ouyang et al., 2017). Thus, this study hypothesizes that:

H3: Perceived usefulness has a positive direct effect on satisfaction with using MOOCs.

H4: Perceived usefulness has a positive direct effect on continuance intention to use MOOCs.

Satisfaction refers to the users' affect with prior MOOC use (Bhattacherjee, 2001). The positive relationship between satisfaction and continuance intention has been confirmed by the majority of previous studies (Alraimi et al., 2015; Daneji et al., 2019; Guo et al., 2016; Jo, 2018; Joo et al., 2018; Lu et al., 2019; Nong et al., 2022; Ouyang et al., 2017; Shanshan & Wenfei, 2022; Zhou, 2017). Users' satisfaction in a MOOC use environment was an essential predictor of an intention of continued use of MOOC (Guo et al., 2016). Thus, this study hypothesizes that:

H5: Satisfaction has a positive direct effect on continuance intention to use MOOCs.

Flow refers to the users' intense concentration on a task without distraction and where behavior and awareness merge in the performance of the activity (Lu et al., 2019). When users were in the flow state, they would learn at total capacity and experience enhanced effectiveness in using MOOCs. Consequently, the flow experience could maximize educational outcomes and enhance users' satisfaction (Lu et al., 2019; Shanshan & Wenfei, 2022). Flow experience, elicited by telepresence and social presence, led to continuance intention among users (Zhao et al., 2020). Thus, this study hypothesizes that:

H6: Flow has a positive direct effect on satisfaction with using MOOCs.
H7: Flow has a positive direct effect on continuance intention to use MOOCs.

Engagement refers to the investment of cognitive, physical, and emotional energies into expressing the ideal self in the context of role performance in MOOCs (Ittersum, 2015). The inclusion of engagement as one of the learning interests in metacognition found a significant and positive relationship between learning interests (liking, enjoyment, engagement) and continuance intention to use MOOCs (Tsai et al., 2018). Thus, this study hypothesizes that:

H8: Engagement has a positive direct effect on continuance intention to use MOOCs.

Social influence refers to the degree to which an individual perceives that essential others believe he or she should use MOOCs (Venkatesh et al., 2003). Users' decisions on whether to continue using MOOCs were affected by word of mouth from the media and the people around them. Furthermore, social influence was a powerful indicator of users' continuance intention of MOOCs (Zhou, 2017). Thus, this study hypothesizes that:

H9: Social influence has a positive direct effect on continuance intention to use MOOCs.

Curiosity refers to the users' desire to seek novelty (Dai et al., 2020). Curiosity is the intrinsic motive to enroll and remain in MOOCs. This passion for learning

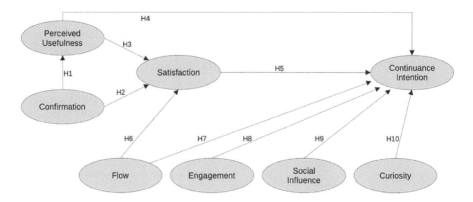

FIGURE 12.2   Theoretical model.

has been reported to be a significant factor in the continuous usage of MOOCs (Dai et al., 2020). Thus, this study hypothesizes that:

H10: Curiosity has a positive direct effect on continuance intention to use MOOCs.

Continuance intention refers to the user's intention to continue using MOOCs (Bhattacherjee, 2001). The proposed ECM is based on the concept that continuance intention would be positively influenced by confirmation, perceived usefulness, and satisfaction. Along with that, it is also positively affected by flow, engagement, social influence, and curiosity. Thus, continuance intention is the dependent variable of this study.

Figure 12.2 shows the theoretical model constructed from the extended ECM constructs and hypotheses.

12.6   RESEARCH METHODOLOGY

This study adopts the SEM approach to test the hypothetical theoretical model according to the guidelines from Kline (2016). Because data collection for SEM is cross-sectional, a survey questionnaire is prepared for this study as in the Appendix. There are two sections in the questionnaire. Section 1 contains a short description of the definition of MOOCs, some examples of popular MOOC platforms, and the personal questions that will be used for profiling the respondents. Section 2 consists of 24 questions covering all the indicators of the variables as shown in the appendix. Each question is listed with five-point Likert-scaled choices ranging from "strongly disagree" to "strongly agree." All 24 questions are adopted from prior research and modified to fit into the MOOC context. Because the target respondents are the general public in Indonesia who have prior MOOC experiences, the questionnaire is translated into Bahasa Indonesia and verified by experts knowledgeable in these two languages.

The survey is carried out online using Google Forms. The target participants are current active MOOC users in Indonesia to whom purposive sampling will sample. Because the population of MOOC users in Indonesia is unknown but expected to be greater than 100,000, the target minimum number of responses is set at 400 per the guideline for minimum sample size (Israel, 1992).

12.7   RESULTS AND DISCUSSIONS

The gross number of responses collected from the survey is 507. After removing invalid data, data with missing values, and outliers, the final set of valid responses is 471, which fulfills the minimum number of samples required for this study.

Table 12.1 shows the characteristics of the respondents based on the valid responses received.

The majority of the respondents belong to the age range between 21 and 35, which accounts for 84.93% of the sample. A similar observation is made about the educational background in which 85.35% of the respondents are holders of a diploma or bachelor's degree. Most of the respondents are new to MOOCs with 95.97% having only 3 years of experience. For the MOOC platforms, it is shown that international platforms make up 73.79% of the platform choices.

The valid responses are then submitted to Statistical Package for the Social Sciences (SPSS) for confirmatory factor analysis. All the factor loadings calculated in the first iteration are above the threshold of 0.4 (Straub et al., 2004), indicating

TABLE 12.1
Respondent Profiling

Group	Item	Frequency	Group	Item	Frequency
Age	≤20	15	**MOOC Experiences**	≤12	105
	21–25	127	**(Months)**	13–24	248
	26–30	164		25–36	99
	31–35	109		37–48	15
	36–40	28		49–60	2
	41–45	19		>60	2
	46–50	8		–	–
	>50	1		–	–
	Total	**471**		**Total**	**471**
Gender	Male	338	**MOOC Platforms**	Coursera	132
	Female	133	**(Multiple Platforms**	Udemy	138
	Total	**471**	**Accepted)**	Udacity	102
Education	Secondary	33		Khan	100
	Diploma	154		EdX	77
	Bachelor	248		Others	195
	Master	35		–	–
	Doctor	1		–	–
	Total	**471**		**Total**	**744**

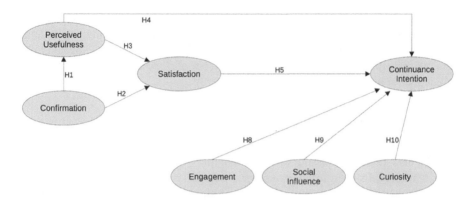

FIGURE 12.3   Modified theoretical model.

acceptance. However, the flow and engagement indicators, even though convergent, are not discriminant as they are grouped under the same factor. Therefore, the construct validity test fails for this iteration.

To improve the model, the latent variable of flow and the related hypotheses (H6 and H7) are dropped. The modified theoretical model is shown in Figure 12.3.

The indicators of the modified theoretical model are then submitted to SPSS for the second iteration of the confirmatory factor analysis. The Bartlett's sphericity test result of 0.000 and the Kaiser-Meyer-Olkin (KMO) test of 0.851 are well accepted. The indicator factor loadings are all well above the threshold of 0.4 (Straub et al., 2004) indicating strong correlations between the indicators and the latent variables. All related indicators are grouped under each of the factors and there is no mixture of indicators across the factors indicating convergent and discriminant. The factor loadings are summarized in Table 12.2.

As shown in Table 12.2, all Cronbach's alpha values are well above the acceptable level of 0.7 (George & Mallery, 2003). Thus, the construct reliability test is passed successfully without dropping any latent variable.

Table 12.3 shows the skewness and kurtosis descriptive statistics of the indicators grouped by the latent variables. All the skewness values fall within the acceptable range of –3 to 3 (Kline, 2016), and kurtosis values within –7 and 7 (Kline, 2016), indicating that the data are pretty suitable for SEM analysis without dropping any of the constructs.

The SEM analysis of the modified theoretical model is conducted by SPSS AMOS software. The results are visualized in Figure 12.4. In summary, six of the eight hypotheses are supported with only hypotheses H3 and H10 not supported.

The model fit statistics that determine how well the theoretical model fits the actual data are summarized in Table 12.4. As Kline (2016) recommended, the results of model fit statistics are satisfactory, which means the theoretical model fits well with the actual data.

In answering the first research question, the SEM results identify six constructs influencing the intention to continue using MOOCs: confirmation, perceived usefulness, satisfaction, continuance intention, engagement, and social influence. As for

TABLE 12.2
Result of Confirmatory Factor Analysis (CFA) and Cronbach's Alpha

Variable	Indicator	Loading	Cronbach's Alpha	Interpretation
Confirmation	CF1	0.867	0.989	Excellent
	CF2	0.865		
	CF3	0.871		
Perceived usefulness	PU1	0.940	0.931	Excellent
	PU2	0.939		
	PU3	0.800		
Satisfaction	SA1	0.811	0.924	Excellent
	SA2	0.845		
	SA3	0.844		
Continuance intention	CI1	0.820	0.928	Excellent
	CI2	0.836		
	CI3	0.833		
Engagement	EG1	0.731	0.817	Good
	EG2	0.825		
	EG3	0.893		
Social influence	SI1	0.908	0.918	Excellent
	SI2	0.910		
	SI3	0.843		
Curiosity	CU1	0.922	0.956	Excellent
	CU2	0.923		
	CU3	0.904		

Notes: Extraction method: Principal component analysis. Rotation method: Equamax with Kaiser normalization. Rotation converged in eight iterations. Kaiser-Meyer-Olkin measure of sampling adequacy = 0.851. Bartlett's test of sphericity: Approximately chi-square = 13,347.546, df = 210, Sig. = 0.000. Only eigenvalues of 1 or more are shown.

TABLE 12.3
Skewness & Kurtosis

Latent	Ind	Skewness	Kurtosis	Latent	Ind	Skewness	Kurtosis
Confirmation	CF1	−0.398	−0.822	Engagement	EG1	−0.153	−0.831
	CF2	−0.387	−0.868		EG2	−0.486	−0.790
	CF3	−0.393	−0.860		EG3	−0.916	−0.346
Perceived usefulness	PU1	−0.067	−0.758	Social Influence	SI1	0.016	−0.610
	PU2	−0.090	−0.682		SI2	0.021	−0.604
	PU3	−0.370	−0.850		SI3	−0.053	−0.632
Satisfaction	SA1	0.221	−1.121	Curiosity	CU1	−0.073	−0.627
	SA2	−0.329	−0.793		CU2	−0.026	−0.552
	SA3	−0.340	−0.809		CU3	−0.224	−0.490
Continuance intention	CI1	−0.385	−0.670				
	CI2	−0.177	−0.973				
	CI3	−0.376	−0.676				

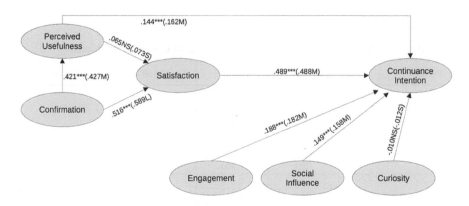

FIGURE 12.4   Result of hypotheses testing.

TABLE 12.4
Model Fit Statistics

N	NC	RMR	GFI	AGFI	NFI	IFI	CFI	RMSEA
471	3.075	0.041	0.899	0.866	0.960	0973	0.973	0.066

the second research question, the SEM results identify the following relationships among the factors that influence the continuance intention in MOOCs:

- Confirmation has a positive direct effect on perceived usefulness (H1/.421***) and satisfaction (H2/.516***)
- Perceived usefulness (H4/.144***) and satisfaction (H5/.489***) have positive direct effects on continuance intention
- Engagement (H8/.188***) and social influence (H9/.149***) have positive direct effects on continuance intention

H1, H2, H4, and H5 are hypotheses from standard ECM constructs that many prior researchers with significant positive results have investigated. The SEM results indicate that when MOOC performance confirms or exceeds the learners' prior expectations, learners will find satisfaction, will feel the system is worth using, and will expect to continue usage in the future (Alraimi et al., 2015; Dai et al., 2020; Daneji et al., 2019; Jo, 2018; Joo et al., 2018; Lu et al., 2019; Nong et al., 2022; Ouyang et al., 2017; Shanshan & Wenfei, 2022; Zhou, 2017).

H8 indicates that when learners invest their cognitive, physical, and emotional energies into expressing their ideal selves in the context of role performance in MOOCs, they tend to enjoy the learning process and be enthusiastic about continuing the usage in the future. This finding is consistent with Tsai et al. (2018) who found that engagement mediating metacognition positively influences continuance intention.

H9 indicates that learners' decision on whether to continue using MOOCs depends on word of mouth from media and the people around them, which is consistent with Zhou (2017) who concluded that social influence was a powerful indicator of users' continuance intention (Zhou, 2017).

The finding on H3 is unexpected, but it can be explained. Even though many prior kinds of research have positively supported H3, there are cases where the same hypothesis is not supported, such as Alraimi et al. (2015) and Daneji et al. (2019). This study has the same opinion as Daneji et al. (2019), where the students are more concerned with the satisfactory result rather than the approach to achieving it, thus limiting the effect of perceived usefulness on satisfaction.

The finding on H10 contradicts Dai et al. (2020) who reported curiosity to be a significant factor in the continuous usage of MOOCs, which to some extent is unexpected, but not surprising. Conventional teacher-based passive learning is prevalent, and the development of curiosity in learning is still infrequent in this part of the world. In such a case, there is not much of a surprise to see that curiosity does not have a positive direct effect on continuance intention.

In terms of theoretical implication, this study reconfirms the robustness of ECM in predicting continuance intention in using MOOCs. Many prior researchers have reported the positive effects of confirmation and satisfaction. This study also extends prior research with additional constructs of engagement and social influence where both constructs positively affect continuance intention in using MOOCs.

Practically, the results of this study are essential for MOOC-platform operators who are faced with the challenge of learners discontinuing their MOOC use. The operators should provide high-quality courses, such as courses from renowned institutions and universities, to increase the level of confirmation and satisfaction of the learners, which will positively affect their intention to continue using MOOCs. Furthermore, the operators should showcase their online peer reviews extensively to improve the effectiveness of social influence. Setting up and encouraging students to join online community forums is another way of improving social influence and engagement to lead to continuance intention in MOOCs.

12.8   CONCLUSION, LIMITATIONS, AND FUTURE STUDIES

The main objectives of this study are to examine the factors that enhance an individual's intention to continue using MOOCs and the relationship among the factors. The model being used is an extended ECM where the standard constructs of confirmation, perceived usefulness, satisfaction, and continuance intention are extended with flow, engagement, social influence, and curiosity. The SEM analysis results concluded that six of eight hypotheses are supported by the data, which is confirmation it has a positive direct effect on perceived usefulness and satisfaction, which in turn has positive direct effects on continuance intention. Engagement and social influence have positive direct effects on continuance intention.

However, this study is associated with some limitations. The current study has not been able to determine the discriminant validity of flow and engagement; thus, it misses the opportunity to study the effect of flow on continuance intention. The constructs, flow and engagement, and the relationship between them are believed to be statistically significant in influencing continuance intention. Thus, future research to confirm this aspect is of much interest.

Due to resource constraints, the respondents' sampling of this study depends heavily on purposive effect, which may, to some extent, influence the final results unfavorably. It is recommended to improve the sampling procedure of future research to increase the sample's representativeness.

The current study focuses solely on the MOOC market of a single country, Indonesia, which might be monotonous in terms of cultural and educational background. It is recommended to conduct similar studies in other Southeast Asian countries as different cultural and educational backgrounds may produce different results. This can help to obtain a clearer picture of the factors affecting the continuance intention in using MOOCs.

REFERENCES

Alraimi, K. M., Zo, H., & Ciganek, A. P. (2015). Understanding the MOOCs continuance: The role of openness and reputation. Computers & Education, 80, 28–38.

Badali, M., Hatami, J., Banihashem, S. K., Rahimi, E., Noroozi, O., & Eslami, Z. (2022). The role of motivation in MOOCs' retention rates: A systematic literature review. Research and Practice in Technology Enhanced Learning, 17(1), 1–20.

Bhattacherjee, A. (2001). Understanding information systems continuance: An expectation-confirmation model. MIS Quarterly, 25, 351–370.

Dai, H. M., Teo, T., Rappa, N. A., & Huang, F. (2020). Explaining Chinese university students' continuance learning intention in the MOOC setting: A modified expectation confirmation model perspective. Computers & Education, 150, 103850.

Daneji, A. A., Ayub, A., & Khambari, M. (2019). The effects of perceived usefulness, confirmation and satisfaction on continuance intention in using massive open online course (MOOC). Knowledge Management & E-Learning, 11(2), 201–214.

George, D., & Mallery, P. (2003). SPSS for Windows Step by Step: A Simple Guide and Reference. 11.0 Update. Boston: Allyn and Bacon.

Guo, Z., Xiao, L., Van Toorn, C., Lai, Y., & Seo, C. (2016). Promoting online learners' continuance intention: An integrated flow framework. Information & Management, 53(2), 279–295.

Impey, C., & Formanek, M. (2021). MOOCS and 100 days of COVID: Enrollment surges in massive open online astronomy classes during the coronavirus pandemic. Social Sciences & Humanities Open, 4(1), 100177.

Israel, G. D. (1992). Determining Sample Size. Program Evaluation and Organizational Development. IFAS, University of Florida. PEOD-6. November.

Ittersum, K. W. V. (2015). The distinctiveness of engagement and flow at work. (Doctoral Thesis). Manhattan: Kansas State University.

Jo, D. (2018). Exploring the determinants of MOOCs continuance intention. KSII Transactions on Internet and Information Systems (TIIS), 12(8), 3992–4005.

Joo, Y. J., So, H. J., & Kim, N. H. (2018). Examination of relationships among students' self-determination, technology acceptance, satisfaction, and continuance intention to use k-MOOCs. Computers & Education, 122, 260–272.

Kline, R. B. (2016). Principles and Practice of Structural Equation Modeling. 4th edition. Guilford Publications.

Lu, Y., Wang, B., & Lu, Y. (2019). Understanding key drivers of MOOC satisfaction and continuance intention to use. Journal of Electronic Commerce Research, 20(2), 105–117.

Meet, R. K., & Kala, D. (2021). Trends and future prospects in MOOC researches: A systematic literature review 2013–2020. Contemporary Educational Technology, 13(3).

Nong, Y., Buavaraporn, N., & Punnakitikashem, P. (2022). Exploring the factors influencing users' satisfaction and continuance intention of MOOCs in China. Kasetsart Journal of Social Sciences, 43(2), 403–408.

Oliver, R. L. (1980). A cognitive model of the antecedents and consequences of satisfaction decisions. Journal of Marketing Research, 17(4), 460–469.

Ouyang, Y., Tang, C., Rong, W., Zhang, L., Yin, C., & Xiong, Z. (2017). Task- technology fit aware expectation-confirmation model towards understanding of MOOCs continued usage intention.

Shanshan, S., & Wenfei, L. (2022). Understanding the impact of quality elements on MOOCs continuance intention. Education and Information Technologies, 27, 10949–10976.

Straub, D., Boudreau, M. C., & Gefen, D. (2004). Validation guidelines for IS positivist research. Communications of the Association for Information Systems, 13(1), 24.

Tsai, Y. H., Lin, C. H., Hong, J. C., & Tai, K. H. (2018). The effects of metacognition on online learning interest and continuance to learn with MOOCs. Computers & Education, 121, 18–29.

Venkatesh, V., Morris, M. G., Davis, G. B., & Davis, F. D. (2003). User acceptance of information technology: Toward a unified view. MIS Quarterly, 27(3), 425–478.

Voss, B. D. (2013). Massive open online courses (MOOCs): A primer for university and college board members. AGB Association of Governing Boards of Universities and Colleges, 1–12.

Xiong, Y., Li, H., Kornhaber, M. L., Suen, H. K., Pursel, B., & Goins, D. D. (2015). Examining the relations among student motivation, engagement, and retention in a MOOC: A structural equation modeling approach. Global Education Review, 2(3), 23–33.

Zhao, Y., Wang, A., & Sun, Y. (2020). Technological environment, virtual experience, and MOOC continuance: A stimulus–organism–response perspective. Computers & Education, 144, 103721.

Zhou, J. (2017). Exploring the factors affecting learners' continuance intention of MOOCs for online collaborative learning: An extended ECM perspective. Australasian Journal of Educational Technology, *33*(5), 123–135.

APPENDIX

APPENDIX

Survey Questionnaire

Variable	Ind	Question	Reference
Confirmation	CF1	My experience with using MOOCs was better than I expected	Bhattacherjee (2001)
	CF2	The service level provided by MOOCs was better than I expected	
	CF3	Overall, most of my expectations from using MOOCs were confirmed	
Perceived usefulness	PU1	Using MOOCs improves my learning performance	Alraimi et al. (2015)
	PU2	Using MOOCs increases my learning effectiveness	
	PU3	I find MOOCs useful for me	

(Continued)

Survey Questionnaire   *(Continued)*

Variable	Ind	Question	Reference
Satisfaction	SA1	MOOCs were well organized	Daneji et al. (2019)
	SA2	My decision to use MOOCs was a wise one	
	SA3	I think I did the right thing by deciding to use MOOCs	
Continuance intention	CI1	I intend to continue using MOOCs rather than discontinue its use	Bhattacherjee (2001)
	CI2	My intention is to continue using MOOCs rather than to use any alternative	
	CI3	If I could, I would like to continue my use of MOOCs	
Flow	FL1	When I used MOOCs, I was not distracted by the disturbances in the environment surrounding me	Lu et al. (2019)
	FL2	When I used MOOCs, I did not feel frustrated or give up	
	FL3	When I used MOOCs, I concentrated on the MOOC and ignored what was happening around me	
Engagement	EG1	No matter whether I answer right or wrong, the course is still fun.	Tsai et al. (2018)
	EG2	I am concentrated on the activities of the course so it makes me feel that time flies.	
	EG3	I think that I'm fully focused on the course.	
Social influence	SI1	People who influence my behavior think that I should continue the use of MOOCs	Venkatesh et al. (2003)
	SI2	People who are important to me think that I should continue the use of MOOCs	
	SI3	The management of my university/ company has been helpful in my continuance use of MOOCs	
Curiosity	CU1	I am interested in discovering how things work	Dai et al. (2020)
	CU2	When I am given an incomplete puzzle, I try and imagine the final solution	
	CU3	When I am given a riddle, I am interested in trying to solve it	

13 Online Supervision for Internship Student During the COVID-19 Pandemic and Beyond

Putu Indah Ciptayani, Putu Manik Prihatini,
Kadek Cahya Dewi, and I Nyoman Eddy Indrayana
Politeknik Negeri Bali
Badung, Indonesia

13.1 INTRODUCTION AND BACKGROUND

By the last of 2019, the COVID-19 virus had spread widely and massively worldwide. The World Health Organization (WHO) declared a Public Health Emergency of International Concern (PHEIC) to prevent and control the spread (Ghani, 2020). This situation forced all countries to isolate and implement social distancing in all activities. Many sectors, such as public health, banking, government, and other businesses, had been affected. By social distancing and the rule of isolation, almost all activities were conducted from home.

Education is one affected sector that carries out all activities from home. A new teaching, supervising, and monitoring approach was urgently needed (Ghani, 2020). At the beginning of the pandemic, many students and teachers had no idea about online learning. Some hoped that COVID-19 would pass and that learning activities could be conducted offline.

The industrial internship program for 3–6 months is a regular offline learning program. This internship program is one of the essential processes for undergraduate students to experience work in the real world. When conducting an internship, the student is usually supervised by the teacher in their college. Mentoring is crucial to increase the student's portfolio success in internship programs (Moeinzadeh et al., 2021). The supervision process is conducted through a face-to-face meeting between the student and the teacher during the internship period. However, the pandemic situation made this method impossible. This chapter aims to elaborate on online supervision. A later section will describe the role of Information and Communication Technology (ICT), the importance of online supervision, the challenge and issue of online supervision, and how to build the online supervision system.

13.2 ONLINE SUPERVISION

Generally, all the internship and supervision processes are conducted face-to-face and offline. The communication between the student and teacher during the supervision process is conducted verbally, by phone, and by email. The offline

DOI: 10.1201/9781003331674-13

supervision process must follow a specific fixed schedule and need a particular place. Consequently, a pile of documents is involved in an offline system. More space and people are needed to manage all documents.

Furthermore, collecting documents from hundreds of students may take days or weeks. The document is likely to be scattered (Ismail et al., 2018); thus, the search process may take time. The manual supervision process makes the system difficult to monitor. This situation forces people to conduct online systems.

The online system has some advantages. All the processes, starting from registration, daily activity reports, supervision, monitoring, and evaluation, can be done in one system. The online system can be integrated with the existing system using Web service technology. The internship program coordinator can record and monitor all the online supervision processes. All documents and data can be saved in one database and downloaded anytime, anywhere, but only by the authorized user. The process of searching and generating information is faster online than offline. Another benefit of online supervision is schedule flexibility (Duraku & Hoxha, 2020) and place compared with the offline system. For social distancing, the online system is the best solution to conduct all the supervision processes, monitoring, and evaluating the internship process. Even though there are various advantages to the online supervision system, this system will not always succeed.

Many people are already accustomed to and comfortable with the face-to-face supervision system. A good relationship between the student and teacher is one of the keys to its success.

A model of participatory alignment (Figure 13.1) describes the relationship between supervisor and student developed online. The model is based on aligned expectations and behaviors, building on the idea of supervision as a partnership.

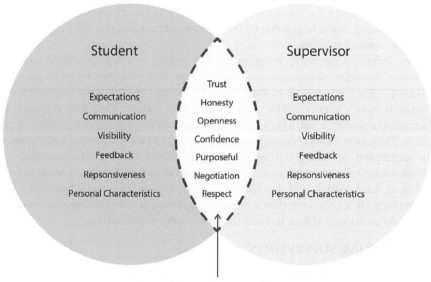

Zone of Participatory Aligment

FIGURE 13.1   Participatory alignment.

A trusting relationship is needed to establish open and honest communication and feedback without removing accountability and ownership from the student. The first supervision process is essential for the rest process, so it is necessary to do it through an online meeting/conference application such as Skype, Google Meet, Zoom, WebEx, Microsoft Team, or other platforms. The student and teacher could see each other by conducting an online meeting, and this initial contact was considered vital in establishing the relationship (Aitken et al., 2022). An excellent online relationship usually begins with open discussions between students and teachers regarding their expectations (Cornelius & Nicol, 2016).

Figure 13.2 shows the supervision process during the final project report written by the students during the internship process. The quality of supervisors' utterances embraces the difference between the application of comments, points of view, instructions, and questions (Augustsson & Jaldemark, 2014). The teacher must be able to observe and provide feedback to the student during the supervision process (Orr, 2010).

Another reason the online supervision system is a success is the knowledge of ICT utilization. Wiyono et al. (2022) found that the teacher's higher knowledge of ICT follows the ICT utilization in the instructional process. Software and hardware access is essential to provide successful online supervision. Technology access factors in supervision include (1) cost and availability; (2) compatibility, maintenance, and upgrading factors; (3) technology skills; (4) comfort and ease of use; (5) technology training; (6) reliable Internet access; and (7) security (Webber & Deroche, 2016). To support the successful online supervision system, the university must train its teachers in related technology and more interaction with students (Duraku &

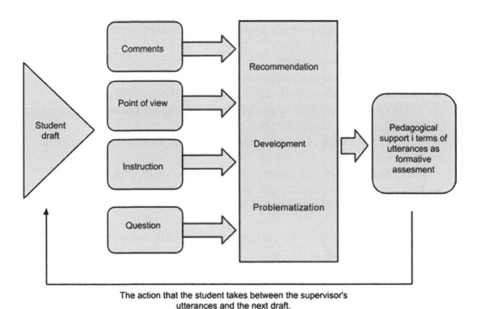

FIGURE 13.2   The supervision process on report draft.

Hoxha, 2020). Webber & Deroche (2016) suggested the following guidelines related to ICT factor in online supervision:

- Learn the technology needed in online supervision application
- Involve both student and teacher in the planning process for technology training
- Please recognize that the perception and attitudes of the student and how they adapt to online supervision is very important
- Assess the discomfort level of students and teachers in using an online supervision system
- Pair the inexperienced and experienced group buddies in transition to using an online supervision system
- Understand that the new students are generally nervous and anxious about performing well with or without the technology.

Online meeting plays a vital role in the online supervision process. It provides synchronous communication, immediate feedback, negotiating, and monitoring reactions to increase motivation and commitment. The study by Könings et al. (2016) found that students with online supervision from online meetings get a better experience than those without online meetings. The frequency and type of this online communication has a great impact, together with the frequent renewal of reciprocal rules and expectations without taking anything for granted. Synchronous feedback is a good practice because it can be mitigated against misinterpretation and the perception that the intended helpful feedback is rather harsh (Gray & Crosta, 2019). The qualities of an effective online supervisor are explained as follows (Gray & Crosta, 2019):

- Has the vision and experience to see ahead, particularly regarding potential online difficulties and strains
- Be creative and work flexibly
- Able to acquire resources generally as well as pertinent online resources
- Able to communicate effectively through the online medium
- Able to motivate students to produce work through the online medium
- Flexible and responsive to student needs
- Can direct the work of students when appropriate using a variety of online resources
- Can monitor and record progress throughout the online program
- Can nurture, create capabilities, and foster the growth of individuals into autonomous practitioners through the online medium

The aspects of effective online student-supervisor relationship rules are regularly reviewed and reaffirmed in the context of online supervision as follows (Gray & Crosta, 2019):

- The supervisor is intrinsically enthusiastic about their topic.
- Supervisor adopts an educative role suitable for the medium of online learning.

- Supervisor cares about them as an individual as well as their research.
- The supervisor is culturally aware and sensitive to the way that the online relationship is developed and progressed.
- The supervisor is readily available and always there when needed.
- The supervisor provides readily understood guidance and is approachable when further clarification is required, using a variety of online resources as appropriate.
- The supervisor provides advice on their work, sending it back as soon as possible with comments and constructive criticism, using a variety of online resources as appropriate.
- Supervisors should provide a coherent structure as well as support within the online supervisor relationship.

13.3   THE CHALLENGE OF ONLINE SUPERVISION

The online supervision system present is not without challenges. Most universities were new to online supervision and were forced by the COVID-19 pandemic to use it. No wonder many students and teachers were confused and not ready to move from face-to-face to online systems, even for people who spend a great deal of time on social media or computers (Strielkowski, 2020).

Common ICT challenges include bandwidth/connectivity, comfort and space, time zones and schedules, noise, and disturbances (Ghani, 2020). In Asian countries, bandwidth issues are always present (Zaheer & Munir, 2020). As Internet speed is not always stable, it may be slower at certain times and delay real-time online supervision (Webber & Deroche, 2016). The lack of ICT knowledge is another challenge (Duraku & Hoxha, 2020).

Other challenges related to social aspects, such as procrastination and personal time management (Strielkowski, 2020), slow down the supervision progress. Time constraints, official restrictions, irregular contacts, and technology are the main issues faced by supervisors, whereas student-supervisor interaction, diversity, perceptions, virtual communities, and academic collaboration are the biggest challenges for supervisors (Zaheer & Munir, 2020). Unclear email communication may lead to misperception. The student sometimes disappoints because the feedback lacks critical and truthful information (Aitken et al., 2022).

The guideline to face the challenges of the online supervision system is as follows:

- Universities provide facilities for high-quality online interaction between supervision and student, such as student centers (Zaheer & Munir, 2020).
- Improving skills in using ICT and the online supervision system by training them or providing the help desk (Webber & Deroche, 2016).
- Collaborate with telecommunication industries to either subsidize the cost of Internet subscriptions or provide free browsing data to the students and instructors as part of their corporate social responsibilities (Adedoyin & Soykan, 2020).

- Text communication should be clear, explicit, and gentle (Aitken et al., 2022).
- Provide good and specific feedback to the student (Aitken et al., 2022).
- Monthly feedback from the supervisor to each student has increased participation by about 50%-100% (Jalili et al., 2017).

13.4   THE ROLE OF ICT IN ONLINE SUPERVISION

Online supervision cannot be separated from technology, especially ICT. The utilization of ICT in the education field was done long before the COVID-19 pandemic, such as e-learning, e-book, or video tutorial. The presence of ICT in the learning process, including supervision, make it more flexible and open (Duraku & Hoxha, 2020). Also the teacher, as a supervisor, can facilitate the student to improve their ability based on their pace (Huang et al., 2020). Some research showed that ICT utilization is effective in the instructional supervision process, both for teachers and students (Kopcha & Alger, 2011; Martin et al., 2017; Suparman, 2013). Even the use of ICT is very effective for implementing supervision in rural, remote areas or during a pandemic (Liu et al., 2018; Matyanga et al., 2020).

Compared with the traditional supervision process, online supervision has a significant benefit; it offers an effective and efficient control for distance education (Vaiz et al., 2021). The online system for supervision can handle the entire internship process, from company registration to the assessment process. During the internship, the entire supervision process and monitoring can be done via the online system.

The list below describes how ICT helps the online supervision implementation:

1. The Database Management System (DBMS) allows all data, including the supervision history, to be saved in a database system (Binti Jaafar et al., 2018). DBMS ensures data integrity and consistency and allows multi-user access. An online information system makes document management more well organized and supports paperless documentation. Information retrieval can be faster and more accurate (Ismail et al., 2018), and the privacy of supervision data can be guaranteed (only authorized users can access the data).
2. Web technology massively changes many businesses around the world. The latest technology makes building a responsive Web-based system became faster and cheaper. Many frameworks are available to help us build an effective and efficient Web-based system. The Web browser and client scripting side development make the Web-based system more attractive and responsive. The Web service technology can integrate the existing academic information system and the new online supervision system. The technology of ICT today brings all the information into our hands, which means that the Web-based system of online supervision can be accessed via mobile phone.
3. Internet technology connects people anywhere, anytime. It is much faster than several years ago, making it easier for people to connect and access the information they need with little effort. Online supervision has become

more common and convenient because all the processes can be flexible, asynchronous, or synchronous.
4. The virtual conference technology supported by both hardware and Internet technology makes everything easier, faster, cheaper (accessible), and more efficient in online supervision.

Based on Wang (2020), the use of ICT in online supervision has some advantages: (1) the supervision process can be done through real-time communication and is more flexible; (2) the student can log onto the system so that the teacher can monitor the internship process; (3) the online system facilitates the student to write a daily activities journal and upload a related resource as needed, while the teacher as a supervisor can give feedback, guidance, and also do assessments; and (4) the electronic materials are easier to collect and convenient to output.

13.5   BUILD AN ONLINE SUPERVISION SYSTEM

An online supervision system, a Web-based or mobile app, is a promising solution to improve the communication and management of the internship supervision process during the COVID-19 pandemic. System development can be implemented in a three-tier architecture. Both conventional methods and the online system can be adapted to the supervision process to boost student research or project outcomes. The teacher can share their feedback with their student through the forum provided by the online system. Also, students can share their opinions through the forum among themselves beyond time and location constraints (Bakar et al., 2016).

The study by Mia et al. (2020) recognized that the common problems related to the internship program included difficulty in finding the best match company for the student, in gaining real-life experience, learning management during the internship, and measuring the learning outcome during and after an internship. Hence, an excellent online system must provide a list of potential companies and an online monitoring process. The supervision process can conduct synchronously or asynchronously based on the discussion purpose. The system must provide a link, email, and forum for task-oriented items (Orr, 2010). A chat or link button to the online meeting must be available for social interaction between teacher and student to help negotiate and develop a supervisory relationship. The teacher should focus on smaller, more easily manageable tasks to help their productivity (Ghani, 2020). Therefore, an online supervision system that provides a progress tracker for the project and discussion related to the project is needed.

All information regarding the applications and host of organizations are safely kept in the database and can be retrieved by the administrator for future reference about other students. Also, industrial supervisors can assess the students using an online system. Another additional feature to be considered is providing the option for the user to provide feedback regarding the system to enhance the usability quality (Binti Jaafar et al., 2018). A robust framework must be easily accessible, user-friendly, transparent, and attractive to students and supervisors (Maor et al., 2016). The user manual and standard operating procedure (SOP) are essential things that must be provided in every system and easily accessed.

One critical success factor of software is usability, which can be measured by conducting usability testing. Psychometric Evaluation and Instructions for Use is an instrument developed by IBM to measure the usability of software (Setiyawan et al., 2021). The characteristics measured in the instrument include understandability, learnability, operability, and attractiveness (Lewis, 2009).

13.6 CONCLUSION

The online system is the best solution to conduct all the registration, supervision processes, monitoring, and evaluating the internship process during the pandemic or distance education. It can be integrated with the existing system, and it is faster and more flexible.

To make the online supervision succeed, a good relationship between the student and teacher is one of the keys to success in the supervision process. The first supervision process, which is essential, must begin with open discussions about their expectations. So an online meeting application plays an important role here to provide synchronous communication, immediate feedback, negotiating, and monitoring reactions to increase motivation and commitment. Also, the knowledge of ICT from both student and supervisor is mandatory. To face a challenge related to bandwidth and space, the university can provide facilities for a high-quality online system or collaborate with telecommunication industries.

An online supervision system can be built by a three-tier architecture. A DBMS keeps data integrity and consistency and allows multi-user access. The system can be accessed by student, supervisor, and internship coordinator. It must provide a list of potential companies, the registration process, supervision process through real time (via linked meeting application), the asynchronous discussion via online forum, the daily activities report and field to provide feedback from the supervisor, and the assessment process. A good system must be equipped by guidance and SOP. The responsive, user-friendly, and high availability of the system can improve the system usability.

REFERENCES

Adedoyin, O. B., & Soykan, E. (2023). Covid-19 Pandemic And Online Learning: The Challenges And Opportunities. *Interactive Learning Environments*, 31(2), 863–875. https://doi.org/10.1080/10494820.2020.1813180

Aitken, G., Smith, K., Fawns, T., & Jones, D. (2022). Participatory Alignment: A Positive Relationship between Educators and Students During Online Masters Dissertation Supervision. *Teaching in Higher Education*, 27(6), 772–786. https://doi.org/10.1080/13562517.2020.1744129

Augustsson, G., & Jaldemark, J. (2014). Online Supervision: A Theory of supervisors' Strategic Communicative Influence on Student Dissertations. *Higher Education*, 67(1), 19–33. https://doi.org/10.1007/s10734-013-9638-4

Bakar, B. A., Isa, N. M., Sani, M. M., & Shahbudin, S. (2016). E-supervision system for undergraduates final year project. *2015 IEEE 7th International Conference on Engineering Education, ICEED 2015*, 155–159. https://doi.org/10.1109/ICEED.2015.7451511

Binti Jaafar, A. N., Binti Rohafauzi, S., Binti Md Enzai, N. I., Bin Mohd Fauzi, F. D. H., Binti Nik Dzulkefli, N. N. S., & Bin Amron, M. T. (2018). Development of internship monitoring and supervising web-based system. *IEEE Student Conference on Research and Development: Inspiring Technology for Humanity, Scored 2017 – Proceedings, 2018-Janua*, 193–197. https://doi.org/10.1109/SCORED.2017.8305395

Cornelius, S., & Nicol, S. (2016). Understanding the needs of Masters Dissertation Supervisors: Supporting students in professional contexts. *Journal of Perspectives in Applied Academic Practice, 4*(1), 2–12.

Duraku, Z. H., & Hoxha, L. (2020). The Impact of COVID-19 on Education and on the Well-Being of Teachers, Parents, and Students: Challenges Related to Remote (online) Learning and Opportunities for Advancing the Quality of Education. *Impact of the COVID-19 Pandemic on Education and Wellbeing*, 17–45.

Ghani, F. (2020). Remote Teaching and Supervision of Graduate Scholars in the Unprecedented and Testing Times. *Journal of the Pakistan Dental Association, 29* (Special Supplement), S36–S42. https://doi.org/10.25301/jpda.29s.s36

Gray, M. A., & Crosta, L. (2019). New Perspectives in Online Doctoral Supervision: A Systematic Literature Review. *Studies in Continuing Education, 41*(2), 173–190. https://doi.org/10.1080/0158037X.2018.1532405

Huang, R. H., Liu, D. J., Tlili, A., Yang, J. F., & Wang, H. H. (2020). *Handbook on Facilitating Flexible Learning During Educational Disruption: The Chinese Experience in Maintaining Undisrupted Learning in COVID-19 Outbreak*. Smart Learning Institute of Beijing Normal University.

Ismail, S. I., Abdullah, R., Kar, S. A. C., Fadzal, N., Husni, H., & Omar, H. M. (2018). Online project evaluation and supervision system (OPENs) for final year project proposal development process. *IEEE Student Conference on Research and Development: Inspiring Technology for Humanity, Scored 2017 – Proceedings, 2018-Janua*, 210–214. https://doi.org/10.1109/SCORED.2017.8305392

Jalili, M., Baker Mafinejad, M., & Gandum Kar, R. (2017). *Principles and Methods of Assessment of Learners in Medical Sciences*. Tehran: Academy of Medical Sciences of the Islamic Republic of Iran.

Könings, K. D., Popa, D., Gerken, M., Giesbers, B., Rienties, B. C., van der Vleuten, C. P. M., & van Merriënboer, J. J. G. (2016). Improving Supervision for Students at a Distance: Videoconferencing for Group Meetings. *Innovations in Education and Teaching International, 53*(4), 388–399. https://doi.org/10.1080/14703297.2015.1004098

Kopcha, T., & Alger, C. (2011). The Impact of Technology-Enhanced Student Teacher Supervision on Student-Teacher Knowledge, Performance, and Self-Efficacy during the Field Experience. *Journal of Computers in Education, 45*, 49–73.

Lewis, J. R. (2009). IBM Computer Usability Satisfaction Questionnaires: Psychometric Evaluation and Instructions for Use. *International Journal of Human – Computer Interaction, 7*, 57–78.

Liu, K., Miller, R., Dickmann, E., & Monday, K. (2018). Virtual Supervision of Student Teachers as a Catalyst of Change for Educational Equity in Rural Areas. *Journal of Design Learning, 2*, 8–19.

Maor, D., Ensor, J. D., & Fraser, B. J. (2016). Doctoral Supervision in Virtual Spaces: A Review of Research of Web-Based Tools to Develop Collaborative Supervision. *Higher Education Research and Development, 35*(1), 172–188. https://doi.org/10.1080/07294360.2015.1121206

Martin, P., Kumar, S., & Lizarondo, L. (2017). Effective Use of Technology in Clinical Supervision. *Internet Interventions, 8*, 35–39.

Matyanga, C. M. J., Dzingirai, B., & Monera-Penduka, T. G. (2020). Virtual Supervision of Pharmacy Undergraduate Research Projects During the COVID-19 Lockdown in Zimbabwe. *Pharmacy Education, 20*, 13–14.

Mia, R., Zahid, A. H., Dev Nath, B. C., & Hoque, A. S. M. L. (2020). A conceptual design of virtual internship system to benchmark software development skills in a blended learning environment. *ICCIT 2020 - 23rd International Conference on Computer and Information Technology, Proceedings*, 19–21. https://doi.org/10.1109/ICCIT51783.2020.9392670

Moeinzadeh, F., Ayati, S. H. R., Iraj, B., Mojgan, M., & Vafamehr, V. (2021). Designing, Implementation, and Evaluation of Internship Comprehensive System for Assessment and Monitoring. *Journal of Education and Health Promotion*, *10*(93), 1–9.

Orr, P. P. (2010). Distance Supervision: Research, Findings, and Considerations for Art Therapy. *Arts in Psychotherapy*, *37*(2), 106–111. https://doi.org/10.1016/j.aip.2010.02.002

Setiyawan, A., Priyanto, Prasetya, T. A., & Hastawan, A. F. (2021). Usability Evaluation of Assignment and Monitoring Information Learning System of Internship Students Based on SMS Gateway With Raspberry Pi. *IOP Conference Series: Earth and Environmental Science*, *700*(1). https://doi.org/10.1088/1755-1315/700/1/012021

Strielkowski, W. (2020). *COVID-19 Pandemic and the Digital Revolution in Academia and Higher Education*. https://doi.org/10.20944/preprints202004.0290.v1

Suparman, U. F. (2013). The implementation of the ICT-based thesis supervision at one postgraduate school in Indonesia. *Proceedings of the International Conference on Education and Language (ICEL)*, Bandar Lampung, Indonesia.

Vaiz, O., Minalay, H., Türe, A., Ülgener, P., Yaşar, H., & Bilir, A. M. (2021). The supervision in distance education: e-supervision. The Online Journal of New Horizons in Education-July, 11(3).

Wang, L. (2020). "Internet + internship management": College internship management optimization. *Proceedings - 2020 International Conference on Computer Engineering and Application, ICCEA 2020*, 312–314. https://doi.org/10.1109/ICCEA50009.2020.00074

Webber, J. M., & Deroche, M. D. (2016). Technology and Accessibility in Clinical Supervision: Challenges and Solutions. In *Using Technology to Enhance Clinical Supervision* (1st ed., pp. 67–85). American Counseling Association.

Wiyono, B. B., Samsudin, Imron, A., & Arifin, I. (2022). The Effectiveness of Utilizing Information and Communication Technology in Instructional Supervision with Collegial Discussion Techniques for the Teacher's Instructional Process and the Student's Learning Outcomes. *Sustainability (Switzerland)*, *14*(9). https://doi.org/10.3390/su14094865

Zaheer, M., & Munir, S. (2020). Research Supervision in Distance Learning: Issues and Challenges. *Asian Association of Open Universities Journal*, *15*(1), 131–143. https://doi.org/10.1108/AAOUJ-01-2020-0003

14 The Lecturer Document Management System in the COVID-19 Pandemic

Benefits, Challenges, Potential, and Difficulties

Ni Gusti Ayu Putu Harry Saptarini,
Putu Indah Ciptayani, I Nyoman Eddy Indrayana,
and I Putu Bagus Arya Pradnyana
Politeknik Negeri Bali
Badung, Indonesia

14.1 INTRODUCTION

The COVID-19 virus at the end of 2019 made several countries impose isolation. In Indonesia, this virus attack began to spread extensively at the beginning of 2020. The Indonesian government issued an appeal for social distancing to minimize the spread of the virus and to minimize direct physical contact. After more than a year and there was no sign that the spread of the virus would stop, this incident was declared a pandemic. Thus, all the COVID-19 prevention protocols that had been carried out before had to continue to be implemented, including minimizing direct contact.

Education was one pandemic-affected area, and learning was automatically carried out online. Administrative staff worked from their homes to minimize direct contact and carry out activities such as managing the lecturer portfolio data, lecturer assessments, and lecturer database for accreditation. All activities related to portfolio management and lecturer performance assessment were previously carried out by collecting printed documents. The pandemic indirectly forced the construction of a system to be able to share data and information online, where all files would be converted into digital documents (paperless).

The concept of the paperless office has been coming for a long time. The first concept was presented as a critique of the management system concept based on a written document (Susanty et al., 2012). When developing a paperless office, actions consist of scanning paper documents into digital forms (Ugale et al., 2017; Indrajit et al., 2018), managing office files electronically (Pasharibu et al., 2019; Indrajit et al., 2018; Genesis & Oluwole, 2018; Onwubere, 2020), and performing a digital or online evaluation of lecturers and staff (Genesis & Oluwole, 2018; Onwubere, 2020).

DOI: 10.1201/9781003331674-14

For this reason, this chapter explores how information systems and information and communication technology (ICT) will assist in managing lecturer portfolio files, their strengths, weaknesses, and success factors.

14.2   ICT FOR PAPERLESS DATA AND INFORMATION SHARING IN EDUCATION

The exchange of data and information is still dominated by hard copies (printouts). However, the idea of minimizing the use of hard copies was put forward 50 years ago. The paperless system is also a significant movement in the education field. Almost all academic activities (except for the documents such as diplomas and transcripts printing final value, as well as the decision letter) can be replaced with digital files and communication between communities using social media applications. (Tarmuji, 2013). This action may improve the possibility of a paperless system achievement.

Paperless file management and sharing at university offers some advantages (Isaeva & Yoon, 2016):

1. Reducing the use of paper will have implications for reducing the cost of purchasing paper, printing paper, and ultimately supporting forest sustainability as a source of paper raw materials.
2. Reduced searching time for documents compared with manually searching through piles of hard copies.
3. Reduces the possibility of duplication of data, thereby reducing storage media and better guaranteeing data consistency.
4. Reduce the need for physical file storage such as cupboards, desks, or drawers.
5. Increase the flexibility of document use and security.
6. Improve the efficiency of the administrative process.
7. It can be accessed anytime and from anywhere.

Based on (Dhumne, 2017) a paperless society uses less physical space when bulky filing cabinets are eliminated or reduced. Thus, the institution can use the existing space for other academic needs, such as a reading room, discussion room, or additional classroom. Renting a smaller building will also benefit the institution financially. The following current development of ICT can help a paperless society in this era of pandemic.

1. The existence of facsimile and email machines can significantly reduce the need to print documents, so this will reduce printing costs and document delivery costs.
2. A scanner machine now commonly found on printers reduces the possibility of losing documents and makes it easier to find documents one day, and this undoubtedly reduces the use of paper to reproduce documents in the future.
3. The current development of ICT allows the simultaneous processing of electronic documents from various places, making it possible for employees to work from home (WFH).

4. The current development of smartphones has provided various features, not only as a means of communication but also as a mini-computer. Thus, using paper can be minimized (Levine, 1999).
5. A backup feature in the cloud network also prevents the loss of essential data and can be accessed from anywhere (Nayyar & Arora, 2019).

Current software development has also supported the paperless exchange of data and information. Several applications for conducting meetings are Google Meet and Zoom, ranging from free to paid. Dropbox or Google Drive provides access to store data on cloud servers and collaborate to modify documents. Access rights can also be set to see only or can make modifications. The program also facilitates tele-conferencing, presentations, file sharing, and video transmission (Harrison, 2013). Therefore, there will be no need for printouts and handouts.

14.3   INFORMATION SYSTEM FOR LECTURER DOCUMENT MANAGEMENT

Recent developments in ICT have presented various choices, from personal computers, laptops, smartphones, notebooks, or tablets. These various choices, especially tablets, provide options that have the opportunity to realize the paperless idea (King & Toland, 2014). The development of ICT to find a tablet like the iPad or Samsung tablet makes the paperless office feel closer.

The tablet is considered well perceived, easy to use, portable, and looks like a book, so it will be straightforward to read or edit documents. However, the tablet still cannot maximize the paperless office. Furthermore, limitations include an inadequate file management system, input, and annotation issues, and it is unsuitable for reading long documents (King & Toland, 2014). For that, we need a system that can overcome this limitation.

A system that can integrate all data and simultaneously process it into the required information and allows simultaneous file management is needed to support the success of a paperless office. Using an integrated information system will significantly benefit the paperless technique, emphasizing the culture of minimizing paper use by working digitally using application servers, portals, and computer systems. The advantages of an information system include cost-effective use, reduced document processing time, guaranteed security, and ease of access (Nayyar & Arora, 2019). Document sharing can also be done quickly, even in real time, between countries so that information exchange can be done quickly, efficiently, and cheaply. Going paperless is essential to implement in new working practices as it makes the workplace and businesses free from the constraints of time and place (Nayyar & Arora, 2019). In the electronic document management system (Susanty et al., 2012), the speed of access to information will be an advantage for users or companies that need fast information.

The existence of this system can make all document processing faster, better, cheaper, and more environmentally friendly. A positive impact on the environment can be achieved due to a reduction in the use of paper (Bagus et al., 2020). Reducing the physical delivery of documents from one place to another will also reduce the carbon footprint, which will positively impact environmental sustainability.

The three-tier document management system offers these advantages: efficiency, better documentation, a better job, better decision, controllable management, improving the organization's image, and eco-friendly (Susanty et al., 2012). Other advantages of an integrated information system include centralized management, efficient services, increased productivity, optimization of resources, reduced errors and costs, total and easy access to information, increased control and security, and elimination of duplicate documents (Orantes-Jimenez et al., 2015).

A document management system that has been created should be able to convert all documents or most documents in an agency into digital form so that a paperless office can be realized. This system should be able to facilitate the entire management process, prevent document placement errors, and speed up access to certain documents needed by users (Selvi et al., 2011). The system must include internal documentation to make it easier for users to use the system (Alenazi et al., 2014).

This information system must prevent duplication/repetition of documents and facilitate the distribution of documents between departments within the institution (DeLone & McLean, 2003). This system can be seen as a combination of mobile and Web applications and services. It should also be able to support document classification to simplify the document maintenance process. In addition, the security side must be guaranteed, where the system should only allow authorized users who can access documents according to the roles set at the beginning of the system (Isaeva & Yoon, 2016). This system will have three roles: lecturer, university staff, and administrator.

14.4   THE DEVELOPING PHASE OF THE LECTURER DOCUMENT MANAGEMENT INFORMATION SYSTEM

The phase of developing an integrated document information system consists of the following stages. The initial stage is to analyze user needs to determine the needs the system must cover. Next is the design stage, where the database and interface design is carried out. The implementation stage implements the system with a programming language and database, in this case, the PHP programming language and the MariaDB database.

The final stage is the testing stage, where alpha and beta testing will be carried out. Alpha testing is done when the program is being developed by checking whether the system works as needed. Checking includes ensuring that the output is correct by the processes that occur in the real world. The beta test is done when the system has been built, and the test is carried out by direct use. Administrators and officers conduct final testing before applying the system (Bagus et al., 2020). This comprehensive test may indicate the performance of a developed system.

14.5   CRITICAL SUCCESS FACTOR OF THE INFORMATION SYSTEM FOR LECTURER DOCUMENT MANAGEMENT

The impact of the rapid development of ICT is found in various aspects, where ICT can automate many processes that were previously done manually. Even with the rapid development of computers a few years ago, paperless has not yet been fully implemented. Until now, the use of paper is still going on quite a lot, so it seems as if the presence of ICT has no significant effect on reducing paper use in offices. (Orantes-Jimenez et al., 2015). The paper domination may be caused by the physical properties of paper, primarily thin, light, and flexible, which enabled quick and efficient cross-referencing and annotation and embodied editorial excellence (Hargrave, 2014). Based on Stöckel & Karlsson (2017), paper's affordances are as follows.

- Flexible navigation: By using paper, the user usually comes into direct contact with the surface of the paper and performs all activities directly on it, whereas by using a computer, most of the input can be done with the keyboard and mouse.
- Cross-document use: Paper allows multiple documents to be used simultaneously, while the computer layer has a size limitation to open multiple windows in one view effectively.
- Direct annotation: Paper allows users to make notes directly by scribbling on a document while actively reading it, without having to use tools such as a keyboard and mouse.
- Switching between reading and writing: Reading and writing at the same time or switching between the two is less cumbersome with paper.

The users' attitude toward the new technology or system is another complex challenge. Until recently, most people felt reluctant or uncomfortable working with electronic devices and were more comfortable using paper. Some people are sometimes not familiar with certain technologies, which is sometimes quite dangerous, and often reject this new system's existence (Al Jaberi et al., 2022). Furthermore, people do not know enough about new technology, proper use, and early rejection and believe printed documents are more valuable than electronic documents (Orantes-Jimenez et al., 2015). Other challenges are poor Internet connectivity and computer skills, lack of Information Technology (IT) professionals and security threats, and lack of managerial support (Dorji, 2018).

Some list the difficulties in implementing the new technology (Orantes-Jimenez et al., 2015) include the following:

- The need for greater investment in hardware and software (such as scanner machines, computer servers, database servers, connectivity, and software)
- Incurring additional costs for training employees/staff
- There are difficulties in installing electronic devices and integrating them with existing systems
- There is a need for updates both in terms of software and hardware
- Difficulty reading documents on a computer screen
- Adapt the designs of processes and services to computer formats with easy handling and adequate accessibility
- The existence of cultural barriers to users in institutions
- There is a habit of printing all documents

All those challenges does not mean that the paperless office cannot be implemented. The pandemic of COVID-19 forced many industries to WFH, which is a great opportunity and a stepping stone to the paperless office (Holman et al, 2003). During WFH, all documents will be shared through digital media, and all documents will be digital so everyone can see them in real time. In addition, the development of communication tool technology in the form of smartphones and tablets, supported by the development of 5G telecommunications, has made data access much more available and fast. By using a tablet, the convenience of using paper can be achieved. Anyone can gain access to the documents needed by using a smartphone. Better support is with cloud computing and cloud-based services, the development of information systems becomes more manageable, and investment can be suppressed. Therefore, implementing a document management information system is much easier in a paperless office and society.

Despite the various technological conveniences, conditioning from the user's side is also essential to support the success of the information system that has been built. The reluctance to switch to a new system or loss of comfort that has been formed is one of the obstacles to being able to switch to a new system. (King & Toland, 2014). Most people will usually resist change at first.

A new policy will be urgently needed here. Research has shown that if a person is given a situation and a problem, they will use their skills and knowledge and eventually produce a policy that is easier to implement because they believe that the policy was developed together to meet current needs (Alenazi et al., 2014). Policymakers should involve system users in making this policy.

The role of the organization's leadership is equally important in being committed to creating a supportive environment and atmosphere and providing policy instruments. They should also be good commanders in implementing this new system (Sugiarto et al., 2022). Support from the IT department is also vital, especially in adapting to the new system.

Research has shown that IT and management departments should be able to provide training and motivation for their workers when switching to a new system so that employees have a good perception and know that the new system is functional and easy to use (Obeidat, 2015). Paperless applications must also be easy to use, and users must be provided with continuous training so that paperless applications can be implemented easier (Prastyo et al., 2020). Developers should make the Graphical User Interface (GUI) more straightforward, understandable, and user-friendly (Isaeva & Yoon, 2016). That is why the organization should:

- Develop a document storage plan before transitioning to a paperless one.
- Determine document storage guidelines.
- Organize documents (using a commercial tool tailored to the company).
- Create a file structure.
- Use date-specific document folders.
- Create a folder for each program within the client drawer.
- Organize the firm's documents.
- Determine drawer-naming conventions.
- Define a structure for document folders.
- Save the money: double-sided printing lets us save money because we spend half of the standard printing paper.

- Save space–less paper, more place.
- Care for the environment: fewer trees felled and less fuel to transport them.

The system that is built should be able to replace the paper properties that have been in the user's mind. For this reason, it is necessary to create a responsive system with high usability that can be accessed compactly on devices such as tablets. Users need to be involved in the creation of the system and its usage policies so that they feel it is what best suits their needs. Companies and users must realize that even though the use of an online system will require large funds at the start, it is an investment for the company to gain work effectiveness and efficiency. Another important thing to maintain the success of the new system is support from management, including establishing clear standard operating procedure and training users.

14.6   CONCLUSION

During the COVID-19 pandemic, the education field was forced online including almost all activities such as lecturer data management for accreditation. All documents related to the lecturer portfolio would be converted into digital documents. Paperless file management and sharing has some advantages: reduce cost (buying paper and print documents), reduce searching time, reduce data duplication, reduce physical storage, and can be accessed anytime and anywhere. This pandemic has been a great opportunity to apply paperless file management.

ICT can help a paperless society in many aspects, such as a scanner to convert hard copy files into digital form, the cloud technology allows simultaneous easy access for document sharing, and rapid development of the smartphone offers mini-computer function in hand. The development of the tablet also gives users a convenient experience that is as good as working with paper, but in a more efficient way. Even so, implementing a paperless office is not always easy. There are several challenges, such as paper properties, convenience, and familiarity compared with digital media; an expensive investment; people's early rejection of changes; and lack of knowledge in technology and Internet connection.

To maximize the paperless office, an integrated information system to manage lecturer files is needed. This system must be responsive and can be accessed via smartphone or tablet to provide a good user experience. The system can support document classification to simplify the document maintenance process and guarantee the data security. The stages of developing an information system include analyzing user needs, designing, implementing, and testing. Therefore, the support from top-level management and providing an infrastructure and training have a big impact on implementing the new information system.

REFERENCES

Al Jaberi, B. H., Sedaghat, M. M., Almallahi, M. N., Alsyouf, I., & Ibrahim, I. A. S. (2022). The role of COVID-19 in moving towards a paperless campus: The case of university of Sharjah. *2022 Advances in Science and Engineering Technology International Conferences, ASET 2022, May.* https://doi.org/10.1109/ASET53988.2022.9734887

Alenazi, S. R. A., Shittu, A. J. K., Al-Matari, E. M. A., & Alanzi, A. R. A. (2014). Paperless Office Management: A Feasibility Analysis for Saudi Arabia Government Offices: Case Study in Ministry of Labor. *Journal of Management Research*, *6*(3), 186. https://doi.org/10.5296/jmr.v6i3.5700

Bagus, Y., Rahman, A., & Sugiantoro, B. (2020). The Development of Web-Based Paperless Office System Using CodeIgniter Framework Case Study of Lembaga Pengembangan Cabang Ranting Muhammadiyah. *Proceeding International Conference on Science and Engineering*, *3*(April), 221–227. https://doi.org/10.14421/icse.v3.501

DeLone, W. H., & McLean, E. R. (1992). Information Systems Success: The Quest for the Dependent Variable. *Information Systems Research*, *3*(1), 1–95.

DeLone, W. H., & McLean, E. R. (2003). *The DeLone and McLean Model of Information Systems Success: A Ten-Year Update.*

Dhumne, K. M. (2017). Paperless Society in Digital Era. *International Journal of Library and Information Studies*, *7*(4), 317–319. http://www.ijlis.org

Dorji, T. (2018). *Going Paperless Office*. Royal Institute of Management, Simtokha.

Genesis, E., & Oluwole, O. (2018). Towards a "Paperless" Higher Education System in Nigeria: Concept, Challenges and Prospects. Journal of Education, Society and Behavioural Science, 24(2), 1–15. https://doi.org/10.9734/JESBS/2018/19913

Hargrave, J. E. (2014). Paperless Mark-up: Editing Educational Texts in a Digital Environment. *Publishing Research Quarterly*, *30*(2), 212–222. https://doi.org/10.1007/s12109-014-9360-9

Harrison, K. (2013). 5 Steps to A (Nearly) Paperless Office. *Forbes*. http://www.forbes

Holman, D., Vertegaal, R., Altosaar, M., Troje, N., & Johns, D. (2005). Paper windows: interaction techniques for digital paper. *Proceedings of the SIGCHI Conference on Human Factors in Computing Systems*, Portland, Oregon, USA, 591–599.

Indrajit, R.E., Saide, Wahyuningsih, R., Tinaria, L. (2018). Implementation of Paperless Office in the Classroom. In: Rocha, Á., Adeli, H., Reis, L.P., Costanzo, S. (eds) Trends and Advances in Information Systems and Technologies. WorldCIST'18 2018. Advances in Intelligent Systems and Computing, vol 745. Springer, Cham. https://doi.org/10.1007/978-3-319-77703-0_50

Isaeva, M., & Yoon, H. Y. (2016). Paperless university -How we can make it work? *2016 15th International Conference on Information Technology Based Higher Education and Training, ITHET 2016*. https://doi.org/10.1109/ITHET.2016.7760717

King, K., & Toland, J. (2014). iPads and the Paperless Office: The Impact of Tablet Devices on Paper Consumption in Higher Education. *Journal of Applied Computing and Information Technology*, *18*(1).

Levine, S. (1999). *U.S. Patent No. 5,974,349* (Patent No. 5,974,349).

Nayyar, N., & Arora, S. (2019). Paperless Technology - A Solution to Global Warming. *2019 2nd International Conference on Power Energy Environment and Intelligent Control, PEEIC 2019*, 486–488. https://doi.org/10.1109/PEEIC47157.2019.8976599

Obeidat, M. A. (2015). Empirical Analysis for the Factors Affecting Realization of Paperless Office. *International Journal of Economics, Commerce and Management United Kingdom*, *III*(6), 773–792. http://ijecm.co.uk/

Onwubere, C. H. (2020). The Imperatives of Information and Communication Technologies in University Administration in Nigeria. Media & Communication Currents, 4(1), 75–90.

Orantes-Jimenez, S. D., Zavala-Galindo, A., & Vazquez-Alvarez, G. (2015). Paperless Office: A New Proposal for Organizations. *IMSCI 2015 - 9th International Multi-Conference on Society, Cybernetics and Informatics, Proceedings*, *13*(3), 70–75.

Pasharibu, Y., Sugiarto, A., Ariarsanti, T., & Wijayant, P. (2019). Dimensions of Green Office Evidence from Regency/City Government Offices in Central Java, Indonesia. Business: Theory and Practice, 20, 391–402. https://doi.org/10.3846/btp.2019.37

Prastyo, P. H., Sumi, A., & Kusumawardani, S., S. S. (2020). A Systematic Literature Review of Application Development to Realize Paperless Application in Indonesia: Sectors, Platforms, Impacts, and Challenges. *Indonesian Journal of Information Systems, 2*(2), 111–129. https://doi.org/10.24002/ijis.v2i2.3168

Selvi, S., Khan, S., Rani, U., Prasad, B. V. N., Paul, A. K., & Biswal, A. K. (2011). Document Management System - Go Green "a Paperless Office" for Steel Plants. *Steel Times International, 35*(8), 39–41.

Stöckel, F., & Karlsson, M. (2017). The Myth of the Paperless Office: Is there a Key Amongst the Clouds? [UMEA Universitet]. In *Electronic Library.* https://doi.org/10.7551/mitpress/4833.001.0001

Sugiarto, A., Lee, C. W., & Huruta, A. D. (2022). A Systematic Review of the Sustainable Campus Concept. *Behavioral Sciences, 12*(5). https://doi.org/10.3390/bs12050130

Susanty, W., Thamrin, T., Erlangga, & Cucus, A. (2012). Document management system based on paperless. *1st International Conference on Engineering and Technology Development*, Bandar Lampung, Indonesia, 135–138.

Tarmuji, A. (2013). Optimization of the use of social media to support the paperless office. *The 2nd International Conference on Green World in Business and Technology*, E121–E128. https://onesearch.id/Record/IOS14805.10350%0Ahttp://eprints.uad.ac.id/10350/2/Int-2013-prosiding icgwbt Optimization of pdf

Ugale, M. K., Patil, S. J., & Musande, V. B. (2017). Document management system: A notion towards paperless office. 2017 1st International Conference on Intelligent Systems and Information Management (ICISIM), 217–224. https://doi.org/10.1109/ICISIM.2017.8122176

15 Fast-Track Program with Recognition of Prior Learning in Post-Pandemic COVID-19

I Made Ari Dwi Suta Atmaja, I Nyoman Gede Arya Astawa, Ni Wayan Wisswani, I Ketut Parnata, and Putu Wijaya Sunu
Politeknik Negeri Bali
Badung, Indonesia

15.1 EDUCATION DURING COVID-19

The COVID-19 outbreak had hit the global education sector, especially universities. During the COVID-19 period, the government imposed restrictions on gathering, social distancing, physical distancing, wearing masks, and constantly washing hands in every activity (Government Policy Briefs, 2020). Through the Ministry of Education, the government has prohibited higher education from carrying out face-to-face (conventional) learning and requires online learning (Kemdikbudristek, 2021). Universities are led to be able to organize online learning processes. Lectures must be held with scenarios that can prevent physical contact between students-lecturers and students-students (Basilaia, 2020).

Digital technology can enable students and lecturers to carry out the learning process even though they are in different places (Haleema et al., 2022). The users of online learning process during the pandemic can access mobile devices such as smartphones or Android phones, laptops, computers, tablets, and iPhones that can be used to access information anytime and anywhere (Gikas & Grant, 2013). Virtual classes using Google Classroom, Google Meet, Zoom, Edmodo, and Schoology services (Enriquez, 2014) and instant messaging applications such as WhatsApp (Adodo, 2016) can be used to support the implementation of the online learning process. Online learning can be done through social media such as Facebook and Instagram (Kumar & Nanda, 2018).

Moreover, students will upload and download many files for safety and convenience. Online learning connects students with learning resources (databases, experts/instructors, libraries) that are physically separated or even far apart but can communicate, interact, or collaborate (directly and indirectly). An online learning process is a form of distance learning that utilizes telecommunications and information technology, such as the Internet (Muhammad, 2020).

DOI: 10.1201/9781003331674-15

15.2   FAST-TRACK EDUCATION POST COVID-19

During the pandemic, online learning was carried out almost worldwide (Goldschmidt, 2020). In other words, in this online learning, all elements of education still are required to facilitate learning so that it remains active without face-to-face interaction. Educators, as the main element in formal education, are encouraged to adapt to the implementation of initially conventional face-to-face methods and switch to online learning (Foo et al., 2021). The problem is not only online learning; another problem is when students have completed their education and face difficulty finding jobs. This happens because the pandemic disrupts industrial operations, so fewer job opportunities exist.

Under normal conditions, the uptake of Vocational High School (SMK) graduates by industry is quite significant because job opportunities are still wide open. However, during an uncertain pandemic, where there are very few job opportunities, recruitment by the industry is significantly reduced. If there are any jobs, the competencies required will be particular for the efficiency and effectiveness of industrial operations.

The Central Bureau of Statistics recorded that the total unemployed as of February 2020 was ±6.88 million. With the open unemployment rate, SMK graduates are still the highest among other education levels, which is 8.49% (Kurniawan et al., 2021). If we talk about the industrial revolution, then the existence of SMK is the front line in welcoming the industrial revolution era we are facing. After the COVID-19 pandemic, the unemployment rate had not decreased even though industrial operations had begun to improve gradually, and there were many reasons for this. One of them could not survive during the pandemic and eventually had to close the company. Therefore, in the post-COVID-19 pandemic, strategic steps or breakthroughs that are still needed must be prepared to increase the workforce's absorption by industry.

The government, through the directorate general of vocational education, has launched a fast-track education program that is intended to link and match formal education (The Republic of Indonesia, 2016), both vocational and higher education, with the business world of the industrial world, as well as increase the absorption of the workforce into the industrial world. This breakthrough and innovative program is called the "Fast-Track Diploma Program in collaboration with SMK and Industry, the Business World, and the World of Work," also known as the "Fast-Track Two Vocational High School Program." This program encourages SMK students to get higher competencies faster through a more practical mechanism (Kemdikbudristek, 2021). To get a Diploma Two (D2), students of the SMK-D2 Fast-Track Program who have been in vocational education for 3 years (including fieldwork practice for 6 months) can freely choose to directly continue 1½ years of education (including 1 year of internship). The fast-track program launched by the government targets SMK graduates who will enter higher education specifically for a D2.

Higher education D2 is the most appropriate to implement a fast-track program that has accommodated the recognition process of past learning and is also free to study on an independent campus, with one of the points being industrial internships. The Ministry of Education, Culture, Research, and Technology stated that the D2 Fast-Track program could reduce unemployment for SMK graduates. Through this program, SMK graduates will be strengthened in terms of technical and non-technical skills that are right on target with the needs of industrial partners.

This program is an option that SMK can implement but is not mandatory. The program carries the spirit of collaboration across education levels. Those involved must have experience developing a link-up system with industry, the business world, and the world of work. Therefore, the initial implementation of this program was started by the SMK-PTV-Industry: 20 PTV, more than 80 vocational high schools, and 35 industries, who are ready to commit to being pioneers in realizing this program. The basic principle is that this program must be based on the real needs of industry and business.

The industry's real needs are competent graduates with a high level of hard skills and soft skills who are mentally ready to work and ready to learn for life. The Fast-Track SMK Program is an integrated vocational and D2 program to increase skilled and superior qualified human resources in a shorter time. The study load of one semester in the D2 program is taken in the last year of SMK, which is equal to five and six semesters.

The total time taken by the SMK and the D2 program is only 4.5 years. The concept of learning for the D2 program is that the total number of credits must be taken (72 credits), of which 12 are obtained when studying at vocational schools, and the remaining 60 are taken for three semesters when taking the D2. The 12 credits taken during this vocational education can be carried out through Recognition of Prior Learning (RPL).

The learning process is designed through a tri-partied collaboration between vocational schools and industry, and the business world, and the world of work. A minimum of one semester during SMK is allocated for the industrial work practice program (industrial internship). Likewise, when in college, to further improve their soft skill and character, students in the eighth and ninth semesters (if calculated from SMK) allocate two semesters for internships at *Dunia Usaha Dunia Industri* (DUDI). With the strengthening of soft skills and character, the hard skills will automatically be honed and mature. The implementation of this program in 2020 is a pilot/test at several universities assigned to implement it. One of them is the Bali State Polytechnic, which opened eight Fast-Track D2 study programs. The fast-track study program adjusts to the work standards of the *Standar Kompetensi Kerja Nasional Indonesia* (SKKNI) and the fields that the industry needs.

15.3   RPL IN EDUCATION PROGRAM

RPL in the education pathway is intended to provide wider opportunities for each individual to pursue education up to higher education. The Ministry of Education issues policies, regulations, guidelines, and standard operating procedures for equivalence assessment related to the implementation of RPL. The program aims to facilitate the community to take formal education at a higher level (Kemdikbudristek, 2021). RPL must also be able to recognize one's past learning achievements without considering the process of increasing one's learning achievements, time, or place.

However, RPL must consider national educational policies such as the obligation to study for 12 years, quality equality, and recognition of nationally recognized learning achievements.

On the other hand, RPL must be accessible to every individual who needs it. Considering that RPL will be different for one field of science and expertise from another, RPL is unique. Thus, RPL can be prepared or developed by considering the educational path (formal, non-formal, informal) and the type of education (vocational education, profession, academic). Therefore, educational institutions need to consider differences in regulations or guidelines for evaluating equality through the RPL scheme (Director General of Vocational Studies, 2022). Recognizing a type of experience or past learning that is not one's own will lead to inefficiency in the educational process. Specifically, RPL in the higher education sector is an acknowledgment or equalization of experience with a student's abilities and or expertise at the previous level of education.

RPL is not the same as recognition of obtaining a degree. In many countries, RPL is used as a consideration for entering an educational program (entry requirement) at a higher level by reducing the number of credits, transferring credits, or releasing some credits for specific courses. A formal educational institution, which the Ministry of Education and Culture declares qualified to conduct RPL, may conduct an RPL assessment process for prospective participants in an education program. Participants of the RPL program must submit a written request and a portfolio prepared under their experience or past Learning Outcomes (LOs) and must be relevant, valid, and recognized evidence by the educational institution that administers the RPL.

A person can use RPL as an acknowledgment to attend formal education at a certain level at a university if the person concerned has obtained a minimum education of the SMA/SMK/C package. Recognition of learning achievements is also carried out in 11 stages, with limited maximum recognition at each level or educational program. This is intended to maintain the quality produced by each level or educational program.

15.4   TYPE A2 RPL ON FAST-TRACK PROGRAM

RPL is one of the educational programs organized by the Ministry of Education. In more detail, the Type A2 RPL program is an acknowledgment of a person's LOs obtained through formal, non-formal, and informal education and work experience in formal education. Thus, all forms of learning achievement outside formal education are recognized. If learning achievement has only been recognized as experience, then the existence of the RPL program is considered a learning experience in formal education.

RPL Type A2 stages of non-formal and informal education, and work experience (Minimum B Accredited Higher Education) are as follows:

a. The applicant consults with the RPL team on the procedures to be followed. The RPL team assists applicants in identifying study program options, which will enable them to find courses that match the LOs they have gained from non-formal and informal education, and work experience.

b. Prepare evidence: The applicant prepares valid, credible, and relevant documents as evidence of the applicant's ability/competence. Collecting evidence generally takes a long time and must be considered by the applicant.

c. Applying for transfer of credit: The applicant fills out the application form provided by the university, accompanied by the collection of supporting evidence, to the Higher Education RPL team.

d. Evaluating the proposal file: The RPL team appoints an RPL assessor from the study program with expertise in the field proposed by the applicant to conduct an evaluation. If the applicant does not meet the requirements in the process of evaluating credit transfer, the process is terminated.

e. Issuing a credit transfer decision letter: RPL assessor sending the results of the credit transfer evaluation, complete with a list of courses and the number of credits obtained by the applicant, to the RPL team as the basis for issuing a credit transfer decision letter issued by an authorized official, at least at the dean level.

15.5   RPL ON D2 FAST-TRACK BALI STATE POLYTECHNIC

In 2022 the Bali State Polytechnic opened a Fast-Track two Diploma Study Program. The two fast-track diploma study programs opened by Politeknik Negeri Bali (PNB) include eight study programs. The D2 Fast-Track Computer Network Administration is among the eight study programs opened. All fast-track study programs with mechanisms for new student admissions use the RPL system, which uses Type A2. The development of this application will later be applied to the D2 Fast-Track Computer Network Administration study program that PNB has opened. Admission of prospective new students for the fast-track study program will be carried out before the new academic year 2022/2023. Prospective students are graduates of SMK partners who have made an Memorandum of Understanding (MoU) with each study program. In the process of selecting prospective students for the fast-track study program, there are obstacles in the current conditions:

i. **Location of High School Partners**
Each fast-track study program opened by PNB already has a high school partner, and the locations of the high school partners are spread across different districts. So it takes time in the selection process for each student from the high school partner.

ii. **Selection Process**
In its implementation, the Type A2 RPL mechanism is still carried out manually and conventionally for each prospective student. This mechanism requires a complicated administrative process and a large amount of funding because it is carried out directly with the respective high school partners by involving the RPL team, assessors, and the school admin.

iii. **No System At All**

Since the RPL scheme was launched, there has been no system to carry out the RPL implementation process directly. Including an online and integrated system to facilitate the implementation of the RPL process will improve the process of implementing RPL for high school partner students. Now it is carried out conventionally and requires quite a long time with partner locations spread across various districts in Bali. PNB does not yet have a Web-based online selection system or Computer Assisted Test (CAT) for the fast-track program.

15.6 REPOSITORY SYSTEM AND RPL ASSESSMENT FAST-TRACK PROGRAM DESIGN

Based on the problems faced in the selection process for prospective students with the Type A2 RPL scheme, a new system design is made, as shown in Figure 15.1.

Translating the RPL system schematic:

1. Translating the RPL System Mechanism: This stage is the process of translating the Type A2 RPL scheme mechanism into a procedure that will be the basis for the stages of implementing the RPL process.
2. Mapping RPL Needs for Prospective Vocational Partner Students: At this stage, the mapping of RPL needs is done for each SMK partner student who will later become a prospective student. This mapping is necessary because each SMK partner has different characteristics, so it is expected to be able to accommodate each SMK partner's needs and readiness.
3. Building a System Per Module According to RPL Needs: In this stage, the divisional system for the RPL scheme is developed. The RPL procedure has many stages that must be passed until the desired final result is reached; therefore, it is crucial to building a divisional system to minimize missed procedures to be implemented.
4. System Integration Becomes for RPL System: After the development of the divisional system is carried out, each module is integrated so that the

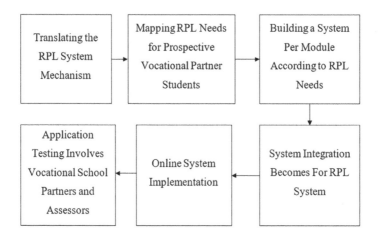

FIGURE 15.1 System design schematic.

system can be used as a whole from the RPL application process until the RPL selection results are issued.

5. Online System Implementation: After integrating each part of the system, the next step is to implement an online application to be accessed from anywhere and anytime. An online system that can be accessed will facilitate the RPL process carried out by prospective students and RPL managers at the organizing college.
6. Application testing involves vocational school partners and assessors.

After implementing the online system, testing will be carried out, including the RPL application process by prospective students, then self-assessment, to the assessment of files conducted by the assessor team. The process of testing this system involves SMK partners, prospective students themselves, and the assessor team. Details of the RPL system design are explained in Figure 15.2.

The detailed mechanism for the system is as follows:

1. The super admin is the head of the Fast-Track D2 Study Program, and he will create an account for the admin of the SMK partner school and the assessor. The number of accounts for school operators depends on the number of SMK partners who work jointly with the D2 study program. Meanwhile, the assessors make up the assessment team according to the assessment team's decree made by the head of the D2 study program. Super admin also plays a role in inputting course names, which are the results of the RPL process assessment. The number of courses resulting from the RPL may vary according to the curriculum of each study program.
2. The school admin is the operator of the SMK and is in charge of creating a default account for SMK students interested in D2 and following the RPL process. Students who have obtained an account then complete their data (biodata).
3. The following process for vocational students is to conduct an independent assessment. Self-assessment is an assessment filled in independently to assess one's readiness for one's competencies.
4. The completeness of the self-assessment is uploading competency files such as competency certificates.
5. If SMK or prospective students have done points 3, 4, and 5, then the appraisal assessor will get a notification. The assessor will provide an assessment and provide recommendations.
6. If the recommendation for the value of the prospective student is still lacking, the assessor can give a test or remediate until the score meets the requirements.
7. Each prospective student will receive notification of the results of the RPL assessment by the appraisal assessor. Those who do not meet the requirements must conduct an RPL supporting assessment. After the RPL supporting assessment has been completed and the results meet the requirements, then assessment of the RPL results courses can be carried out.

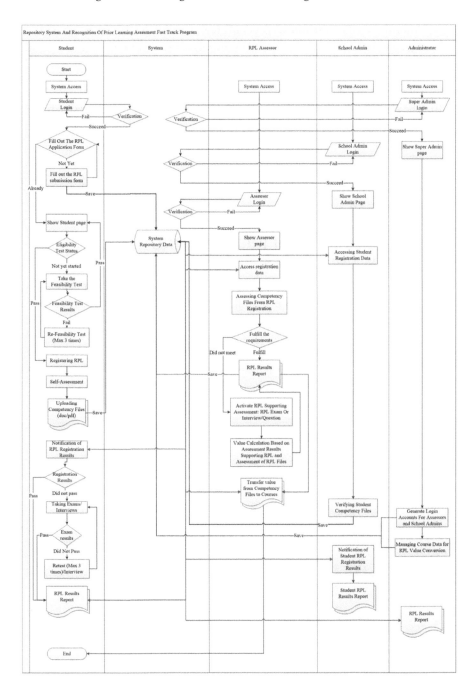

FIGURE 15.2 Flowchart detailing repository system and assessment RPL.

8. After the course assessment is completed, the assessor will print an RPL report to be submitted to the head of the D2 Study Program.
9. The school operator also gets a notification and can print a report on the results of their respective school's RPL, including notifications that will be sent to the prospective student's account.
10. The results of the RPL is printed and submitted to the head of the respective study programs. The task of the head of the study program is to re-verify the results of the RPL. It remains to be submitted to the head of higher education if appropriate.
11. The results of this RPL report can also be in the form of a decree, which the director of PNB will later sign as a decision letter on the results of the RPL for prospective students.

15.7   IMPLEMENTATION OF PRIOR LEARNING SYSTEM APPLICATIONS

RPL applicants can access the website page at https://rplpnb.id/. For RPL applicants, please register first to be able to use the system. Applicants prepare all files so that the RPL process can be carried out. Applicants can continue the RPL process according to the instructions from the system. The system display is shown in Figure 15.3.

Figure 15.3 shows the front page of the RPL system. This system is made only for RPL applicants, heads of study programs, assessors, and assessment teams from SMKs. Each entity has access rights according to its function. After the prospective

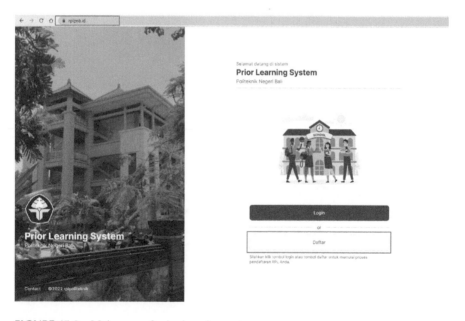

FIGURE 15.3   Main page of prior learning system.

student registers, they will be verified by the assessor team to continue carrying out the next RPL process, such as the independent assessment process and uploading files for RPL assessment. After completing the assessment process, each prospective student will receive notification of the results of the RPL and the results of the RPL used in issuing a decision letter on the RPL results of the D2 fast-track program.

Based on the previous description, it can be concluded that the system was made to make it easier for users to carry out the RPL process without having to come to the location of each SMK. The online system can be accessed anytime and anywhere without being limited by place and time. In the COVID-19 condition, the RPL system that was built greatly assisted the competency assessment process for prospective D2 *Asesor Jaminan Kualitas* (AJK) students by eliminating the face-to-face process. This can help to prevent transmission for prospective students who were sick or indicated that they had contracted COVID-19.

Then the RPL assessment process is carried out by the assessment team, which is determined by the organizing study program and can be added or removed by the system admin, namely the head of the Fast-Track D2 Study Program. The process of verifying and authenticating the RPL file collaborates with the SMK because the files submitted were as long as they were SMK students. In the end, the output of the RPL results can be used as an attachment in making the SK results of the RPL to be announced by the academic section of the tertiary institution.

For suggestions for future system development, registration facilities and at the same time a selection system can be added for prospective students of the D2 Fast-Track study program. Also suggested is the addition of an assessment system by field lecturers from industry for industrial internship courses, which will be carried out by students in the next second and third semesters.

REFERENCES

Adodo, S. O. (2016). Effect of Mind-Mapping as a Self-Regulated Learning Strategy on Students' Achievement in Basic Science and Technology. *Mediterranean Journal of Social Sciences*, *4*(6), 30–41.

Basilaia, G. (2020). Replacing the Classic Learning Form at Universities as an Immediate Response to the COVID-19 Virus Infection in Georgia. *International Journal for Research in Applied Science and Engineering Technology*, *8*(3), 101–108. https://doi.org/10.22214/ijraset.2020.3021

Director General of Vocational Studies. (2022). Regulation of the Director General of Vocational Studies number 18 of 2022 concerning Guidelines for Implementing Recognition of Past Learning in Vocational Higher Education. Jakarta

Government Policy Briefs (2020). Circular of the Ministry of Education, Culture, Research, and Technology Number 4 of 2020. 2020. Implementation of Education During Coronavirus Disease (COVID-19) Emergency.

Enriquez, M. A. S. (2014). Students' Perceptions on the Effectiveness of the Use of Edmodo as a Supplementary Tool for Learning. DLSU Research Congress, *2*(6), 1–6.

Foo, C., Cheung, B., & Chu, K. (2021). A Comparative Study Regarding Distance Learning and the Conventional Face-to-Face Approach Conducted Problem-Based Learning Tutorial During the COVID-19 Pandemic. *BMC Medical Education*, *21*(141). https://doi.org/10.1186/s12909-021-02575-1

Gikas, J., & Grant, M. M. (2013). Mobile Computing Devices in Higher Education: Student Perspectives on Learning With Cellphones, Smartphones & Social Media. *Internet and Higher Education*, 19, 18–26. http://dx.doi.org/10.1016/j.iheduc.2013.06.002

Goldschmidt, K. (2020). The COVID-19 Pandemic: Technology Use to Support the Wellbeing of Children. *Journal of Pediatric Nursing, 53*:88–90.

Haleema, A., Javaida, M., Qadri, M. A., & Suman, R. (2022). Understanding the Role of Digital Technologies in Education: A Review. *Journal Sustainable Operations and Computers*, 3(2022), 275–285. http://dx.doi.org/10.1016/j.susoc.2022.05.004

Kemdikbudristek. (2021). Regulation of the Minister of Education, Culture, Research, and Technology of the Republic of Indonesia Number 41 of 2021 concerning Recognition of Past Learning. Jakarta.

Kumar, V., & Nanda, P. (2018). Social Media in Higher Education. *International Journal of Information and Communication Technology Education*, *15*(1), 12. https://doi.org/10.4018/ijicte.2019010107

Kurniawan, R., Jaedun, A., Mutohhari, F., & Kusuma, W. M. (2021). The Absorption of Vocational Education Graduates in The Automotive Sector in The Industrial World. Journal of Education Technology, 5(3). https://doi.org/10.23887/jet.v5i3.35365

Muhammad, N. A. K. (2020). The role of digital technology in sustaining online learning during the pandemic Covid19. *UHAMKA International Conference on ELT and CALL (UICELL) 2020*, Jakarta, Indonesia

The Republic of Indonesia. (2016). President Instruction Number 9. Year 2016 on Revitalization of Vocational Education to Improve Quality and Human Resource Competitiveness. The Republic of Indonesia.

16 Student Satisfaction with Distance Learning During Pandemic Era Using Machine Learning Methods

Erry Fuadillah and Lala Septem Riza
Universitas Pendidikan Indonesia
Bandung Indonesia

16.1 INTRODUCTION

The COVID-19 pandemic had impacted all sectors, one of which is education. The COVID-19 pandemic had driven everyone to learn how to adapt all the various activities in stopping the spread of COVID-19. This outbreak forced the government to close schools and encourage Distance learning (DL) (online) from home (Wijayanti & Fauziah, 2020). Diverse ways ensure that learning activities continue even n the absence of ace-to-face sessions.

Education is essential to continue even in a pandemic. To keep everyone from getting infected with COVID-19, the Indonesian government made a policy through Circular Number 4 of 2020 concerning the Implementation of Education Policies in the Emergency Period of the Spread of COVID-19, namely conducting online learning or DL. It is a learning activity in which students are separated from educators, and learning uses various learning resources through communication technology, information, and other media (Yuangga & Denok, 2020). DL aims to meet educational standards by utilizing information technology by using computers or gadgets that are interconnected between students and teachers as well as between students and lecturers so that through the use of technology, the teaching and learning process can still be carried out correctly (Pakpahan & Fitriani, 2020).

The implementation of DL significantly depends on the use of technology. The implementation of DL was essential during the COVID-19 pandemic to limit outdoor activities and to maintain the transmission of the COVID-19 virus (Wijayanti & Fauziah, 2020). DL provides a different challenge from conventional learning activities. Therefore maintaining the quality of education becomes more complex (Al-Rahmi et al., 2020). Various studies were carried out to maintain the quality of education during the implementation of DL by creating student involvement (Bismala & Manurung, 2021) by conducting a student satisfaction survey implementation of DL (Moh et al., 2020). Student satisfaction can be seen in the success of

DOI: 10.1201/9781003331674-16

students doing DL. Student success becomes the central point in implementing DL because students are encouraged to rely on most of their own abilities during DL.

DL has many advantages, such as increasing the creativity of teachers and students and encouraging teachers and students to continue to use the latest technology related to learning activities. Apart from that, all DL activities also have drawbacks (Wijayanti & Fauziah, 2020). Therefore, it is essential to learn about student satisfaction with DL activities (Sujatha et al., 2021) to indicate academic quality (Al-Rahmi et al., 2020). Understanding student satisfaction helps the teacher when preparing learning materials, media, content, and interactions for students (Bismala & Manurung, 2021) (Muzammil et al., 2020).

There have been many surveys on DL satisfaction in recent years (Kornpitack & Sawmong, 2022), and a survey has been conducted to see the factors influencing student satisfaction and happiness when implementing DL (Baber, 2020). However, surveys have changed from conventional surveys with simple methods to surveys using the latest technology to improve analysis results (Hew et al., 2020). Data analysis is a data processing process that includes examining data, cleaning data, changing data, and making appropriate models so that the process results are defined as the basis for decisions. The analysis has evolved over the years, and data analysis using machine learning methods is a hot topic discussed and continues to be developed all the time.

The application of machine learning in the world of education is often called educational data mining (EDM), which is the process of data processing and information retrieval (Chrisnanto & Abdullah, 2021). Machine learning has many techniques that can be used according to the data analysis required. It can be used to identify learning styles (Rasheed & Wahid, 2021), predict learning success (Altaf et al., 2019; Chrisnanto & Abdullah, 2021), make graduation predictions (Aydoğ, 2019), and analyze student satisfaction (Radhakrishnan & Sujatha, 2021).

Previous research was conducted to analyze student satisfaction data on the results of the DL implementation using the Massive Open Online Course (MOOC) tool (Hew et al., 2020) involving 249 randomly selected students. The study showed that subject teachers, content, assessments, and schedules played an essential role in explaining student satisfaction, whereas subject structure, course, duration, video, interaction, perceived course workload, and perceived difficulty had no significant role. Another study with 91 students utilized the EDM technique and cluttering algorithm (K-Means, K-Medoids) (Chrisnanto & Abdullah, 2021). Furthermore, student satisfaction survey results are classified to determine the average, good, and bad groups (Radhakrishnan & Sujatha, 2021).

In this chapter, data analysis on student satisfaction at all levels of education was carried out by as many as 699 participants from various schools to investigate student satisfaction with DL during the pandemic era at each level of education. Data analysis was carried out using the machine learning method to improve the results.

16.2   RESEARCH METHOD

This section discusses the stage in research that applies data analysis by applying machine learning methods to determine student satisfaction in implementing DL.The research method in this Chapter shown in Figure 16.1.

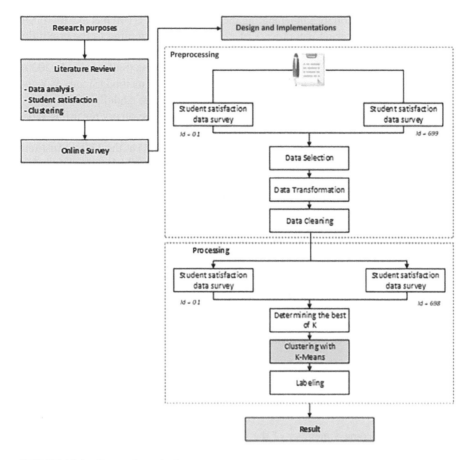

FIGURE 16.1 Research method.

The research method shows the stages carried out systematically, and in this study, five stages were carried out. First, determine the formulation, and research objectives. The formulation in this study is how to analyze data on student satisfaction regarding the implementation of DL by applying machine learning. Researchers feel this research needs to be done to maintain the quality of special education in the conditions of the COVID-19 pandemic. However, data analysis requires skills and abilities, so the application of machine learning methods is essential.

Second, literature studies were conducted to see related research on data analysis, student satisfaction, and clustering. Data analysis in education aims to find information that can positively impact teachers, students, and educational institutions (Altaf et al., 2019). Data analysis is closely related to data mining (Chrisnanto & Abdullah, 2021), and in the education domain, it is called educational data mining (Shrestha & Pokharel, 2019). Student satisfaction in learning shows the quality of existing education (Bismala & Manurung, 2021). Student satisfaction became more challenging to improve during the COVID-19 pandemic, and they tent to be dissatisfied. The learning process is different from the social distancing rules. The implementation of DL is a permanent solution for implementing the learning process (Moh et al., 2020). On the other hand, clustering is a process of grouping data according to the proximity of the characters of each data group. In education, clustering has been widely used to predict graduation, student placement, and student success (Salloum et al., 2020). K-Means is the most widely and commonly used clustering method (Sinaga & Yang, 2020), and has been widely used in education (Chrisnanto & Abdullah, 2021).

The third stage is collecting data by conducting an online survey regarding satisfaction with the implementation of DL. The survey was carried out following a similar study conducted by Sujatha in 2021 (Sujatha et al., 2021) at the Vellore Institute of Technology Periyar Central Library (VIT University) in which the validation of survey questions had been carried out previously.

Fourth, designs and implementation at this stage are divided into two stages, namely the preprocessing and processing stages. The central part of processing at this stage is data clustering using the K-Means clustering method. K-Means is a data analysis method or data mining method that performs an unsupervised learning modeling process (Ashma Nurmeila et al., 2020) and uses methods that group data across various partitions. In simple terms, K-Means measures the average proximity to the cluster's center so that the similarity of members in one cluster is high while the proximity to other clusters is low.

The Euclidian distance formula can be used to calculate the distance of the ith data (x_i) to the center of the k-cluster (c_k), named (d_{ik}) (Sinaga & Yang, 2020).

$$d_{ij} = \sqrt{\sum_{j=1}^{m}\left(x_{ij} - c_{kj}\right)^2} \tag{16.1}$$

Data will become a member of the j-cluster if the distance between the data to the jth cluster center is the smallest value compared with the distance to other cluster centers.

Finally, reports from the study are grouped with students with good, average, and bad clusters. With these groups, it is hoped that schools will know the policies that must be implemented in the DL process.

16.3   RESULTS AND DISCUSSION

This research was conducted to analyze student satisfaction survey data on the implementation of DL. There are 699 respondents from all levels of education in elementary school, junior high school, senior high, and university. The survey consisted of 25 questions previously conducted by (Sujatha et al., 2021) to determine the satisfaction of implementing DL at VIT University. The distance learning data can be seen in Table 16.1.

Preprocessing is the stage before processing data so that the data are ready for use. The first stage, data selection, is the stage for selecting the attributes to match what is needed. At this stage, the attributes to be deleted are email, name, school origin, and class.

The second stage is data transformation, a step to convert nominal data into numeric data based on the data that has been selected. The K-Means algorithm is

TABLE 16.1

Distance Learning Data

Gender	Home Location	Education Level	...	...	Average Score	Learning Activities	The Success of the DL
Woman	Rural	Bachelor			85.5	Practice	8
Woman	Urban	Student			85.5	Both of them	2
Man	Urban	Student			95.5	Practice	10
Woman	Rural	Student			85.5	Theory	5
Man	Urban	Student			85.5	Both of them	5

TABLE 16.2

Numerical Transformation Distance Learning Data

Gender	Home Location	Education Level	...	...	Average Score	Learning Activities	The Success of the DL
2	1	2			85.5	2	8
2	2	1			85.5	3	2
1	2	1			95.5	2	10
2	1	1			85.5	1	5
1	2	1			85.5	3	5

theoretically better at accepting numerical data (Purnama et al., 2022). The result for numerical transformation distance learning data can be seen in Table 16.2.

Third, data cleaning is a step to clean data outside the range. It is expected that data cleaning can improve the accuracy of data clustering.

The spread of data indicates the existence of data outside the data group, which should be seen in Figure 16.2. The age attribute has 71 years of data. The results of preprocessing produce data that will be used for the primary process and the steps that have been carried out are expected to increase the success of data clustering.

Processing is the main stage in data analysis. Data analysis performs data processing to obtain the expected information. The data analysis process is used as the basis for building knowledge using the clustering method. The clustering method is used to obtain dataset information, which cannot be done manually.

16.3.1 DETERMINATION OF THE NUMBER OF CLUSTERS

Before clustering with the K-Means method, the number of clusters was determined to obtain the most optimal number of clusters. The method used is the *silhouette coefficient* method.

Figure 16.3 shows that the highest cluster values are 2 = 0.38039 and 3 = 0.37853. This shows that the most optimal number of clusters is 2 and 3. In a similar study by Radhakrishnan and Sujatha (2021), the number of selected clusters was 3 for the good, average, and bad.

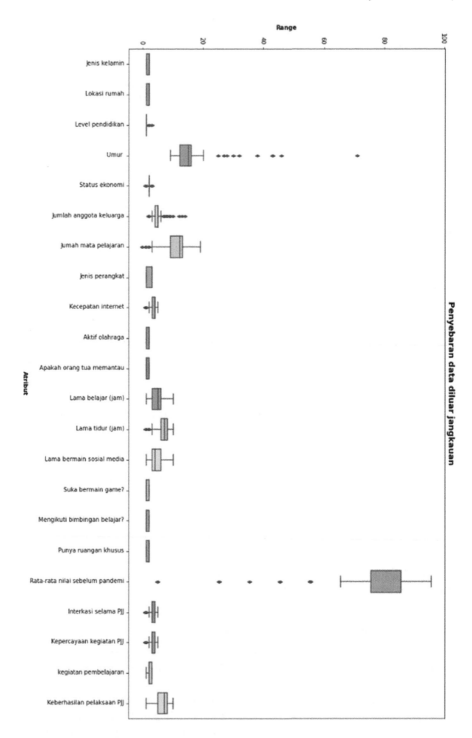

FIGURE 16.2   Data spread.

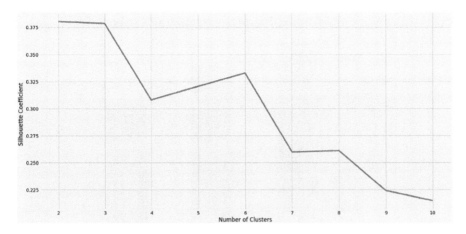

FIGURE 16.3   Silhouette coefficient visual.

16.3.2   K-Means Clustering

After the number of clusters is known, the student satisfaction data is clustered using the K-Means method. This method has several stages, namely determining the number of centroids, determining the initial centroid randomly, looking for the closest distance to each centroid, and doing this continuously until the cluster does not change (Figure 16.4).

The data used includes 698 respondents consisting of elementary school, junior high school, senior high, and university. The data are divided into three clusters:

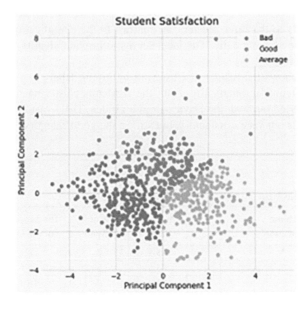

FIGURE 16.4   Student satisfaction data clustering results.

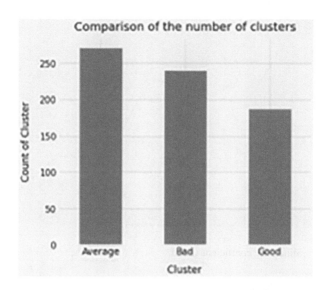

FIGURE 16.5   Comparison of the number of clusters.

good, bad, and average. To facilitate the visualization of clustered data, principal component analysis (PCA) was used (Figure 16.5). The classification results show 271 students are in the average cluster, 187 are exemplary, and 240 feel bad.

16.3.3   LABELING

The clustering process is carried out by applying the K-Means method to student satisfaction data to the three clusters. In contrast to the classification in clustering, labeling is done automatically. The label serves to provide identity to the data that have been processed.

Table 16.3 shows the results of clustering by giving labels to 698 respondents. Labels are assigned automatically using the K-Means clustering method. Further testing was carried out with the Davies-Bouldin index (DBI), resulting in a value of 3.0609, which is not very satisfactory, but still in the good category.

TABLE 16.3
Student Satisfaction Survey Cluster Data

Gender	Home Location	...	...	Average Score	Learning Activities	The Success of the DL	Cluster
2	1			85.5	2	8	Good
2	2			85.5	3	2	Bad
1	2			95.5	2	10	Average
2	1			85.5	1	5	Bad
1	2			85.5	3	5	Bad

TABLE 16.4

Average Features for Each Cluster

N.	Feature	Cluster		
		Bad	Average	Good
1	Gender	1.5750	1.5092	1.6043
2	Home location	1.4667	1.9151	1.2193
3	Education level	1.0000	1.0000	1.0802
4	Age	15.5125	11.9816	17.0267
5	Economic status	2.1708	1.6863	2.2460
6	Number of family members	4.7000	4.6347	4.9626
7	Number of subjects	11.9125	10.6162	10.8289
8	Device type	2.8208	1.7860	2.8449
9	Internet speed	3.2542	4.1218	3.5562
10	Active sports	1.6625	1.4982	1.5668
11	Do parents monitor	1.3458	1.3911	1.1230
12	Study time (hours)	4.3000	5.0886	4.9572
13	Sleep duration (hours)	6.6625	7.1771	7.2193
14	Long time playing social media	5.2208	3.8967	4.4332
15	Like to play games?	1.4333	1.1808	1.6257
16	Following tutoring?	1.6417	1.2804	1.4652
17	Have a special room	1.8500	1.5277	1.5401
18	Average score before the pandemic	77.8708	86.1605	79.2968
19	Interaction during DL	2.4875	3.5646	3.6150
20	Trust DL activities	2.2958	3.6199	3.9144
21	Learning Activities	2.3708	2.2030	2.2941
22	The success of the implementation of DL	4.8583	7.5904	7.9786

The analysis was carried out descriptively to find out more about the results of the student satisfaction survey on the implementation of DL.

Table 16.4 shows the average value for each feature against the bad, average, and good classes. It can be seen that the average score before the pandemic is not a reference that students will be satisfied with the implementation of DL. It is shown that the Average cluster shows a higher average value. Students about 17 years old or entering high school/vocational school are relatively more mature and can maximize DL activities.

Figure 16.6(a–d) shows the comparison for each cluster at each level of education. There are significant differences at the elementary, junior, high school, and university levels. Each level of education has different psychological conditions and is influenced by many factors, such as the equipment used, location of residence, and economic status.

The highest percentage of good clusters occurred at the university education level with a total of 100%. In terms of the highest number of good cluster data, they were at the high school and vocational school education levels, namely 162 respondents (40.7%) as shown in Table 16.5.

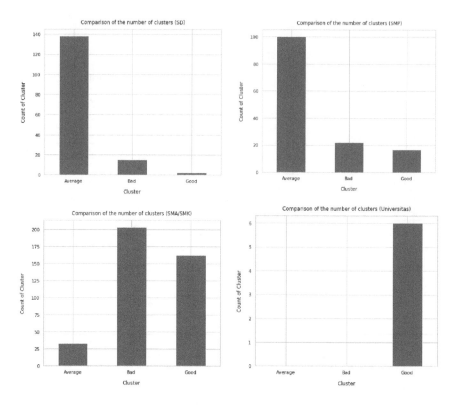

FIGURE 16.6   (a–d) Comparison of the number of clusters (education level).

TABLE 16.5

Percentage and Number of Cluster Data for Each Level

	Percentage				Amount			
Cluster	Elementary School	Junior High School	Senior High School	University	Elementary School	Junior High School	Senior High School	University
Average	89.03	71.94	8.29	0	138	100	33	0
Bad	9.67	15.82	51	0	15	22	203	0
Good	1.29	12.23	40.7	100	2	17	162	6

16.4   CONCLUSION

The COVID-19 pandemic hit every country worldwide and resulted in social activity restrictions. Restrictions on social activities result in the inability to carry out normal school activities. DL activities are a permanent solution for implementing learning activities in schools. However, DL activities have more significant challenges so maintaining the quality of education is a concern in all countries. Maintaining the quality of education requires direct student involvement and can be done by measuring the level of student satisfaction. Analysis of student satisfaction survey data has been successfully carried out by using the K-Means clustering method. The clustering results show that the highest good clusters are at the high school and vocational school education levels, with 162 respondents.

REFERENCES

Al-Rahmi, A. M., Shamsuddin, A., & Alismaiel, O. A. (2020). Unified Theory of Acceptance and Use of Technology (UTAUT) Theory: The Factors Affecting Students' Academic Performance in Higher Education. *Psychology and Education*, *57*(9), 2839–2848. Retrieved from www.psychologyandeducation.net

Altaf, S., Soomro, W., & Rawi, M. I. M. (2019). Student Performance Prediction using Multi-Layers Artificial Neural Networks: A Case Study on Educational Data Mining. *ICISDM 2019: Proceedings of the 2019 3rd International Conference on Information System and Data Mining*, 59–64. https://doi.org/10.1145/3325917.3325919

Ashma Nurmeila, S., Witanti, W., & Sabrina Nurul, P. (2020). Segmentasi Pelanggan Berdasarkan Keluhan dengan Menggunakan K-Means Cluster Analysis Pada PT Infomedia Nusantara. *Prosiding Seminar Nasional Sistem Informasi Dan Teknologi (SISFOTEK)*, 276–280.

Aydoğdu, Ş. (2019). Predicting Student Final Performance Using Artificial Neural Networks in Online Learning Environments. *Education and Information Technologies*, *25*, 1913–1927. https://doi.org/10.1007/s10639-019-10053-x

Baber, H. (2020). Determinants of Students' Perceived Learning Outcome and Satisfaction in Online Learning During the Pandemic of COVID19. *Journal of Education and E-Learning Research*, *7*(3), 285–292. https://doi.org/10.20448/JOURNAL.509.2020.73.285.292

Bismala, L., & Manurung, Y. H. (2021). Student Satisfaction in e-Learning Along the COVID-19 Pandemic With Importance Performance Analysis. *International Journal of Evaluation and Research in Education*, *10*(3), 753–759. https://doi.org/10.11591/ijere.v10i3.21467

Chrisnanto, Y. H., & Abdullah, G. (2021). The Uses of Educational Data Mining in Academic Performance Analysis at Higher Education Institutions (case study at UNJANI), *Matrix*, *11*(1), 26–35. https://doi.org/http://dx.doi.org/10.31940/matrix.v11i1.2330

Hew, K. F., Hu, X., Qiao, C., & Tang, Y. (2020). What Predicts Student Satisfaction With MOOCs: A Gradient Boosting Trees Supervised Machine Learning and Sentiment Analysis Approach. *Computers and Education*, *145*, 103724. https://doi.org/10.1016/j.compedu.2019.103724

Kornpitack, P., & Sawmong, S. (2022). Empirical Analysis of Factors Influencing Student Satisfaction With Online Learning Systems During the COVID-19 Pandemic in Thailand. *Heliyon*, *8*(3), e09183. https://doi.org/10.1016/j.heliyon.2022.e09183

Moh, M., Sutawijaya, A., & Harsasi, M. (2020). Investigating Student Satisfaction in Online Learning: The Role of Student Interaction and Engagement in. Turkish Online Journal of Distance Education, 21(Special Issue, July), 88–96. https://doi.org/10.17718/tojde.770928

Pakpahan, R., & Fitriani, Y. (2020). Analisa Pemanfaatan Teknologi Informasi Dalam Pembelajaran Jarak Jauh Di Tengah Pandemi Virus Corona COVID-19. *Journal of Information System, Applied, Management, Accounting and Research*, *4*(2), 30–36.

Purnama, C., Witanti, W., & Nurul Sabrina, P. (2022). Klasterisasi Penjualan Pakaian untuk Meningkatkan Strategi Penjualan Barang Menggunakan K-Means. *Journal of Information Technology*, *4*(1), 35–38.

Rasheed, F., & Wahid, A. (2021). Learning Style Detection in E-Learning Systems Using Machine Learning Techniques. *Expert Systems With Applications*, *174*(February), 114774. https://doi.org/10.1016/j.eswa.2021.114774

Salloum, S. A., Alshurideh, M., & Shaalan, K. (2020). *Mining in Educational Data: Review and Future Directions Mining in Educational Data: Review and Future Directions.* Springer International Publishing. https://doi.org/10.1007/978-3-030-44289-7

Shrestha, S., & Pokharel, M. (2019). Machine Learning Algorithm in Educational Data. *2019 Artificial Intelligence for Transforming Business and Society (AITB)*, *1*, 1–11. https://doi.org/10.1109/AITB48515.2019.8947443.

Sinaga, K. P., & Yang, M. (2020). Unsupervised K-Means Clustering Algorithm. *IEEE Access*, *8*. https://doi.org/10.1109/ACCESS.2020.2988796

Sujatha, R., Chatterjee, J. M., Jhanjhi, N., & Brohi, S. N. (2021). Performance of Deep Learning vs Machine Learning in Plant Leaf Disease Detection. *Microprocessors and Microsystems*, *80*, 103615. https://doi.org/10.1016/j.micpro.2020.103615

Wijayanti, R. M., & Fauziah, P. Y. (2020). Perspektif dan Peran Orangtua dalam Program PJJ Masa Pandemi COVID-19 di PAUD. *Jurnal Obsesi : Jurnal Pendidikan Anak Usia Dini*, *5*(2), 1304–1312. https://doi.org/10.31004/obsesi.v5i2.768

Yuangga, K. D., & Denok, S. (2020). Pengembangan Media Dan Strategi Pembelajaran Untuk Mengatasi Permasalahan Pembelajaran Jarak Jauh Di Pandemi COVID- 19. *Guru Kita*, *4*(3), 51–58.

17 Food Security Clustering in Indonesia around the COVID-19 Pandemic

Imam Mukhlis, Aji Prasetya Wibawa,
and Agung Winarno
Universitas Negeri Malang
Malang, Indonesia

Özlem Sökmen Gürçam
Iğdir University
Iğdır, Turkey

17.1 INTRODUCTION

A coronavirus (COVID-19) arrived in late 2019 [1]. The virus spread quickly and had no treatment. In March 2020, the World Health Organization (WHO) declared COVID-19 a global pandemic due to its rapid spread [2]. Many parties had tried to battle the pandemic, but the world was unprepared for it. Physical or social distancing helped stop the virus [3]. Schools, factories, and houses of worship were closed. Cooperation required everyone to stay well and at home. Staying home during the COVID-19 pandemic was advised due to stress [4], panic [5], and health concerns [6]. Some countries had protested social distancing orders because not everyone can work under them.

Lockdowns had been ordered in regions with high COVID-19 rates to stop the spread. Wuhan, China, where COVID-19 began, was successfully locked down [7]. Lockdowns were harder for economically weaker and demographically distinct countries, which will risk their economies. Instead, they have leveraged social distancing to slow the virus's transmission. The COVID-19 pandemic had made daily life challenging, especially in lockdown areas. Some experts believed that self-isolation [8], travel prohibitions [9], and social restrictions [10] had risked numerous people's professions due to the COVID-19 pandemic. Panic buying had also affected the food supply [11]. The pandemic hit agriculture and harmed food security in many countries, especially developing ones.

Sustainable development depends mainly on food security. The agricultural sector supports the economy and employs many developing nations [12]. Thus, food security and agriculture sector disruptions will affect these regions significantly. Food sovereignty can help achieve a people-centered nation-building agenda. Thus, food security must be built over time. Food sovereignty and independence are necessary [13], which requires the government to overcome various obstacles. One is national

DOI: 10.1201/9781003331674-17

food supply and demand data discrepancies. Of course, public food consumption expenditure affects food security. The lower the public food consumption expenditure, the higher the food security and well-being of a region. The research maps the area cluster to food security.

In computer science, the mapping process can be done using clustering techniques [14]. Clustering divides a dataset into classes with strong intra-cluster and low inter-cluster similarity. K-means and its variations are among many clustering methods [15–17]. Others use minimal spanning trees, density analysis, spectral analysis, subspace clustering, and other methods [18–23]. K-Means reduces the sum of squared Euclidean distances between each sample point and its nearest grouping center [24]. Kernel K-Means [25] uses kernel functions to find nonlinearly separable structures. The kernel is radial basis function (RBF), polynomial, sigmoid, and gaussian.

This chapter proposes the application of K-Means with kernel modification. The goals of this research are

1. To improve the consistency of the analysis of cluster results using K-Means with the kernel mechanism.
2. To Implement an adaptive K-Means clustering model on various food security datasets from various districts.
3. To build better cluster results, experimental investigations, and validation of the proposed model against the K-Means, K-Means (RBF) kernel, K-Means (polynomial) kernel, K-Means (sigmoid) kernel, and K-Means (sigmoid) kernel Means (gaussian) Kernels.

The chapter is organized as follows: Section 17.1 introduces the background of the research, state of the art, and contribution statements. Section 17.2 presents the method. Section 17.3 contains the experiment's results and discussion. Conclusions and future work are mentioned in Section 17.4.

17.2   METHOD

The food security dataset is from Kediri, Tulungagung, Nganjuk, and Trenggalek in East Java, Indonesia. Figure 17.1 shows the map of the four cities. The datasets were obtained by employing a survey of food security and agriculture. The data period is taken in mid-2022. The dataset contains information on food data consisting of commodities, prices, availability, consumer response, inflation, income, market size, population, and real wages.

One of the most important and commonly utilized strategies in the preprocessing step is feature selection. This strategy decreases the number of features that must be considered when calculating a target class value [26]. Irrelevant characteristics and data overload are frequently missed features. The primary goal of feature selection is to choose the best feature among a group of features [27]. Four of nine attributes are correlated after preprocessing using feature selection. The four attributes are commodities, prices, availability, and consumer response. Table 17.1 shows the dataset that will be used for the following process.

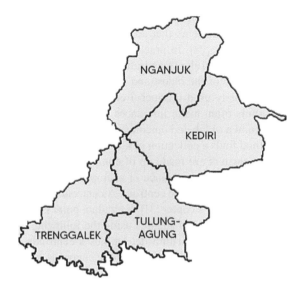

FIGURE 17.1   Research areas.

TABLE 17.1
Kediri Dataset Sample

No.	Commodities	Prices	Availability (ton)	Consumer Response
1	Cooking oil	Rp 19,666/L	123.01	Cheap
2	Soya bean	Rp 14,333/kg	1080	Expensive
3	Chicken eggs	Rp 26,333/kg	48	Expensive
4	Rice	Rp 10,666/kg	94547	Cheap
5	Chicken meat	Rp 37,333/kg	2823.989	Expensive
6	Beef	Rp 106,666/kg	413	Affordable
7	Red onion	Rp 56,666/kg	18271.3	Expensive
8	Garlic	Rp 19,333/kg	277.06	Expensive
9	Flour	Rp 6833/kg	90	Cheap
10	Chili	Rp 76,110/kg	74442.9	Expensive
11	Sugar	Rp 12,666/kg	2234730	Affordable
12	Corn	Rp 6166/kg	92158	Cheap
13	Tomatoes	Rp 5333/kg	8398.8	Affordable
14	Beans	Rp 9333/kg	2526.1	Expensive
15	Cauliflower	Rp 8000/kg	1108.2	Affordable
16	Cassava	Rp 1250/kg	175.957	Cheap
17	Peanuts	Rp 14,000/kg	90.14	Cheap
18	Mung beans	Rp 11,000/kg	60.47	Cheap
19	Potato	Rp 9000/kg	75.77	Cheap
20	Carrot	Rp 20,000/kg	26.59	Expensive

Clustering is a collection of strategies for grouping or clustering data. Clusters are roughly described as data items that are more comparable to each other than data objects in other clusters [28]. In practice, clustering aids in the identification of two data qualities: meaningfulness and utility. There are other clustering algorithms, but K-Means is one of the oldest and most often used. K-Means clustering is a fundamental and widely used unsupervised machine-learning technique [29]. Unsupervised algorithms often make inferences from datasets using input vectors without reference to known or labeled outcomes.

The K-Means method finds a collection of k-clusters and assigns each example to one of them [30]. The clusters are made up of comparable examples. The distance between them determines the resemblance of examples. The "means" in K-Means refers to data averaging or locating the centroid. A centroid is an imagined or actual point that represents the cluster's center [31]. Each data point is assigned to a cluster by minimizing the in-cluster sum of squares using the following objective function Equation (17.1). The K-Means algorithm determines k-centroids and then assigns every data point to the closest cluster by keeping the centroids as small as possible.

$$J = \sum_{j=1}^{k} \sum_{i=1}^{n} \left\| x_i^{(j)} - c_j \right\|^2 \tag{17.1}$$

where J is the objective function, k is the number of clusters, n is the number of cases, $\left\| x_i^{(j)} - c_j \right\|^2$ is distance function, x_i is case i, and c_j is centroid for cluster j.

The K-Means technique in data mining begins with the initial set of randomly picked centroids, which serve as the starting points for each cluster, and then performs iterative (repetitive) computations to optimize the centroids' placements [32]. It stops forming and optimizing clusters after the centroids have stabilized (no change in their values because the clustering was successful) or the specified number of iterations has been reached. The algorithm's core component operates in a two-step procedure known as expectation maximization. Each data point is assigned to its nearest centroid during the expectation stage. The maximizing stage following computes the mean of all the points in each cluster and establishes the new centroid, as explained in the following algorithms.

K-Means algorithm pseudocode

1: Specify the number k of the cluster to assign,
2: Randomly initialize k centroids,
3: **repeat**
4: **expectation:** Assign each point to its closest centroid,
5: **maximization:** Compute the new centroid (mean) of each cluster,
6: **until** The centroid positions do not change,

Kernel K-Means estimates the distance between items and clusters using kernels [33]. K-Means is an exclusive clustering approach, which implies that each item is assigned to one of a set of clusters. Objects in the same cluster are comparable to one another. The distance between them determines the resemblance between the two items. Because of the nature of kernels, one distance must be calculated by adding all cluster members.

In contrast to the K-Means operator, this technique has a quadratic number of samples and does not produce a centroid cluster model. The kernel type is only available in K-Means when the numerical measure parameter is set to "kernel Euclidean distance." Euclidean distance is a square root of the sum of quadratic differences over all attributes as seen in Equation (17.2). This option determines the type of kernel function.

$$Dist_{XY} = \sqrt{\sum_{k=1}^{m} \left(X_{ik} - X_{jk} \right)^2} \tag{17.2}$$

Kernel functions enable the implementation of a model in a higher-dimensional space (feature space) without the need to define a mapping function from the input space to the feature space. The kernel function effectively determines the dot product in higher dimensions by transforming n-dimensional input to m-dimensional data, where m is substantially more than n [34]. The basic principle behind employing kernel is that a linear classifier or regression curve in higher dimensions is transformed into a nonlinear classifier or regression curve in lower dimensions, which is explained as follows [35].

a. Radial Basis Function (RBF)

RBF kernel is a kernel function used in machine learning to find a nonlinear classifier or regression line. The RBF is the most popular kind of kernel function, as it responds locally and infinitely throughout the whole x-axis, The RBF kernel is defined by Equation (17.3) where the kernel gamma parameter specifies γ, the gamma. The kernel's performance is greatly influenced by the variable gamma parameter, which should be carefully tailored to the particular issue.

$$k\left(x_i,\ x_j \right) = \exp\left(-\gamma \| x_i - x_j \|^2 \right) \tag{17.3}$$

b. Polynomial

The polynomial kernel function is a kernel function that is used when the data are not linearly separated. The polynomial kernel is defined by Equation (17.4), where d is the degree of the polynomial and is specified by the kernel degree parameter. Parameter degree (d) serves to find the optimal value in each dataset. The parameter d is the degree of the polynomial kernel function with a default value of $d = 2$. The greater the value of d, the less accuracy of the resulting system will be volatile and less stable; due to the higher the parameter value d, the more curved the resulting hyperplane line.

$$k\left(x_i,\ x_j \right) = \left(x_i,\ x_j + 1 \right)^d \tag{17.4}$$

In machine learning, the kernel polynomial is a function suitable for other kernelizations. It happened because the polynomial kernel represents the similarity of the training sample vectors in the feature space. Polynomial kernels are well suited for problems where all the training data is normalized.

c. Sigmoid

Sigmoid is a hyperbolic tangent sigmoid kernel. When employed as an activation function for artificial neurons, this function is comparable to a two-layer perceptron model of the neural network. The distance is calculated as Equation (17.5), where x^T, y is the inner product of the attribute vector of the two examples, and α and c can be adjusted using the kernel a and kernel c parameters. A typical value for α is $1/N$, where N is the data dimension. Note that not all choices of α and c lead to a valid kernel function.

$$k(x,y) = \tanh(\alpha x^T, y + c) \tag{17.5}$$

d. Gaussian

When data transformation requires no prior knowledge, a gaussian kernel is utilized, where x is the distance from the origin in the horizontal axis, y is the distance from the origin in the vertical axis, and σ is the standard deviation of the gaussian, as in Equation (17.6).

$$k(x,y) = \exp\left(-\frac{\|x - y\|^2}{2\sigma^2}\right) \tag{17.6}$$

17.3   RESULT AND DISCUSSION

From the results of preprocessing, the existing dataset will be clustered using K-Means. The cluster consists of three scenarios based on price, availability, and consumer response to 20 commodities in Table 17.1. Each scenario is divided into three clusters: cluster_0, cluster_1, and cluster_2. The results of each cluster are in Tables 17.2–17.4.

Price clustering resulted in Table 17.2. Prices are expensive (cluster_0), affordable (cluster_1), and low (cluster_2). K-Means has the most diverse price cluster outputs compared with kernel K-Means, as seen in Table 17.2. K-Means places Tulungagung and Nganjuk in the same cluster of expensive commodity prices. It is affordable for Trenggalek. Kediri's commodity prices are low. RBF and polynomial K-Means

---

TABLE 17.2

Clustering by Price

Method	Kediri	Tulungagung	Nganjuk	Trenggalek
K-Means	cluster_2	cluster_0	cluster_0	cluster_1
K-Means (Kernel) RBF	clsuter_0	cluster_1	cluster_1	cluster_0
K-Means (Kernel) Polynomial	clsuter_0	cluster_1	cluster_1	cluster_0
K-Means (Kernel) Sigmoid	clsuter_0	cluster_0	cluster_0	cluster_0
K-Means (Kernel) Gaussian	clsuter_0	cluster_0	cluster_0	cluster_0

TABLE 17.3

Clustering by Availability

Method	Kediri	Tulungagung	Nganjuk	Trenggalek
K-Means	cluster_1	cluster_2	cluster_0	cluster_0
K-Means (Kernel) RBF	clsuter_0	cluster_1	cluster_1	cluster_0
K-Means (Kernel) Polynomial	clsuter_0	cluster_1	cluster_1	cluster_1
K-Means (Kernel) Sigmoid	clsuter_0	cluster_0	cluster_0	cluster_0
K-Means (Kernel) Gaussian	clsuter_0	cluster_0	cluster_0	cluster_0

TABLE 17.4

Clustering by Consumer Response

Method	Kediri	Tulungagung	Nganjuk	Trenggalek
K-Means	cluster_1	cluster_2	cluster_0	cluster_0
K-Means (Kernel) RBF	clsuter_0	cluster_1	cluster_1	cluster_0
K-Means (Kernel) Polynomial	clsuter_0	cluster_1	cluster_1	cluster_0
K-Means (Kernel) Sigmoid	clsuter_0	cluster_0	cluster_0	cluster_0
K-Means (Kernel) Gaussian	clsuter_0	cluster_1	cluster_1	cluster_0

both produce comparable clustering results. Kediri and Trenggalek are more expensive than Tulungagung and Nganjuk. The K-Means cluster with sigmoid kernel and gaussian has only one cluster, and all districts are located within clusters of expensive commodities. Price-based K-Means with kernels offers more consistent results than K-Means, as shown in Table 17.2. Figure 17.2(a) demonstrates that all commodity-priced neighborhoods are expensive.

Cluster-based availability results are seen in Table 17.3. The availability cluster has small (cluster_0), medium (cluster_1), and many (cluster_2). Table 17.3 demonstrates that K-Means yields more diversified availability cluster results than kernel-based methods. K-Means places Nganjuk and Trenggalek into a small cluster of commodity availability. Kediri has a medium availability of commodities, whereas Tulungagung has many combinations. RBF and polynomial K-Means both produce two clusters. According to RBF, Kediri, and Trenggalek commodities, K-Means kernel cluster is in the small availability cluster, whereas Tulungagung and Nganjuk commodities are in the medium availability cluster. The K-Means cluster with a polynomial kernel reveals that only Kediri is in the small availability cluster, whereas the rest are in the medium availability of commodities cluster.

Regarding commodity availability, all districts belong to a tiny K-Means cluster with sigmoid and gaussian kernels. Table 17.3 demonstrates that K-Means with kernels generates more consistent results than K-Means based on availability. All districts fall into the small category for commodity availability, whereas only Tulungagung falls into the medium category, as in Figure 17.2(b).

Consumer response clusters are produced in Table 17.4. The consumer response cluster includes cheap (cluster_0), affordable (cluster_1), and expensive (cluster_2).

(a)

(b)

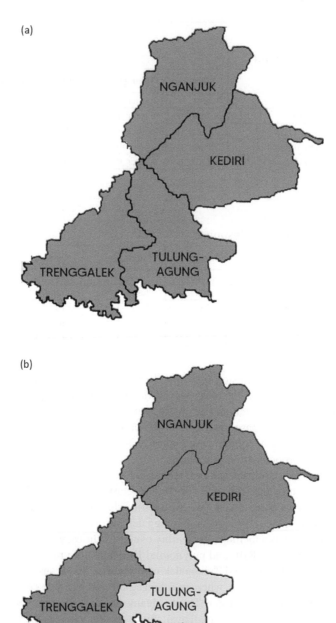

FIGURE 17.2 Clustering area by (a) price, (b) availability, and (c) consumer response. *(Continued)*

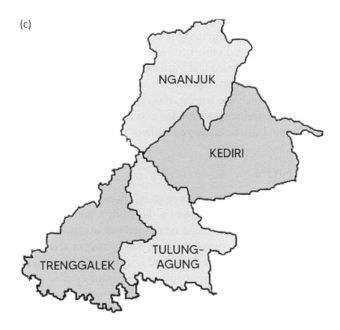

FIGURE 17.2   *(Continued)*

From Table 17.4, K-Means has the most distinct consumer response cluster outcomes than kernel-based K-Means. K-Means clusters Nganjuk and Trenggalek as cheap consumer responses. Consumer response is affordable cluster for Kediri. The expensive consumer response cluster includes Tulungagung. K-Means with kernel RBF, polynomial, and gaussian cluster similarly. Kediri and Trenggalek are in the cheap consumer response cluster, whereas Tulungagung and Nganjuk are in the affordable cluster. All districts are in a cheap commodity response cluster for the K-Means cluster with sigmoid kernels. Table 17.4 shows that the cluster based on consumer reaction with kernels is more consistent than K-Means. Figure 17.2(c) shows that Kediri and Trenggalek are cheap, whereas Tulungagung and Nganjuk are affordable.

From Figure 17.2, due to insufficient supply, Nganjuk commodity prices are in the pricey cluster. Since it is in an affordable cluster, the neighborhood does not consider this condition to be heavy. Food costs will rise as people's high purchasing power reduces commodity availability. If food prices rise too much, the community will revolt. Kediri's exorbitant food prices match its scarce food supply. The affordable cluster includes people's purchasing power response from these two things. However, the availability of middle-priced goods makes the community's response affordable. High commodity costs do not decrease public response while there is plenty of availability. Food commodity prices place Trenggalek as expensive. On the other hand, Trenggalek is in a cheap food cluster. Low-cost public response is unaffected.

Based on the results, kernel-based K-Means clusters are more consistent than K-Means. The kernel in K-Means clustering may successfully perform unsupervised learning operations from nonlinear data. This kernel function maps data points to higher dimensions. RBF, polynomial, sigmoid, and gaussian cluster findings are similar. RBF and polynomial can do this because they both process nonlinear data well. According to the input data, price and availability variables have nonlinear nominal data values, whereas consumer response attributes have categorical data. Because sigmoid and gaussian kernels are similar, this can happen. The sigmoid kernel, like a two-layer perceptron neural network model, acts as an activation function for gaussian-aligned neurons and can be employed without prior dataset information.

17.4   CONCLUSION

To ensure food security in Kediri, Tulungagung, Nganjuk, and Trenggalek regions during the COVID-19 pandemic, based on the study's findings, one can conclude that applying the K-Means method can be carried out in regional mapping clusters where the case raised is the price, availability, and consumer response to commodities for food needs, which is highly correlated to food security. This conclusion can be reached as a result of the study's findings. According to the research findings, K-Means with the kernel can produce more consistent values than regular K-Means. This is a possibility because the Kernel used in K-Means clustering can effectively perform unsupervised learning operations from several nonlinear datasets. This kernel function also enables the mapping of data points to a new dimension higher in magnitude. A bigger amount of data, namely data from all of the cities and districts in the East Java province or Indonesia, can be used in further study to improve the results that have already been obtained.

REFERENCES

1. S. Muhammad, X. Long, and M. Salman, "COVID-19 pandemic and environmental pollution: A blessing in disguise?" *Sci. Total Environ.*, vol. 728, p. 138820, Aug. 2020, doi: 10.1016/j.scitotenv.2020.138820.
2. R. Djalante *et al.*, "Review and analysis of current responses to COVID-19 in Indonesia: Period of January to March 2020," *Prog. Disaster Sci.*, vol. 6, p. 100091, Apr. 2020, doi: 10.1016/j.pdisas.2020.100091.
3. I. Ahmed, M. Ahmad, C. Rodrigues, G. Jeon, and S. Din, "A deep learning-based social distance monitoring framework for COVID-19," *Sustain. Cities Soc.*, vol. 65, p. 102571, Feb. 2021, doi: 10.1016/j.scs.2020.102571.
4. T. Galanti, G. Guidetti, E. Mazzei, S. Zappalà, and F. Toscano, "Work from home during the COVID-19 outbreak," *J. Occup. Environ. Med.*, vol. 63, no. 7, pp. e426–e432, Apr. 2021, doi: 10.1097/JOM.0000000000002236.
5. J. Yue, X. Zang, Y. Le, and Y. An, "Anxiety, depression and PTSD among children and their parent during 2019 novel coronavirus disease (COVID-19) outbreak in China," *Curr. Psychol*, vol. 41, no. 8, pp. 5723–5730, 2022, doi: 10.1007/s12144-020-01191-4.
6. S. Baradaran Mahdavi, and R. Kelishadi, "Impact of sedentary behavior on bodily pain while staying at home in COVID-19 pandemic and potential preventive strategies," *Asian J. Sports Med.*, vol. 11, no. 2, May 2020, doi: 10.5812/asjsm.103511.
7. K. E. C. Ainslie *et al.*, "Evidence of initial success for China exiting COVID-19 social distancing policy after achieving containment," *Wellcome Open Res.*, vol. 5, p. 81, Oct. 2020, doi: 10.12688/wellcomeopenres.15843.2.

8. J. Li, R. Ghosh, and S. Nachmias, "In a time of COVID-19 pandemic, stay healthy, connected, productive, and learning: Words from the editorial team of HRDI," *Hum. Resour. Dev. Int.*, vol. 23, no. 3, pp. 199–207, 2020, doi: 10.1080/13678868.2020. 1752493.

9. T. Villacé-Molinero, J. J. Fernández-Muñoz, A. Orea-Giner, and L. Fuentes-Moraleda, "Understanding the new post-COVID-19 risk scenario: Outlooks and challenges for a new era of tourism," *Tour. Manag.*, vol. 86, p. 104324, Oct. 2021, doi: 10.1016/j.tourman.2021.104324.

10. M. Hossain, "The effect of the covid-19 on sharing economy activities," *J. Clean. Prod.*, vol. 280, p. 124782, Jan. 2021, doi: 10.1016/j.jclepro.2020.124782.

11. H. H. Wang, and N. Hao, "Panic buying? Food hoarding during the pandemic period with city lockdown," *J. Integr. Agric.*, vol. 19, no. 12, pp. 2916–2925, 2020, doi: 10.1016/S2095-3119(20)63448-7.

12. A. Khan, S. Bibi, A. Lorenzo, J. Lyu, and Z. U. Babar, "Tourism and development in developing economies: A policy implication perspective," *Sustainability*, vol. 12, no. 4, p. 1618, 2020, doi: 10.3390/su12041618.

13. A. García-Sempere, H. Morales, M. Hidalgo, B. G. Ferguson, P. Rosset, and A. Nazar-Beutelspacher, "Food sovereignty in the City?: A methodological proposal for evaluating food sovereignty in urban settings," *Agroecol. Sustain. Food Syst.*, vol. 43, no. 10, pp. 1145–1173, 2019, doi: 10.1080/21683565.2019.1578719.

14. A. Abu Saa, M. Al-Emran, and K. Shaalan, "Factors affecting students' performance in higher education: A systematic review of predictive data mining techniques," *Technol. Knowl. Learn*, vol. 24, no. 4, pp. 567–598, 2019, doi: 10.1007/s10758-019-09408-7.

15. J. Heil, V. Häring, B. Marschner, and B. Stumpe, "Advantages of fuzzy k-means over k-means clustering in the classification of diffuse reflectance soil spectra: A case study with West African soils," *Geoderma*, vol. 337, pp. 11–21, Mar. 2019, doi: 10.1016/j.geoderma.2018.09.004.

16. M. T. Islam, P. Kumar Basak, P. Bhowmik, and M. Khan, "Data Clustering Using Hybrid Genetic Algorithm with k-Means and k-Medoids Algorithms," in *2019 23rd International Computer Science and Engineering Conference (ICSEC)*, Oct. 2019, pp. 123–128, doi: 10.1109/ICSEC47112.2019.8974797.

17. S. Askari, "Fuzzy c-means clustering algorithm for data with unequal cluster sizes and contaminated with noise and outliers: Review and development," *Expert Syst. Appl.*, vol. 165, p. 113856, Mar. 2021, doi: 10.1016/j.eswa.2020.113856.

18. D. Cheng, Q. Zhu, J. Huang, Q. Wu, and L. Yang, "Clustering with local density peaks-based minimum spanning tree," *IEEE Trans. Knowl. Data Eng.*, vol. 33, no. 2, pp. 374–387, 2021, doi: 10.1109/TKDE.2019.2930056.

19. P. C. Pop, "The generalized minimum spanning tree problem: An overview of formulations, solution procedures and latest advances," *Eur. J. Oper. Res.*, vol. 283, no. 1, pp. 1–15, 2020, doi: 10.1016/j.ejor.2019.05.017.

20. P. Bhattacharjee, and P. Mitra, "A survey of density based clustering algorithms," *Front. Comput. Sci.*, vol. 15, no. 1, p. 151308, 2021, doi: 10.1007/s11704-019-9059-3.

21. S. Wang, Q. Li, C. Zhao, X. Zhu, H. Yuan, and T. Dai, "Extreme clustering – A clustering method via density extreme points," *Inf. Sci. (NY).*, vol. 542, pp. 24–39, Jan. 2021, doi: 10.1016/j.ins.2020.06.069.

22. X. Zhu, S. Zhang, W. He, R. Hu, C. Lei, and P. Zhu, "One-step multi-view spectral clustering," *IEEE Trans. Knowl. Data Eng.*, vol. 31, no. 10, pp. 2022–2034, 2019, doi: 10.1109/TKDE.2018.2873378.

23. D. Huang, C.-D. Wang, J.-S. Wu, J.-H. Lai, and C.-K. Kwoh, "Ultra-scalable spectral clustering and ensemble clustering," *IEEE Trans. Knowl. Data Eng*, vol. 32, no. 6, pp. 1212–1226, 2020, doi: 10.1109/TKDE.2019.2903410.

24. C. Yuan, and H. Yang, "Research on K-value selection method of K-Means clustering algorithm," *J – Multidiscip. Sci. J.*, vol. 2, no. 2, pp. 226–235, 2019, doi: 10.3390/j2020016.

25. B. Nguyen, and B. De Baets, "Kernel-based distance metric learning for supervised k-means clustering," *IEEE Trans. Neural Networks Learn. Syst.*, vol. 30, no. 10, pp. 3084–3095, 2019, doi: 10.1109/TNNLS.2018.2890021.

26. M. Rostami, K. Berahmand, E. Nasiri, and S. Forouzandeh, "Review of swarm intelligence-based feature selection methods," *Eng. Appl. Artif. Intell.*, vol. 100, p. 104210, Apr. 2021, doi: 10.1016/j.engappai.2021.104210.

27. V. Bolón-Canedo, and A. Alonso-Betanzos, "Ensembles for feature selection: A review and future trends," *Inf. Fusion*, vol. 52, pp. 1–12, Dec. 2019, doi: 10.1016/j.inffus.2018.11.008.

28. J. Xiong *et al.*, "Enhancing privacy and availability for data clustering in intelligent electrical service of IoT," *IEEE Internet Things J.*, vol. 6, no. 2, pp. 1530–1540, Apr. 2019, doi: 10.1109/JIOT.2018.2842773.

29. K. P. Sinaga, and M.-S. Yang, "Unsupervised k-means clustering algorithm," *IEEE Access*, vol. 8, pp. 80716–80727, 2020, doi: 10.1109/ACCESS.2020.2988796.

30. L. Bai, J. Liang, and F. Cao, "A multiple k-means clustering ensemble algorithm to find nonlinearly separable clusters," *Inf. Fusion*, vol. 61, pp. 36–47, Sep. 2020, doi: 10.1016/j.inffus.2020.03.009.

31. D. Kumalasari, A. B. W. Putra, and A. F. O. Gaffar, "Speech classification using combination virtual center of gravity and k-means clustering based on audio feature extraction," *J. Inform*, vol. 14, no. 2, p. 85, 2020, doi: 10.26555/jifo.v14i2.a17390.

32. S. Manochandar, M. Punniyamoorthy, and R. K. Jeyachitra, "Development of new seed with modified validity measures for k-means clustering," *Comput. Ind. Eng.*, vol. 141, p. 106290, Mar. 2020, doi: 10.1016/j.cie.2020.106290.

33. M. Shutaywi, and N. N. Kachouie, "Silhouette analysis for performance evaluation in machine learning with applications to clustering," *Entropy*, vol. 23, no. 6, p. 759, 2021, doi: 10.3390/e23060759.

34. V. Kutateladze, "The kernel trick for nonlinear factor modeling," *Int. J. Forecast*, vol. 38, no. 1, pp. 165–177, 2022, doi: 10.1016/j.ijforecast.2021.05.002.

35. B. Liu, T. Zhang, Y. Li, Z. Liu, and Z. Zhang, "Kernel probabilistic k-means clustering," *Sensors*, vol. 21, no. 5, p. 1892, 2021, doi: 10.3390/s21051892.

18 Support Vector Machine for Sentiment Analysis of COVID-19 Vaccine

Poetri Lestari Lokapitasari Belluano, Audi Faathirmansyah Mashar, Andi Widya Mufila Gaffar, Abdul Rachman Manga, and Purnawansyah
Universitas Muslim Indonesia
Makassar, Indonesia

18.1 INTRODUCTION: COVID-19 VACCINE SENTIMENT

Social media, such as Twitter, is a popular place to share various positive, negative, and neutral sentiments (Ariwibowo & Indra, 2021). The frequency of monthly usage of social media applications in Indonesia is highest in order from YouTube, followed by WhatsApp, Instagram, Facebook, and Twitter, with a percentage of 63.6% or 108.12 million users (Kemp, 2021). Millions of Twitter comments generate vast amounts of digital information on various topics, including the COVID-19 vaccine (Danang & Jorgi, 2021).

The COVID-19 vaccine was one of the trending topics on Twitter. The vaccine could be acceptable in combating the long-running epidemic, which raises various sentiments, so Twitter is an appropriate place for various sentiments about the topic. Data from social media such as Twitter can be used to conduct sentiment analysis on the COVID-19 vaccine by classifying sentiment into three labels: negative, positive, and neutral.

Many algorithms can be used to analyze sentiment on social media, one of which is a Support Vector Machine (SVM) (Romadoni et al., 2020). The SVM algorithm is widely used in automatic classification, such as text classification, image recognition, medical analysis, or prediction (Susilowati et al., 2015). The SVM method has kernel techniques, including the linear, polynomial, Radial Basis Function (RBF), gaussian, and sigmoid kernel (Aditia et al., 2021). This kernel is related to algorithm efficiency.

This sentiment analysis was intended for group sentiment divided into three classes: positive, negative, and neutral. This chapter compares RBF and the sigmoid kernel for SVM sentiment analysis. The best result could be used for educating people regarding the COVID-19 vaccine.

18.2 METHOD

The research method can be seen in Figure 18.1, which begins with data collection, which is then transferred to a Comma Separated Value (CSV) format file, preprocessing, sentiment labeling, statement weighting, training model creation, and then classified using the SVM method and an evaluation is carried out.

DOI: 10.1201/9781003331674-18

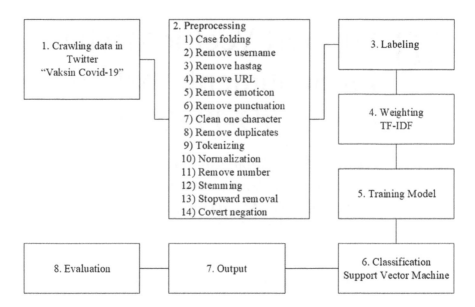

FIGURE 18.1 Research method.

Data was first collected from Twitter with the help of a library twin. Table 18.1 shows data collected using the keyword "Covid Vaccine" with a range of 3800 data stored in *.csv format files, from a period between November 2 and November 7, 2021. Later, the data will be re-selected. The same data and less relevant data will also be removed later. From this data, a total of 1200 data will be selected.

There are several steps involved in the preprocessing process. First, case folding converts all capital to lowercase (Ikasari et al., 2020). Second, remove the username and the user name that begins with the "@" symbol on the sentiment, because it is considered unnecessary (Octavianus et al., 2022). Third, remove hashtags, namely removing only the hashtag or hashtag "#" because it is considered unnecessary. Usually, the topics discussed by Twitter have similar topics marking them

TABLE 18.1

Twitter Data

Tweet
- Kasus covid-19 yang sudah turun dan lengkapnya dosis vaksin bukan berarti kita abai prokes ya, tetap jaga prokes untuk melindungi lingkungan sekitar #AkselerasiVaksinasiPolri Ciptakan Herd Immunity https://t.co/y4MpKfdxeP
- @TedHilbert Dan semua pasiennya akan tetap disebut sebagai korban covid. Padahal korban vaksin! 😖
- WHO Izinkan Penggunaan Covaxin, Vaksin Covid-19 Buatan India https://t.co/QIGVPBms2l Sinovac #JagoOngkirMurah Wattpad Hybe Siti Nurbaya Webtoon Abu Dhabi Kota Jayapura #nctdream #DAY6_OneAndOnly

with hashtags so only the word after the hashtag and not the hashtag is needed (Arenggoasih & Wijayanti, 2020). Fourth, remove the URL often found in an unnecessary sentiment because it is infective and has no meaning (Nursyiah et al., 2021); thus, it needs to be removed.

Fifth, remove emoticons, as they sometimes give rise to ambiguity because they are less specific than words. Sixth, remove punctuation because it is not needed in the sentiment analysis process. Seventh, clean one character, namely by the process of cleaning text. Sometimes there is only one character left, and it is considered meaningless, so it needs to be removed (Pratama & Trilaksono, 2015). Eighth, remove duplicates where Twitter has a retweet, which may cause repeated data (Bugis et al., 2022). Ninth, during tokenizing the sentence will be broken down into various words according to the collection of words that make up the sentence.

Tenth, normalization converts non-standard words into standard words, including words from foreign languages, whereas changing the words is done manually. Eleventh, sometimes numeric characters that are found are not needed, so at this stage the numeric characters will be deleted. Twelfth, stemming is a refinement of the normalization stage carried out previously. The library is Sastrawi Stemmer Factory with 30342 basic sentences. It is considered suitable for perfecting the normalization stages carried out previously. Thirteenth, stopword removal removes words that often appear and have no meaning, such as prepositions, compound words, and others. And finally, convert negation converts negative words into a sentence. The word negation can change the meaning of the sentiment of a sentence so that the word negation will be combined with the following word (Najiyah & Haryanti, 2021). The final result of preprocessing can be seen in Table 18.2.

In this process, labeling is done manually by labeling each sentence based on the sentiment generated based on the data that has been preprocessed previously. The labeling process can be seen in Table 18.3.

At this stage, the weighting is carried out using Term Frequency - Inverse Document Frequency (TF-IDF) with the help of the library sklearn by doing import TfidfVectorizer, which helps convert data into vectors. Data that has gone through the preprocessing stage by cleaning the entire data are still qualitative. In the TF-IDF, the qualitative data will be converted into quantitative data. The following is the result of the calculation from the document, and the example given previously can be seen in Table 18.4.

TABLE 18.2
Result of Preprocessing

Tweet (Convert Negation)
- kasus covid sudah turun lengkap dosis vaksin bukanarti abai protokol sehat iya tetap jaga protokol sehat lindung lingkung akselerasi vaksin polri cipta kawan imun
- semua pasien tetap sebut bagai korban covid padahal korban vaksin
- who izin covaxin vaksin covid buat india sinovac jago ongkos kirim murah wattpad senang siti nurbaya webtoon abu dhabi kota jayapura mimpi nct hari satu hanya

TABLE 18.3

Labeling

Tweet (Labeling)	Sentiment
kasus covid sudah turun lengkap dosis vaksin bukanarti abai protokol sehat iya tetap jaga protokol sehat lindung lingkung akselerasi vaksin polri cipta kawan imun	Positive
semua pasien tetap sebut bagai korban covid padahal korban vaksin	Negative
who izin covaxin vaksin covid buat india sinovac jago ongkos kirim murah wattpad senang siti nurbaya webtoon abu dhabi kota jayapura mimpi nct hari satu hanya	Neutral

The model algorithm SVM with sigmoid kernel and RBF is used. At this stage, the library scikit-learn is used to import the class Support Vector Classifier (SVC), which is a version of SVM for classification.

At the classification stage, the model will then be used, and the test will be classified into various sentiments: positive, negative, or neutral sentiment. Based on this, we can evaluate the performance of the model.

The overall prediction results can be used to evaluate the model by using the confusion matrix and K-fold cross-validation. Based on this, performance can be seen based on precision, recall, F1 score, and the model's accuracy can be evaluated.

TABLE 18.4

TF-IDF

Term	TF-IDF
imun	1.6931471805599454
kawan	1.6931471805599454
cipta	1.6931471805599454
polri	1.6931471805599454
akselerasi	1.6931471805599454
lingkung	1.6931471805599454
lindung	1.6931471805599454
jaga	1.6931471805599454
tetap	1.2876820724517808
iya	1.6931471805599454
sehat	3.386294361119891
protokol	3.386294361119891
abai	1.6931471805599454
bukanarti	1.6931471805599454
vaksin	2.0
dosis	1.6931471805599454
lengkap	1.6931471805599454
turun	1.6931471805599454
sudah	1.6931471805599454
covid	1.0
kasus	1.6931471805599454

18.3   RESULT AND DISCUSSION

With the evaluation of the K-fold cross-validation, data will be divided according to the number of folds used with a balanced proportion of testing. This study used six folds. The following accuracy is obtained from the first to the sixth iteration using the sigmoid kernel and RBF, which can be seen in Table 18.5.

Based on Table 18.6, the RBF kernel obtained an average of 0.8075, while the sigmoid kernel was 0.8075. Visualization of K-fold cross-validation in the form of a line diagram shows that the two kernels achieved the highest accuracy in the second iteration with an accuracy of 0.845 from the sigmoid kernel and an accuracy of 0.875 from the RBF kernel (Figure 18.2).

Evaluation of the model based on the second iteration, which has the highest accuracy, using the confusion matrix can be shown in Figures 18.3 and 18.4.

Based on Table 18.7, the performance of the second iteration RBF kernel with a total of 1200 data on sentiment analysis on the COVID-19 vaccine via Twitter data is shown. The accuracy of RBF kernel is 0.875.

TABLE 18.5

Accuracy

	Accuracy	
Iteration	Sigmoid Kernel	RBF Kernel
1	0.785	0.79
2	0.845	0.875
3	0.825	0.8
4	0.8	0.795
5	0.785	0.78
6	0.8	0.805
Avg	0.8075	0.8075

TABLE 18.6

Second Iteration RBF Kernel Average Calculation

	Positive	Negative	Neutral
Precision	$\frac{55}{55+3+3} = \frac{55}{61} = 0.90$	$\frac{53}{16+53+10} = \frac{53}{79} = 0.67$	$\frac{50}{7+3+50} = \frac{50}{60} = 0.83$
Recall	$\frac{55}{55+16+7} = \frac{55}{78} = 0.70$	$\frac{53}{3+53+3} = \frac{53}{59} = 0.90$	$\frac{50}{3+10+50} = \frac{50}{63} = 0.79$
F1 score	$\frac{2*0,90*0,70}{0,90+0,70} = \frac{1.26}{1.60} = 0.79$	$\frac{2*0,67*0,90}{0,67+0,90} = \frac{1.206}{1.57} = 0.77$	$\frac{2*0,83*0,79}{0,83+0,79} = \frac{1.3114}{1.62} = 0.81$
Accuracy			$\frac{55+53+50}{200} = \frac{158}{200} = 0.875$

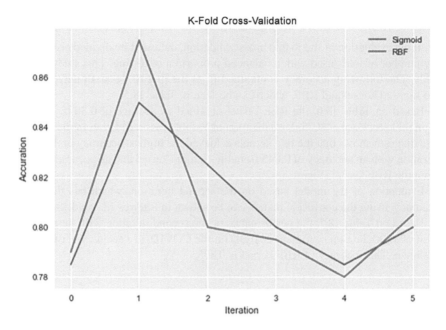

FIGURE 18.2   K-Fold cross validation.

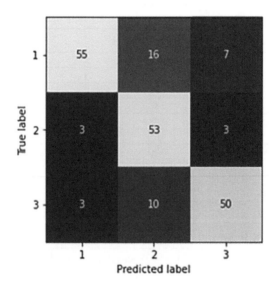

FIGURE 18.3   The second iteration of the confusion matrix RBF kernel.

Based on Table 18.8, the performance of the second iteration sigmoid kernel with a total of 1200 data on sentiment analysis on the COVID-19 vaccine via Twitter data is shown. The accuracy the sigmoid kernel has an accuracy of 0.785, 0.85, 0.825, 0.80, 0.785, 0.80 0.785.

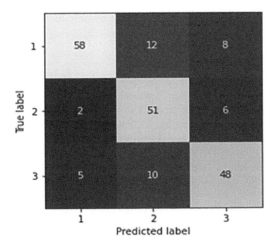

FIGURE 18.4   The second iteration of the confusion matrix sigmoid kernel.

TABLE 18.7
Second Iteration RBF Kernel Performance

	Precision	Recall	F1 Score
Positive	0.90	0.70	0.79
Negative	0.67	0.90	0.77
Neutral	0.83	0.79	0.81
Accuracy			**0.875**

TABLE 18.8
Second Iteration Sigmoid Kernel Performance

	Precision	Recall	F1 Score
Positive	0.89	0.74	0.81
Negative	0.70	0.86	0.77
Neutral	0.77	0.76	0.76
Accuracy			**0.785**

18.4   CONCLUSION

After going through various steps based on the system design that was built, the SVM method comparing the RBF kernel and sigmoid kernel was used to analyze sentiment toward the COVID-19 vaccine. Sentiment analysis was carried out on positive, negative, and neutral sentiment tweets, which have the same accuracy of 0.8075 using the RBF and sigmoid kernels. There was a difference in the second iteration, which is the iteration with the highest accuracy, namely the RBF kernel, which has a better accuracy of 0.009 compared with the sigmoid kernel.

REFERENCES

Aditia, I. I., Latuconsina, R., & Dinimaharawati, A. (2021). Decision Support System for Selection of Workplaces Decision Support System of Internship Workplace Selection for Electrical Engineering Faculty Students of Telkom University. eProceedings of Engineering. Bandung: Telkom University.

Arenggoasih, W., & Raisa, W. C. (2020). Pesan kementerian agama dalam moderasi melalui media sosial instagram. *Jurnalisa*, *06*(1), 160–176.

Ariwibowo, P., & Indra, I. (2021). Detect Trending Topics Related to Covid-19 in Indonesian Tweets Using the Maximum Capturing Method. *SENAMIKA: Student National Seminar on Computer Science and Its Applications*. Jakarta: Pembangunan Nasional Veteran Jakarta University.

Bugis, I. W., Hutagulung, J. E., & Harahap, I. R. (2022). Expert System for Diagnosing Lupus with the Forward Chaining Method Using Web. *Building of Informatics, Technology and Science*. Sumatera Utara.

Kemp, S. (2021). *Digital 2021: the latest insights into the 'state of digital' - We Are Social UK*. Retrieved from We Are Social, (2021).

Kurniawan, D., & Sutan, A. J. (2021). Penggunaan Sosial Media Dalam Menyebarkan Program Vaksinasi Covid-19 Di Indonesia. *Kebijakan Publik*, *12*(1), 27–34.

Najiyah, I., & Haryanti, I. (2021). Sentiment Analysis of Covid-19 Using the Probabilistic Neural Network and Tf-Idf Methods. *Jurnal Responsif: Science and Informatics Research*, *3*(1), 100–111. https://doi.org/10.51977/jti.v3i1.488

Nursyiah, S. Y., Erfina, A., & Warman, C. (2021). New Normal Sentiment Analysis During Covid-19 Using the Naive Bayes Classifier Algorithm. *SISMATIK (Seminar Nasional Sistem Informasi dan Manajemen Informatika)*.

Sari, D. I., Wati, Y. F., & Widiastuti. (2020). Analisis Sentimen Dan Klasifikasi Tweets Berbahasa Indonesia Terhadap Transportasi Umum Mrt Jakarta Menggunakan Naïve Bayes Classifier. *Jurnal Ilmiah Informatika Komputer*, *25*(1), 64–75. https://doi.org/10.35760/ik.2020.v25i1.2427

Octavianus, R. C., Robbi, D., Ervintyana, L., & Toba, H. (2022). Pengembangan Perangkat Microservices untuk Analisis Media Sosial sebagai Pendukung Pelacakan Penyebaran Tuberculosis. *JLK (Jurnal Linguistik Komputasional)*, *5*(1), 24–33.

Pratama, E. E., & Trilaksono, B. R. (2015). Klasifikasi Topik Keluhan Pelanggan Berdasarkan Tweet dengan Menggunakan Penggabungan Feature Hasil Ekstraksi pada Metode Support Vector Machine (SVM). Jurnal Edukasi Dan Penelitian Informatika (JEPIN), 1(2), 53–59. https://doi.org/10.26418/jp.v1i2.11023

Romadoni, F., Umaidah, Y., & Sari, B. N. (2020). Text Mining for Customer Sentiment Analysis of Electronic Money Services Using the Support Vector Machine Algorithm. *SISFOKOM: Information Systems and Computers*. Pangkalpinang: LPPM ISB Atma Luhur University.

Susilowati, E., Sabariah, M. K., & Gazali, A. A. (2015 Implementasi Metode Support Vector Machine untuk Melakukan Klasifikasi Kemacetan Lalu Lintas Pada Twitter. E-Proceeding of Engineering, 2(1), 1478–1484.

19 Seasonal and Trend Forecasting of COVID-19 Cases Using Deep Learning

Agung Bella Putra Utama
Universitas Negeri Malang
Malang, Indonesia

Haviluddin
Universitas Mulawarman
Samarinda, Indonesia

Andri Pranolo
Hohai University,
Nanjing, China and
Universitas Ahmad Dahlan
Yogyakarta, Indonesia

Xiaofeng Zhou and Yingchi Mao
Hohai University
Nanjing, China

19.1 INTRODUCTION

In late 2019, the city of Wuhan in China was the epicenter of an outbreak of a novel virus called COVID-19. The World Health Organization (WHO) declared COVID-19 a pandemic on March 11, 2020, after the virus reached 118,000 cases in over 110 nations within that period [1, 2]. The disease has rapidly expanded across the entire world and is significantly negatively affecting the healthcare systems of many countries, including the United States of America [3], India [4], Brazil [5], France [6], and Germany [7]. The growing demand for medical care causes a significant increase in the number of people seeking treatment, which results in a scarcity of hospital beds and tense circumstances within healthcare facilities. The development of a model and an accurate forecast of the spread of verified COVID-19 cases and deaths is essential to understanding the virus and assisting decision makers in bringing it under control.

Due to the tremendously detrimental COVID-19 effect had on people's health, the pandemic is currently considered one of the most dangerous challenges experienced in the modern world. The impact was observed in susceptible populations, and affected asthmatics [8], the elderly, and persons who suffer from chronic conditions. As a result, it transformed into a problem that requires expertise in multiple fields, including epidemiologists [9], the pharmaceutical business [10], professionals

DOI: 10.1201/9781003331674-19

specializing in modeling diagnosis systems [11], and municipal authorities [12]. This chapter was part of a larger project that models and forecasts COVID-19 time-series data. A significant research challenge had been observed in several different scientific areas worldwide due to the appearance and dissemination of COVID-19. This challenge aimed to halt or contain the increasing spread of this disease. Consequently, numerous time-series modeling, estimating, and forecasting methodologies are presented to comprehend and control this pandemic.

Time-series forecasting is a study involving analyzing time-series data to develop a model that will be used as the basis for forecasting [13]. This model can then be used to make predictions. There are four distinct types of data patterns: horizontal, seasonal, trend, and cyclical. Horizontal patterns are unanticipated and random occurrences, yet the fact that they can exist at all might influence oscillations in time-series data [14]. Variations in the data that occur regularly during a single year, such as quarterly, quarterly, monthly, weekly, or daily, are seasonal patterns [15]. The trend pattern describes the direction the data will take over a more extended period; this tendency can take the form of an increase or a decrease in the data [16]. On the other hand, the cyclical pattern is a variation in the data over more than one year.

One of the most critical challenges encountered in various industries is analyzing time-oriented data and attempting to forecast the future value of a dataset organized as a time series. The foundation for facilitating the use of existing resources in hospitals and improving management techniques to manage infected patients optimally was an accurate forecast of the number of COVID-19 cases. This forecast must be made as soon as possible. In recent years, machine learning and deep learning have emerged as potentially fruitful study subjects for various applications in academic institutions and the private sector. Arun Kumar et al. [17]. compared Recurrent Neural Network (RNN), Gated Recurrent Unit (GRU), Long Short-Term Memory (LSTM), and statistical strategies Autoregressive Integrated Moving Average (ARIMA) and Seasonal Autoregressive Integrated Moving Average (SARIMA) to forecast cumulative confirmed, recovered, and deaths. The best model has the lowest Mean Squared Error (MSE), Root Mean Square Error (RMSE). LSTM and GRU beat statistical ARIMA and SARIMA models with 40 times lower RMSE. Pal et al. [18] predicted active cases using deep learning (Multilayer Perceptron [MLP], Convolutional Neural Network [CNN], LSTM). The MLP model has an MSE of 25401.804 and MAE of 105.945. Zain and Alturki [19] constructed a CNN-LSTM model to predict COVID-19 instances. A suggested model was compared with17 baseline models using test and forecast data (two deep-learning models, two statistical techniques, three linear models, five ensemble learning models, and five machine-learning models). CNN-LSTM had the lowest test and predicted Mean Absolute Percentage Error (MAPE), RMSE, and Relative Root Mean Square Error (RRMSE). The results also imply that CNN and LSTM models made accurate predictions for the COVID-19 time series. Oshinubi et al. [20] used Extreme Machine Learning (ELM), MLP, LSTM, GRU, CNN, and deep neural network (DNN) on time-series data from the start of the epidemic in France, Russia, Turkey, India, the USA, Brazil, and the UK to forecast daily new cases and daily fatalities. These approaches were evaluated using MAPE and RMSE. They converted time (days) to frequency to examine data peaks and periodicity while predicting the pandemic evolution using ELM, MLP, and spectral analysis. MLP had the most daily cases and deaths, according to evaluations.

Continuing with the theme of deep-learning approaches, the purpose of this article is to present a comparative analysis comparing the three most advanced data-based forecasting algorithms in terms of their performance in predicting COVID-19 cases. In essence, to predict the time series of the number of new COVID-19 cases and deaths, three deep-learning models, namely MLP, LSTM, and CNN, are implemented and compared. These models deal with temporal dependencies in time-series data [21], have distribution-free learning models [22], and are flexible in how they model nonlinear features [23]. These are just a few of these models' many intriguing characteristics. The deep-learning model was evaluated using a WHO statistical dataset consisting of COVID-19 patients recorded from the beginning of COVID-19 to August 1, 2022. This dataset is available to the public. The USA, India, Brazil, France, Germany, the UK, Italy, Korea, Russia, Turkey, Spain, and Japan were selected as the 12 nations whose data were analyzed for this study because they had the highest number of cases. This study might contribute to compare the differences between seasonal and trend COVID-19 data forecasting using deep-learning approaches.

In Section 19.2 of this chapter, the methodologies utilized in this research are explained. These methods include a brief explanation of MLP, LSTM, and CNN and how they might be applied to forecasting. The findings are presented in Section 19.3, with a discussion of those results and a comparison of relevant models. The last part, the conclusion, can be found in Section 19.4.

19.2   METHOD

19.2.1   DATASET

This research applied a COVID-19 dataset, which had information from 12 nations that collectively had the most number of cases in the world. The dataset was taken from the public WHO website, which may be accessed and downloaded at https://covid19.who.int/WHO-COVID-19-global-data.csv. The WHO website is also a source of information. Table 19.1 contains information about the 12 nations mentioned previously. The period covered by the analysis begins on January 3, 2020, and ends on August 1, 2022. The procedure is split into two parts: training data, which covers the period from January 3, 2020, to March 25, 2022, and testing data, which covers the period from March 26, 2022, to August 1, 2022. Based on data collected by the WHO, the split began on January 3, 2020, and will end on March 25, 2022, following the WHO's established timeline. According to the findings of this study, the post-pandemic era started on March 26, 2020.

The attributes that make up the dataset are as follows: date reported, country code, country, WHO region, new cases, cumulative cases, new deaths, and cumulative deaths. Within the scope of this investigation, we will be focusing primarily on the following four attributes: new cases, cumulative cases, new deaths, and cumulative deaths. The new cases attribute stores information on the number of new cases that occur each day, the cumulative cases attribute stores the cumulative number of additional cases, the new deaths attribute stores information on the number of deaths

TABLE 19.1

Twelve Countries with the Most COVID-19 Cases

Number	Country	Summary
1	USA	90,213,060
2	India	44,036,275
3	Brazil	33,813,587
4	France	32,881,176
5	Germany	30,903,673
6	UK	23,348,263
7	Italy	21,040,025
8	Korea	19,820,650
9	Russia	18,612,543
10	Turkey	15,889,495
11	Spain	13,226,579
12	Japan	12,749,822

that take place each day, and the cumulative deaths attribute stores information on the total number of deaths that have taken place. Figure 19.1 provides a visual representation of the data utilized in this research.

Figure 19.1 shows that the properties of the dataset used possess varying characteristics of the various forms of time-series data. There are two types of time-series data: the sessional data type for the new cases and new deaths attributes and the trend data type for the cumulative cases and cumulative deaths attributes. The sessional data type for the new cases and deaths attributes is used to record the most recent information.

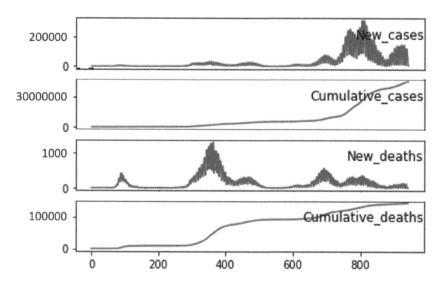

FIGURE 19.1   Dataset visualization.

19.2.2 DATA PREPROCESSING

The quality of the input can be improved by preprocessing, which allows for better performance values to be produced [24]. The normalization of the data was done as part of the preprocessing for this study. The goal of data normalization is to reduce the number of errors that are introduced into the forecasting process [25]. The data are normalized to ensure that the network's output agrees with the applied activation function. The method of normalizing the data employed is called min-max normalization, which involves converting the actual number to a value that falls somewhere in the range of 0 to 1 [26]. The equation for min-max normalization can be found at Equation (19.1) [27].

$$x' = \frac{(x - min_x)}{(max_x - min_x)} \tag{19.1}$$

where x' is the outcome of normalizing the data, x is the data that has to be normalized, min_x is the minimum value of all the data, and max_x is the maximum value of all the data.

19.2.3 FORECASTING PROCESS

This chapter presents a deep-learning framework for the time-series forecasting of the COVID-19 dataset. To forecast daily cases and deaths, three different deep-learning models have been applied. Figure 19.2 illustrates the overall structure of the offered forecasting systems.

From Figure 19.2, the forecasting for COVID-19 has been completed in two primary stages: training and testing. After the raw data have been preprocessed and normalized at the first stage, it is then incorporated into the construction of the deep-learning model. During the training process, the values of the parameters of deep-learning models are chosen to reduce the loss function to its smallest possible value. The Adam optimizer is employed for this particular purpose. After that, in the testing stage, the previously developed models are utilized, together with the chosen parameters, to predict the amount of COVID cases. MAPE and RMSE will check the correctness of the model. This study's primary objective is to investigate the capacity of the deep-learning model's MLP, LSTM and CNN forecast the number of COVID-19 cases according to the time-series data type of each attribute in the dataset. Specifically, this investigation will focus on whether or not these models can accurately predict the number of cases.

19.2.4 MULTILAYER PERCEPTRON (MLP)

The study of artificial neural networks is a fascinating area of investigation. A neural network's most fundamental and fundamentally important functional unit is the model of a single neuron. The term "perceptron" refers to this one neuron in particular. Because of this, the name "multilayer perceptron" indicates a large network produced by connecting many layers, each of which is further composed

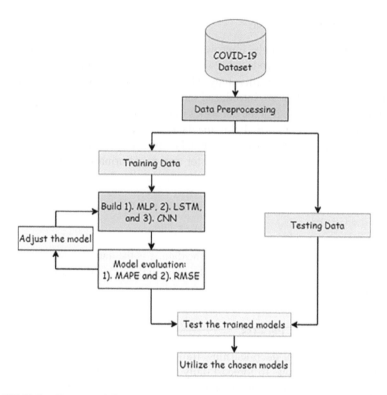

FIGURE 19.2   Conceptual framework of the forecasting methods.

of many perceptrons [28]. These dense layers, which are all fully coupled to one another, perform the transformation that converts a dimensional input into the appropriate one-dimensional output. As can be seen in Figure 19.3, an MLP network consists of at least three layers, which are labeled as input, hidden, and output, respectively.

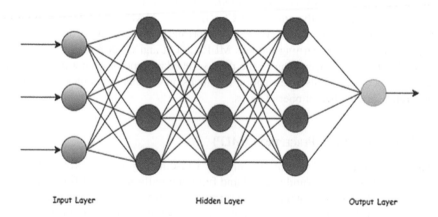

FIGURE 19.3   MLP structure.

From Figure 19.3, these three layers of nodes make up the MLP model's architecture. Each layer has a connection to the nodes that make up the network architecture. The nodes in the input layer are connected to those in the hidden layer. The nodes in the hidden layer are connected directly to the nodes in the output layer. MLP can be broken into parts, including activation functions, learning algorithms, and network design [29]. Each of the nodes that make up the hidden layer has an activation function built into it, which gives the output of these nodes a nonlinear quality. Activation function for an ith in a hidden neuron could be defined as in Equation (19.2).

$$h_i = f(u_i) = f\left(\sum_{k=0}^{K} w_{ki} x_k\right) \tag{19.2}$$

where h_i is a hidden neuron of ith, $f(u_i)$ describes a link function that creates a nonlinear relationship between the visible layers and those that are hidden, w_{ki} denotes $(k,i)^{th}$ input weight in a weight $(K \times N)$ matrix, x_k is Kth indicates an input value, and y_j is j^{ith} output values according to Equation (19.3).

$$y_j = f(u_j') = f\left(\sum_{i=0}^{N} w_{ij}' h_i\right) \tag{19.3}$$

These artificial neural networks reflect the model of our biological brains and how they are utilized to perform challenging computer tasks, such as predictive modeling in machine learning. The objective is to build algorithms and data structures that can aid models in solving complex problems. Neural networks may learn the representation in the training dataset and then relate it to the best form of the output variable. MLP networks may mathematically learn any mapping function related to the universal approximation technique using this philosophy [30]. Due to their ability to handle issues stochastically, MLPs can be applied in research. MLP is a regularly employed forecasting tool in research. MLP characteristics provide a greater predicting value.

19.2.5   LONG SHORT-TERM MEMORY (LSTM)

LSTM is a complex gated memory unit that was developed to solve the vanishing gradient concerns that inhibit the effectiveness of a straightforward RNN [31]. To be more exact, when the important time step is considered, the gradient either becomes excessively tiny or excessively large, which causes an issue known as a vanishing gradient. This issue manifests itself during the training phase. The optimizer backpropagates and causes the method to run, even though the weights seldom ever alter in any way. In its most basic form, LSTM comprises three gates that govern the flow of information, as in Figure 19.4.

From Figure 19.4, these gates are referred to as input, forget, and output gates. In their most fundamental form, these gates are produced only by applying logistic functions to weighted sums; the weights themselves can be derived through backpropagation during the training process [24]. The input gate and the forget gate are

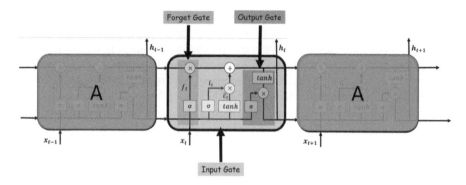

FIGURE 19.4   LSTM cell structure.

responsible for managing the state of the cell. The output can be generated either by
the output gate or by the hidden state, which reflects the memory that is being used
in a certain way. This method enables the network to memorize information for
an extended period of time, something that the traditional single RNN cannot do.
The extended capability of LSTM models to capture long-term dependencies and
the remarkable ability of these models to deal with time-series data are, of course,
two of its most attractive properties. Given the input time series x_t and the number
of hidden units h_t, the gates contain the following equations for forget gates, input
gate, intermediate cell state, cell state, output gate, and hidden state, as shown in
Equations (19.4)–(19.9) [32].

$$f_t = \sigma\left(w_f.[h_{t-1},x_t] + b_f\right) \tag{19.4}$$

$$i_t = \sigma\left(w_i.[h_{t-1},x_t] + b_i\right) \tag{19.5}$$

$$\tilde{c}_t = \tanh\left(w_c.[h_{t-1},x_t] + b_c\right) \tag{19.6}$$

$$c_t = f_t . c_{t-1} + i_t. \tilde{c}_t \tag{19.7}$$

$$o_t = \sigma\left(w_o.[h_{t-1},x_t] + b_o\right) \tag{19.8}$$

$$h_t = o_t . \tanh(c_t) \tag{19.9}$$

with σ and tanh as the activation function; w_f, w_i, w_c, w_o are the weight values;
b_f, b_i, b_c, and b_o are the bias values; h_{t-1} is the previous period input value; and c_{t-1}
is the old state.

19.2.6   CONVOLUTIONAL NEURAL NETWORK (CNN)

CNN is one of the most often employed neural networks in deep learning. Due to
local connectivity and shared weights, the number of parameters that must be trained
has drastically decreased. Unlike other neural network models, such as the MLP,
CNN is designed to accept multiple arrays as input and then process the input using
convolution operators in local areas by imitating how humans perceive [33]. In other

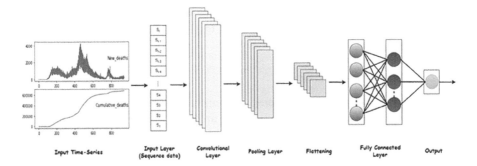

FIGURE 19.5 CNN structure.

words, the CNN seeks to discover the relationship between the input and the output and to include this information in the filter weights. Figure 19.5 demonstrates the CNN architecture.

As depicted in Figure 19.5, a simple CNN model consists of an input layer, a convolutional layer, a pooling layer, a flattening, a fully connected layer, and an output layer [34]. A top-notch CNN is built as a sequence of steps. The initial stages consist of two types of layers: convolutional and pooling. The convolutional and pooling layers play a significant role in CNN models, which are directly influenced by the basic concepts of simple and complicated cells in visual neuroscience. Each convolutional layer consists of numerous convolution filters to extract unique characteristics. The units in a convolutional layer are connected to local patches of the preceding layer by a set of weights; these local weighted sum results are then passed via an activation function, which is a nonlinearity function. There are two typical activation functions. This pair consists of the sigmoid function and the rectified linear unit (ReLU). Both of them can be expressed mathematically using Equations (19.10) and (19.11), respectively [35].

$$\sigma(z) = \frac{1}{1 - e^{-z}} \tag{19.10}$$

$$f(x) = \max(0, x) \tag{19.11}$$

In addition, the pooling layer is primarily utilized to lower the spatial dimension, minimizing the number of calculations required for network training. Two or three stages of convolution, nonlinearity, and pooling are stacked, then more convolutional layers are added. The features finally move through the fully connected layers and reach the output layer.

CNN can perform representation learning and automatically extract features from unprocessed input. With transform invariance, CNN recovers features regardless of how they appear in the data, which is essential for Computer Vision (CV) [36] and Natural Language Processing (NLP) [37]. CNN is also suitable for data analysis due to its efficient feature extraction, especially spatial feature extraction. Considering a succession of observations as image shapes, CNNs are typically employed for classification issues in which the network is trained to classify the observations, but they may also be trained to solve regression problems to be utilized for prediction [38]. In recent years, researchers have used CNN to predict time series accurately and attained high prediction accuracy.

19.2.7 EVALUATION METRICS

For evaluating and comparing different implemented models, we have developed a set of metrics upon which model comparisons are based. It is prudent to compare the model's performance and outcomes to determine which one is superior. The metrics, MAPE and RMSE, were utilized to analyze the forecasting results. The RMSE and MAPE equation looks at Equations (19.12) and (19.13).

$$\text{MAPE} = \frac{1}{N}\sum_{i=1}^{N}\frac{|yi - \widehat{yi}|}{yi} \times 100\% \tag{19.12}$$

$$\text{RMSE} = \sqrt{\frac{1}{N}\sum_{i=1}^{N}(yi - \widehat{yi})^2} \tag{19.13}$$

The MAPE statistic is utilized to display errors indicative of accuracy [39]. RMSE is a tool that can be utilized to identify abnormalities or outliers in the designed prediction system [40]. More accurate predicting results are represented by MAPE and RMSE values closer to 1 and lower. Histograms are going to be used for the next part of our investigation, which will focus on the distribution of forecasting errors.

19.3 RESULTS AND DISCUSSION

Based on the dataset gathered, it is known that the values in each attribute contain time-series data types, along with seasonal and trend types. These types were obtained from the dataset. The forecasting process uses three deep-learning methods: MLP, LSTM, and CNN. Each method's parameters are set to the same value of some parameter derived from the outcomes of random search-based hyperparameter tuning. The purpose of using the same parameter values is to enable comparisons between them. The parameter setting value can be seen in Table 19.2.

TABLE 19.2
Parameter Setting Value

Parameters	MLP	LSTM	CNN
Hidden layer	2	2	2
Unit (Neuron)	64	64	64
Activation function output	Sigmoid	tanh	ReLU
Loss function	MSE	MSE	MSE
Optimizer	Adam	Adam	Adam
Epoch	100	100	100
Batch size	64	64	64
Dropout	0.2	0.2	0.2

In this research, all of these dataset attributes are considered. The goal is to find out how well the deep-learning method can predict based on the data already existing. Tables 19.3 and 19.4 show the forecasting results obtained from the 12 nations that have seen the most significant number of COVID-19 instances.

From Table 19.3, it can be seen that MAPE and RMSE are the types of seasonal data on new cases and new deaths of COVID-19. The MLP method has the best MAPE and RMSE values when processing UK COVID-19 data for both new cases (MAPE 9.93234 and RMSE 0.027376) and new deaths (MAPE 8.60027 and RMSE 0.01829). This is possible due to the fact that the UK's COVID-19 data includes a big and different cumulative number of new cases and new deaths, consistent with one of the benefits of MLP, which can produce accurate forecasts for diverse values. The best results in MLP are different from the other two methods used. In LSTM and CNN, the best MAPE and RMSE are when processing Korean COVID-19 data. In LSTM, the best MAPE and RMSE are generated when processing new death data. The MAPE value of 5.83125 and RMSE of 0.00409 is also the best compared with the MAPE and RMSE of MLP and CNN in new cases and deaths. For CNN, the best MAPE and RMSE values in new cases were 8.54987 and 0.00871, while in new deaths, 7.1419 and 0.01594. This is possible because the data on Korean COVID-19 new cases and new deaths exhibit strong seasonal patterns relative to data from other nations, allowing LSTM and CNN to handle it by producing good values.

According to Table 19.4, MLP and LSTM have good MAPE and RMSE values when processing cumulative cases and cumulative fatalities of COVID-19 in France. The cumulative cases and cumulative fatalities of COVID-19 in France tend to exhibit a nonlinear trend pattern, allowing MLP and LSTM to process and produce a good performance. The optimal MAPE and RMSE MLP for cumulative cases (11.12727 and 0.26167) and fatalities (13.29925 and 0.22861). Similar to seasonal data, the best values for MAPE and RMSE produced by LSTM on cumulative deaths are 11.12454 and 0.12389 in this trend data. Unlike the previous two approaches, processing Korean COVID-19 data yielded the best MAPE and RMSE results for CNN because the data on cumulative cases and cumulative deaths exhibits an upward trending tendency. In cumulative cases, the MAPE was 12.07164, and the RMSE was 0.16649, whereas in cumulative deaths, the MAPE was 12.99613, and the RMSE was 0.16036.

As seen in Figure 19.6, the LSTM has the lowest MAPE value across the board compared with any currently used approach. With a MAPE of 8.02212, LSTM outperforms MLP and CNN when analyzing seasonal data. The MAPE LSTM has a score of 11.20960 in the trend data type, which is higher than the scores achieved by other approaches. From Figure 19.7, the LSTM has the best RMSE across the board for all kinds of data. Compared with the other approaches, the RMSE in the seasonal data belonging to LSTM, which is 0.04841, has the best value. The RMSE produced by the LSTM model is the best in the trend data type, coming in at 0.13224. This figure is lower than the RMSE produced by other models. To put it another way, the RMSE value that LSTM achieves is superior to that of the other methods when applied to all three types of deep-learning data.

According to the results, there was a substantial difference between the MAPE and RMSE results derived from seasonal and trend data types. MAPE and RMSE

TABLE 19.3
Seasonal Data

Country	MLP				LSTM				CNN			
	New Cases		New Deaths		New Cases		New Deaths		New Cases		New Deaths	
	MAPE	RMSE	MAPE	RMSE	MAPE	RMSE	MAPE	RMSE	MAPE	RMSE	MAPE	RMSE
America	10.89307	0.04216	9.98084	0.06035	9.00988	0.04023	9.00302	0.03044	10.27329	0.04432	9.63332	0.04343
India	11.03957	0.08075	10.53226	0.05984	7.16802	0.01313	6.17888	0.05148	8.99909	0.05729	10.54785	0.05912
Brazil	11.43842	0.06661	8.92754	0.05168	9.10144	0.06503	7.19898	0.03773	11.21862	0.06584	8.26811	0.03601
France	10.55344	0.10599	10.05038	0.02171	8.63108	0.09979	9.33978	0.02298	13.20352	0.10013	9.96236	0.02918
Germany	12.80597	0.37783	12.48664	0.03544	8.12163	0.15103	8.43923	0.03806	12.094871	0.15242	10.93915	0.04066
United Kingdom	**9.93234**	**0.02376**	**8.60027**	**0.01829**	7.16509	0.0182	8.62081	0.02581	8.68536	0.02352	10.10707	0.07297
Italy	11.22891	0.1125	10.68542	0.03446	9.41835	0.10331	9.87176	0.0353	10.75517	0.10804	10.09518	0.03585
Korea	13.29673	0.52369	10.04296	0.58924	**5.9295**	**0.00415**	5.83125[1]	0.00409[2]	**8.54987**	**0.00871**	**7.1419**	**0.01594**
Russia	10.41234	0.0368	10.78993	0.04897	7.27899	0.05688	8.0287	0.09183	10.02889	0.01124	9.50368	0.02755
Turkey	11.40883	0.13127	12.80635	0.08907	8.21758	0.13472	6.84598	0.06171	10.19621	0.13758	9.10839	0.06113
Spain	14.3182	0.15023	15.2268	0.11893	9.32365	0.13136	9.58382	0.11306	12.807	0.14867	13.92797	0.12674
Japan	13.51474	0.10768	12.43096	0.14353	8.54655	0.09641	7.32325	0.05939	12.02785	0.13119	12.05099	0.06112

[1] MAPE best results on Seasonal Data.
[2] RMSE best results on Seasonal Data.

TABLE 19.4
Trend Data

Country	MLP				LSTM				CNN			
	Cumulative Cases		Cumulative Deaths		Cumulative Cases		Cumulative Deaths		Cumulative Cases		Cumulative Deaths	
	MAPE	RMSE	MAPE	RMSE	MAPE	RMSE	MAPE	RMSE	MAPE	RMSE	MAPE	RMSE
America	14.36209	0.26676	14.28944	0.25388	11.18382	0.12701	11.14462	0.13471	13.59837	0.27182	13.89936	0.26929
India	14.53234	0.29475	14.30747	0.25791	11.21824	0.13917	11.20732	0.12822	13.68303	0.24758	13.71795	0.25461
Brazil	14.80594	0.1305	14.14847	0.23997	11.21372	0.13841	11.21165	0.14039	13.73982	0.23961	13.53819	0.23135
France	**11.12727**	**0.26167**	**13.29925**	**0.22861**	**11.12454**	**0.11151**	**11.03899**[1]	**0.12389**[2]	13.28743	0.17981	13.64664	0.22707
Germany	14.41686	0.1646	14.2518	0.24812	11.26642	0.13661	11.20403	0.14946	13.80545	0.22696	13.07289	0.17205
United Kingdom	14.3767	0.26834	14.38706	0.27147	11.32475	0.13397	11.18218	0.12907	13.71775	0.24467	13.87212	0.26191
Italy	14.56554	0.2942	14.18993	0.23714	11.25348	0.15846	11.35489	0.13688	13.24861	0.21427	13.18879	0.18509
Korea	14.20165	0.41215	14.20423	0.37667	11.19348	0.15928	11.31906	0.13703	**12.07164**	**0.16649**	**12.99613**	**0.16036**
Russia	14.68113	0.11783	14.3238	0.26066	11.17062	0.14906	11.26263	0.13264	13.50101	0.2268	13.01716	0.16699
Turkey	14.55654	0.29604	14.28608	0.25393	11.18228	0.12386	11.12698	0.135	13.62652	0.23393	13.07075	0.1755
Spain	14.33361	0.27486	14.20613	0.24082	11.15891	0.13811	11.20762	0.13006	13.36072	0.20035	13.1073	0.17601
Japan	14.90283	0.1181	14.67326	0.11236	11.5282	0.14126	11.25524	0.10957	13.64923	0.17181	13.54804	0.22017

[1] MAPE best results on Trend Data.
[2] RMSE best results on Trend Data.

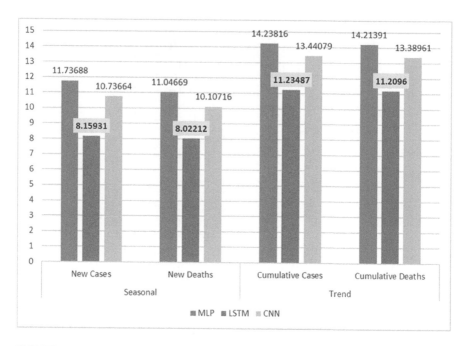

FIGURE 19.6   Average MAPE in all data types.

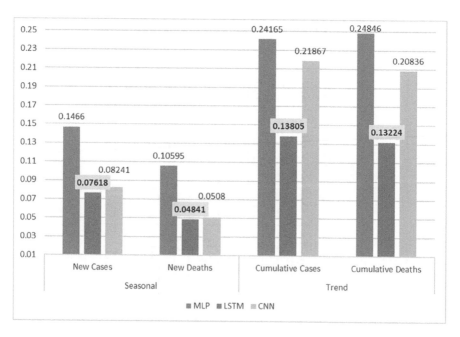

FIGURE 19.7   Average RMSE in all data types.

values derived from seasonal data are superior to trend data types using all known algorithms. These outcomes are possible because the current approaches in deep learning are the product of constructing a neural network, which has the benefit of processing nonlinear input. One of these nonlinear data types is seasonal data because seasonal data exhibits a periodic fluctuation pattern. On the other hand, trend data does not have a pattern of oscillations because it tends to data direction, which might take the form of an increasing or decreasing linear trend. Typically, machine-learning forecasting algorithms such as linear regression and ARIMA can be used for linear data types.

From the overall results, it is known that LSTM has better performance in seasonal data compared with CNN and MLP. This can happen because of the advantages of LSTM, which has memory and can store the previous time step information for learning compared with CNN and MLP. CNN also has a reasonably good value when compared with MLP because CNN can detect important features automatically and can model nonlinear data. MLP has poor results because each data is processed alternately with other data in this study. After all, it has interdependence between data so that it is under the shortcomings of MLP, which cannot be used for sequential data modeling, causing the resulting MAPE and RMSE to be less good.

Finally, the deep-learning method is unsuitable for long-term and high-density trend data types. Even though those data are normalized, the model sensitivity cannot sense the time-series fluctuations properly. As a result, the MAPE and RMSE of those data are higher than the seasonal data. For future performance, a mechanism to improve the forecasting sensitivity to data trends with deep learning is required.

19.4 CONCLUSION

The effectiveness of the deep-learning MLP, LSTM, and CNN was evaluated compared with the 12 countries worldwide with the highest number of COVID-19 cases. In seasonal and trend data, the LSTM deep-learning method's performance was superior to all other methods. On the other hand, compared with other trend data types, the MAPE and RMSE for deep learning using seasonal data are pretty good. The outcome of the deep-learning experiment for the COVID-19 forecasts motivated extending this study and covering trend data time series utilizing the innovative model produced for subsequent research. Even though the deep-learning model was more accurate regarding the COVID-19 seasonal data, this model still has room for additional development. An optimizer for the data trend parameter is required for a deep-learning system to function correctly. Consequently, future research may offer hybrid deep learning and an optimized method to enhance the generalization and prediction performance of the model, such as DNN. Further, adding more data and external factors to the COVID-19 datasets, such as changes in season, vaccination plans, additional lockdowns, another resampling, and restructuring forecasting methods, will be used to improve the accuracy of the COVID-19 forecasting system.

REFERENCES

1. Y. Kanipakam, V. Nagaraja, B. M. Gandla, and S. D. Arumugam, "A review on COVID-19 outbreak: An unprecedented threat to the globe," *J. Sci. Dent.*, vol. 11, no. 1, pp. 37–41, 2021, doi: 10.5005/jp-journals-10083-0942.

2. P. Holloway, R. Bergeron, and L. E. Connealy, and C. Fetters, "Viral pandemic: A review of integrative medicine treatment considerations," *Proceedings of ACIM Research.*, vol. 2, no. 2, pp. 1–14, 2020.

3. E. Bojdani *et al.*, "COVID-19 pandemic: Impact on psychiatric care in the United States," *Psychiatry Res.*, vol. 289, p. 113069, Jul. 2020, doi: 10.1016/j.psychres.2020.113069.

4. D. Roy, S. Tripathy, S. K. Kar, N. Sharma, S. K. Verma, and V. Kaushal, "Study of knowledge, attitude, anxiety & Perceived mental healthcare need in Indian population during COVID-19 pandemic," *Asian J. Psychiatr.*, vol. 51, p. 102083, Jun. 2020, doi: 10.1016/j.ajp.2020.102083.

5. R. Rocha *et al.*, "Effect of socioeconomic inequalities and vulnerabilities on health-system preparedness and response to COVID-19 in Brazil: A comprehensive analysis," *Lancet Glob. Heal.*, vol. 9, no. 6, pp. e782–e792, Jun. 2021, doi: 10.1016/S2214-109X(21)00081-4.

6. A. Chevance *et al.*, "Ensuring mental health care during the SARS-CoV-2 epidemic in France: A narrative review," *Encephale.*, vol. 46, no. 3, pp. 193–201, Jun. 2020, doi: 10.1016/j.encep.2020.04.005.

7. A. Bäuerle *et al.*, "Increased generalized anxiety, depression and distress during the COVID-19 pandemic: A cross-sectional study in Germany," *J. Public Health (Bangkok).*, vol. 42, no. 4, pp. 672–678, Nov. 2020, doi: 10.1093/pubmed/fdaa106.

8. Y. Gao *et al.*, "Risk factors for severe and critically ill COVID-19 patients: A review," *Allergy*, vol. 76, no. 2, pp. 428–455, Feb. 2021, doi: 10.1111/all.14657.

9. E. J. Murray, "Epidemiology's time of need: COVID-19 calls for epidemic-related economics," *J. Econ. Perspect.*, vol. 34, no. 4, pp. 105–120, 2020, doi: 10.1257/jep.34.4.105.

10. N. Bragazzi, M. Mansour, A. Bonsignore, and R. Ciliberti, "The role of Hospital and community pharmacists in the management of COVID-19: Towards an expanded definition of the roles, responsibilities, and duties of the pharmacist," *Pharmacy*, vol. 8, no. 3, p. 140, 2020, doi: 10.3390/pharmacy8030140.

11. K. H. Abdulkareem *et al.*, "Realizing an effective COVID-19 diagnosis system based on machine learning and IoT in smart Hospital environment," *IEEE Internet Things J.*, vol. 8, no. 21, pp. 15919–15928, Nov. 2021, doi: 10.1109/JIOT.2021.3050775.

12. M. Scott, "Covid-19, place-making and health," *Plan. Theory Pract.*, vol. 21, no. 3, pp. 343–348, 2020, doi: 10.1080/14649357.2020.1781445.

13. S. M. Idrees, M. A. Alam, and P. Agarwal, "A prediction approach for stock market volatility based on time series data," *IEEE Access*, vol. 7, pp. 17287–17298, 2019, doi: 10.1109/ACCESS.2019.2895252.

14. A. Yadav, C. K. Jha, and A. Sharan, "Optimizing LSTM for time series prediction in Indian stock market," *Procedia Comput. Sci.*, vol. 167, pp. 2091–2100, 2020, doi: 10.1016/j.procs.2020.03.257.

15. I. Naim, T. Mahara, and A. R. Idrisi, "Effective short-term forecasting for daily time series with complex seasonal patterns," *Procedia Comput. Sci.*, vol. 132, pp. 1832–1841, 2018, doi: 10.1016/j.procs.2018.05.136.

16. A. Asfaw, B. Simane, A. Hassen, and A. Bantider, "Variability and time series trend analysis of rainfall and temperature in northcentral Ethiopia: A case study in Woleka sub-basin," *Weather Clim. Extrem.*, vol. 19, pp. 29–41, Mar. 2018, doi: 10.1016/j.wace.2017.12.002.

17. K. E. ArunKumar, D. V. Kalaga, C. Mohan Sai Kumar, M. Kawaji, and T. M. Brenza, "Comparative analysis of gated recurrent units (GRU), long short-term memory

(LSTM) cells, autoregressive integrated moving average (ARIMA), seasonal autoregressive integrated moving average (SARIMA) for forecasting COVID-19 trends," *Alexandria Eng. J.*, vol. 61, no. 10, pp. 7585–7603, 2022, doi: 10.1016/j.aej.2022.01.011.

18. H. O. Pal, J. Rohith Sundar, A. Deepanshu, and Chauhan, "A Deep Learning Based Safe Travel Advisory Tool for COVID-19," in *2022 3rd International Conference for Emerging Technology (INCET)*, May 2022, pp. 1–7, doi: 10.1109/INCET54531. 2022.9824039.

19. Z. M. Zain, and N. M. Alturki, "COVID-19 pandemic forecasting using CNN-LSTM: A hybrid approach," *J. Control Sci. Eng.*, vol. 2021, pp. 1–23, Jul. 2021, doi: 10.1155/2021/8785636.

20. K. Oshinubi, A. Amakor, O. J. Peter, M. Rachdi, and J. Demongeot, "Approach to COVID-19 time series data using deep learning and spectral analysis methods," *AIMS Bioeng.*, vol. 9, no. 1, pp. 1–21, 2021, doi: 10.3934/bioeng.2022001.

21. K. Choi, J. Yi, C. Park, and S. Yoon, "Deep learning for anomaly detection in time-series data: Review, analysis, and guidelines," *IEEE Access*, vol. 9, pp. 120043–120065, 2021, doi: 10.1109/ACCESS.2021.3107975.

22. T. Hu, Q. Guo, Z. Li, X. Shen, and H. Sun, "Distribution-free probability density forecast through deep neural networks," *IEEE Trans. Neural Networks Learn. Syst*, vol. 31, no. 2, pp. 612–625, 2020, doi: 10.1109/TNNLS.2019.2907305.

23. A. Zeroual, F. Harrou, A. Dairi, and Y. Sun, "Deep learning methods for forecasting COVID-19 time-series data: A comparative study," *Chaos, Solitons & Fractals*, vol. 140, p. 110121, Nov. 2020, doi: 10.1016/j.chaos.2020.110121.

24. A. Pranolo, Y. Mao, A. P. Wibawa, A. B. P. Utama, and F. A. Dwiyanto, "Robust LSTM with tuned-PSO and bifold-attention mechanism for analyzing multivariate time-series," *IEEE Access*, vol. 10, pp. 78423–78434, 2022, doi: 10.1109/ACCESS.2022.3193643.

25. T. Ouyang, Y. He, H. Li, Z. Sun, and S. Baek, "Modeling and forecasting short-term power load with copula model and deep belief network," *IEEE Trans. Emerg. Top. Comput. Intell.*, vol. 3, no. 2, pp. 127–136, 2019, doi: 10.1109/TETCI.2018.2880511.

26. T. Shintate, and L. Pichl, "Trend prediction classification for high frequency bitcoin time series with deep learning," *J. Risk Financ. Manag.*, vol. 12, no. 1, p. 17, 2019, doi: 10.3390/jrfm12010017.

27. A. P. Wibawa, R. R. Ula, A. B. P. Utama, M. Y. Chuttur, A. Pranolo, and Haviluddin, "Forecasting e-Journal Unique Visitors using Smoothed Long Short-Term Memory," in *2021 7th International Conference on Electrical, Electronics and Information Engineering (ICEEIE)*, Oct. 2021, pp. 609–613, doi: 10.1109/ICEEIE52663.2021. 9616628.

28. H.-J. Chiu, T.-H. S. Li, and P.-H. Kuo, "Breast Cancer–Detection system using PCA, multilayer perceptron, transfer learning, and support vector machine," *IEEE Access*, vol. 8, pp. 204309–204324, 2020, doi: 10.1109/ACCESS.2020.3036912.

29. N. Calik, M. A. Belen, and P. Mahouti, "Deep learning base modified MLP model for precise scattering parameter prediction of capacitive feed antenna," *Int. J. Numer. Model. Electron. Networks, Devices Fields*, vol. 33, no. 2, Mar. 2020, doi: 10.1002/ jnm.2682.

30. J. García Cabello, "Mathematical neural networks," *Axioms*, vol. 11, no. 2, p. 80, 2022, doi: 10.3390/axioms11020080.

31. A. P. Wibawa, I. T. Saputra, A. B. P. Utama, W. Lestari, and Z. N. Izdihar, "Long Short-Term Memory to Predict Unique Visitors of an Electronic Journal," in *2020 6th International Conference on Science in Information Technology (ICSITech)*, Oct. 2020, pp. 176–179, doi: 10.1109/ICSITech49800.2020.9392031.

32. A. W. Saputra, A. P. Wibawa, U. Pujianto, A. B. P. Utama, and A. Nafalski, "LSTM-based multivariate time-series analysis: A case of journal visitors forecasting," *Ilk. J. Ilm*, vol. 14, no. 1, pp. 57–62, 2022, doi: 10.33096/ilkom.v14i1.1106.57-62.

33. Q. Zhang, M. Zhang, T. Chen, Z. Sun, Y. Ma, and B. Yu, "Recent advances in convolutional neural network acceleration," *Neurocomputing*, vol. 323, pp. 37–51, Jan. 2019, doi: 10.1016/j.neucom.2018.09.038.

34. R. F. Dewandra, A. P. Wibawa, U. Pujianto, A. B. P. Utama, and A. Nafalski, "Journal unique visitors forecasting based on multivariate attributes using CNN," *Int. J. Artif. Intell. Res.*, vol. 6, no. 1, 2022, doi: https://doi.org/10.29099/ijair.v6i1.274.

35. Z. Shen, X. Fan, L. Zhang, and H. Yu, "Wind speed prediction of unmanned sailboat based on CNN and LSTM hybrid neural network," *Ocean Eng.*, vol. 254, p. 111352, Jun. 2022, doi: 10.1016/j.oceaneng.2022.111352.

36. E. Setyati, S. Az, S. P. Hudiono, and F. Kurniawan, "CNN based face recognition system for patients with down and William syndrome," *Knowl. Eng. Data Sci.*, vol. 4, no. 2, p. 138, 2021, doi: 10.17977/um018v4i22021p138-144.

37. B. Sun *et al.*, "Demonstration of Applications in Computer Vision and NLP on Ultra Power-Efficient CNN Domain Specific Accelerator with 9.3TOPS/Watt," in *2019 IEEE International Conference on Multimedia & Expo Workshops (ICMEW)*, Jul. 2019, pp. 611–611, doi: 10.1109/ICMEW.2019.00115.

38. A. P. Wibawa, A. B. P. Utama, H. Elmunsyah, U. Pujianto, F. A. Dwiyanto, and L. Hernandez, "Time-series analysis with smoothed convolutional neural network," *J. Big Data*, vol. 9, no. 1, p. 44, 2022, doi: 10.1186/s40537-022-00599-y.

39. H. A. Rosyid, M. W. Aniendya, and H. W. Herwanto, "Comparison of Indonesian imports forecasting by limited period using SARIMA method," *Knowl. Eng. Data Sci.*, vol. 2, no. 2, p. 90, 2019, doi: 10.17977/um018v2i22019p90-100.

40. P. Purnawansyah, H. Haviluddin, H. Darwis, H. Azis, and Y. Salim, "Backpropagation neural network with combination of activation functions for inbound traffic prediction," *Knowl. Eng. Data Sci.*, vol. 4, no. 1, p. 14, 2021, doi: 10.17977/um018v4i12021p14-28.

20 Immunology and Microbiology Journals Quartile Classification Using Decision Tree (ID3) Ensemble Models

Nastiti Susetyo Fanany Putri, Aji Prasetya Wibawa, and Harits Ar Rosyid
Universitas Negeri Malang
Malang, Indonesia

Andrew Nafalski
University of South Australia
Adelaide, Australia

Eisuke Hanada
Saga University
Saga, Japan

20.1 INTRODUCTION

Coronavirus emerged in late 2019 (COVID-19) with its epicenter in Wuhan, China. After 118,000 cases were reported in over a 110 countries by March 11, 2020, the World Health Organization (WHO) declared COVID-19 a pandemic [1, 2]. The disease spread quickly over the entire planet. This condition gives scholars new research topics published in various scientific journals. Table 20.1 provides the number of journals in the category of immunology and microbiology at SCImago Journal Rank (SJR) over the past 3 years. The SJR report is categorized into four groups or quartiles [3]. The journal's quality is displayed throughout the most excellent quartile Q1 and the lowest Q4 [4]. Researchers use these classes as a selection basis to publish their research.

In immunology and microbiology, this classification technique can recognize the classes. The technique finds models or functions that explain and differentiate ideas or classes of data [5, 6]. This classification predicts the class label of an object whose label is unknown [7].

This chapter attempts to utilize a classification technique with ensemble approaches. The ensemble model is a further development of the basics classification

TABLE 20.1

Quantity of Immunology and Microbiology Journals for 3 Years

Year	Q1	Q2	Q3	Q4	–	Quantity
2019	140	150	140	136	39	605
2020	135	146	136	131	30	578
2021	143	142	145	135	9	574

method [8] by combining the same two algorithms with a specific pattern [9, 10] and then deciding the final result by the voting system [11, 12]. The fundamental objective of using an ensemble is to overcome the conventional single classifier [13] through overfitting [14] and data noise reduction [15]. This study examines the performance of the ensemble method in immunology and microbiology journals from 2019 to 2021.

Methods are discussed in Section 20.2 of this chapter. We use Bagging and Boosting for the ensemble classification approach. The findings are provided and discussed in Section 20.3. Finally, Section 20.4 comprehensively discusses the previous sections.

20.2 METHOD

This study has four phases: data collection, preprocessing, classification, and evaluation. The research method is depicted in Figure 20.1.

The first step in this research is data collection. The data of journal and country rankings are retrieved from the SCImago website (https://www.scimagojr.com/) with specific subjects: immunology and microbiology. The attributes of September 2022 data are shown in Table 20.2. Nine of 20 attributes are used for classification because the selected approaches will only process the numerical data types [16, 17]. This study is classified as multiclass because it contains four classes, Q1, Q2, Q3, and Q4, where the SJR Best Quartile is the class label. The other eight attributes, H index, Total Docs (2020), Total Docs (3 Years), Total Refs, Total Cites (3 Years), City Docs (3 Years), Cite/Doc (2 Years), and Ref.Doc, are the independent labels.

Preprocessing, the data preparation stage, is necessary for classification [18, 19]. The data must be prepared to get a precise classification. Preprocessing can improve the predictive classification performance [20]. Data cleansing, integration, transformation, reduction, feature selection, and resampling are examples of preprocessing [21, 22]. This study only uses data cleaning due to the data characteristic and the selected classification method.

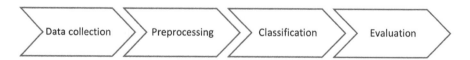

FIGURE 20.1   Research method.

TABLE 20.2

List of Dataset Attributes

Attribute	Data Type	Range
Rank	Integer	1-2164
Sourceid	Real	12016-21101020133
Title	Nominal	Annual Review of Plant Biology, Ecology Letters, ISME Journal, etc.
Type	Nominal	Journal
Issn	Nominal	995444, 00015342, etc.
SJR	Real	0.1-11695
SJR Best Quartile	Nominal	Q1, Q2, Q3, Q4, NQ
H index	Integer	0-342
Total Docs (2020)	Integer	0-3921
Total Docs (3 Years)	Integer	0-6917
Total Refs	Integer	0-251461
Total Cites (3 years)	Integer	0-42304
Citable Docs (3 years)	Integer	0-6322
Cite/Doc (2 years)	Real	0-25.28
Ref.Doc	Real	0-326.27
Country	Nominal	Indonesia, Hungary, Poland, etc.
Region	Nominal	Northern America, Western Europe, the Asiatic region, etc.
Publisher	Nominal	SEJANI Ltd, CSIC, EM International, etc.
Coverage	Nominal	1988–2020, 1978–2020, 1977, 1996–2020, etc.
Categories	Nominal	Agricultural and Biological Sciences, Ecology. Evolution Behavior and Systematic Cell Biology etc.

Data cleaning eliminates missing values and noise [23]. Several instances are removed to prevent incorrect classification [24]. After this process, 1679 instances in the dataset are used. Table 20.3 contains information on each class label after preprocessing.

This study uses the meta-ensemble for Boosting by merging a group of weak algorithms to form a more robust algorithm [25, 26]. The two Boosting types applied are AdaBoost and XGBoost. AdaBoost was initially designed to enhance

TABLE 20.3

Data Cleaning Result

Class Label	Before Cleaning	After Cleaning
q1	418	418
q2	438	438
q3	421	421
q4	402	402
–	120	–
Sum	1799	1679

the performance of binary classifiers [27]. XGBoost is an enhanced version of the gradient boosting machine (GBM) [28] that incorporates parallel preprocessing at the node level [29]. XGBoost also implements several regularization approaches to prevent overfitting [30].

Another applied ensemble model is Bagging, an ensemble strategy that combines many learners trained on different subsamples of the original data [31]. A Bagging model produces many datasets by bootstrapping the training data, developing models based on the various datasets, and then using these models to make predictions [32]. Depending on the problem being solved, all the predictions are merged to produce a representative value (mean, median, or majority vote) for classification and an average for regression. Because a single learner is frequently sensitive to noise in the training data, Bagging combines many outcomes into a single prediction, which should produce more consistent and accurate results based on reduced variation [33].

A confusion matrix is used for evaluation [34]. It [35] consists of predictive classification results and actual values utilizing the classification scheme. Six criteria are used to assess classification performance: accuracy, precision, recall, specificity, F1 score, and error rate [36]. However, this study only investigated the accuracy, precision, and recall values, which are recognized fundamental metrics for the classification method.

20.3 RESULTS AND DISCUSSION

Parameter setting was carried out regarding the value of n estimates and n depth. Table 20.4 includes a list of the classification's outcomes for Bagging.

From Table 20.4, the best value of the bagging method is in the 100 estimators starting from depth 100 with an accuracy value of 86.82%, 82.6%, and 82.53% for precision and recall. With the addition of the estimator value at depth 10, the accuracy value tends to fluctuate. Whereas at a depth value of 100 and greater, the classification performance value produces the same value if the estimator value is the same. The t-test is declared significantly related if the t value is <0.05.

Paired sample t-test was conducted to determine the relationship between depth and estimator on classification performance. The addition of the depth value does not significantly impact the classification performance because the t-test value is 0. In contrast, the addition of the estimators' value significantly affects the t-test result of 0.0028. Table 20.5 shows the AdaBoost classification result.

The highest accuracy value of the AdaBoost method is 87.05%, with a depth value of 50 and an estimator of 100. AdaBoost's performance is more stable than other methods applied. Adding depth and estimator values to the AdaBoost method significantly affects the t-test values of 0.0001 and 0.0013, respectively. The XGBoost classification result is presented in Table 20.6.

In the third method, XGBoost, the best performance is at 87.17% for accuracy, 82.15%, and 81.94% for precision and recall. XGBoost produces the same value at the same estimator value at each depth value. The addition of the depth value does not significantly impact the t-test value 0 and the addition of the estimator value because the t-test value is 0.058. Table 20.7 compares the best performance

TABLE 20.4

Bagging Classification Result

Method	N_Depth	N_Estimators	Accuracy	Precision	Recall
Bagging		50	82.6	81.56	81.28
		100	83.14	81.15	80.89
Decision	10	150	82.96	81.02	80.69
		200	83.32	81.26	80.87
Tree		500	83.38	81.01	80.49
		1000	83.56	81.62	81.1
		50	86.45	82.32	82.32
		100	86.82	82.6	82.53
	50	150	86.64	82.56	82.55
		200	86.69	83.29	83.13
		500	86.57	82.89	82.74
		1000	86.45	83.03	82.96
		50	86.45	82.32	82.32
		100	86.82	82.6	82.53
	100	150	86.64	82.56	82.55
		200	86.69	83.29	83.13
		500	86.57	82.89	82.74
		1000	86.45	83.03	82.96
		50	86.45	82.32	82.32
		100	86.82	82.6	82.53
	500	150	86.64	82.56	82.54
		200	86.69	83.29	83.13
		500	86.57	82.89	82.74
		1000	86.45	83.03	82.96
		50	86.45	82.32	82.32
		100	86.82	82.6	82.53
	1000	150	86.63	82.56	82.55
		200	86.69	83.29	83.13
		500	86.57	82.89	82.74
		1000	86.45	83.03	82.96

of the three methods applied. In general, the Boosting algorithm outperforms the Bagging approach. XGBoost has the highest accuracy, whereas AdaBoost has the highest precision.

20.4   CONCLUSION

This chapter concluded that the XGBoost classification produced a reasonably acceptable score near the SCImago category because XGBoost's built-in optimization system used a regularization technique. N_ estimator is the most used parameter in the ensemble because the incorrect prediction in the first estimator is regenerated

TABLE 20.5
AdaBoost Classification Result

Method	N_Depth	N_Estimators	Accuracy	Precision	Recall
AdaBoost		50	86.94	83.16	82.91
		100	86.45	82.32	82.09
Decision	10	150	86.69	82.73	82.26
		200	86.63	82.59	82.29
Tree		500	86.51	82.59	82.29
		1000	86.45	83.78	83.49
		50	86.51	81.78	81.57
		100	87.05	84.33	83.9
	50	150	86.81	84.17	83.89
		200	86.51	84.86	84.47
		500	86.39	84.14	83.88
		1000	86.69	85.19	84.83
		50	86.45	81.78	81.57
		100	86.93	84.33	83.9
	100	150	86.69	84.17	83.89
		200	86.51	84.86	84.47
		500	86.39	84.38	84.07
		1000	86.69	84.05	84.67
		50	86.45	81.78	81.57
		100	86.45	81.78	81.57
	500	150	86.69	84.17	83.89
		200	86.51	84.86	84.47
		500	86.39	84.38	84.07
		1000	86.69	84.05	83.67
		50	86.45	81.78	81.57
		100	86.93	84.33	83.9
	1000	150	86.69	84.17	83.89
		200	86.51	84.86	84.47
		500	86.39	84.39	84.07
		1000	86.69	84.05	83.67

in the following estimator to make the method work optimally. However, the ID3 has several weaknesses, including a longer training time and a calculation process that can be significantly more complex than other algorithms. A minor change in the data can result in a substantial change in the decision tree's structure, resulting in instability.

For future research, scientists can use different fundamental algorithms or more renewable meta-ensemble variations. Some potential methods that can be used are support vectors, naïve Bayes, and even neural networks.

TABLE 20.6

XGBoost Classification Result

Method	N_Depth	N_Estimators	Accuracy	Precision	Recall
XGBoost		50	87.17	82.15	81.94
		100	87.12	81.72	81.54
Decision		150	86.99	81.32	81.16
	10	200	86.75	81.45	81.35
Tree		500	86.33	81.43	81.35
		1000	86.09	81.04	80.97
		50	87.17	82.17	81.94
		100	87.12	81.72	81.54
		150	86.99	81.32	81.16
	50	200	86.75	81.45	81.35
		500	86.33	81.43	81.35
		1000	86.09	81.07	80.97
		50	87.17	82.15	81.94
		100	87.12	81.72	81.54
		150	86.99	81.32	81.16
	100	200	86.75	81.45	81.35
		500	86.33	81.43	81.35
		1000	86.09	81.04	80.97
		50	87.17	82.15	81.94
		100	87.12	81.72	81.54
	500	150	86.99	81.32	81.16
		200	86.75	81.45	81.35
		500	86.33	81.43	81.35
		1000	86.09	81.04	80.97
		50	87.17	82.15	81.94
		100	87.12	81.72	81.54
		150	86.99	81.32	81.16
	1000	200	86.75	81.45	81.35
		500	86.33	81.45	81.35
		1000	86.09	81.04	80.97

TABLE 20.7

Comparison of the Best Result of Each Classification Method

Method	N_Depth	N_Estimators	Accuracy	Precision	Recall
Bagging	50	100	86.82	82.6	82.53
AdaBoost	50	100	87.05	84.33	83.9
XGBoost	10	50	87.17	82.15	81.94

REFERENCES

1. S. A. Sarkodie, and P. A. Owusu, "Global assessment of environment, health and economic impact of the novel coronavirus (COVID-19)," *Environ. Dev. Sustain.*, vol. 23, no. 4, pp. 5005–5015, 2021, doi: 10.1007/s10668-020-00801-2.

2. O. Jamsheela, "A study of the correlation between the dates of the first Covid case and the first Covid death of 25 selected countries to know the virulence of the Covid-19 in different tropical conditions," *Ethics, Med. Public Heal.*, vol. 19, p. 100707, Dec. 2021, doi: 10.1016/j.jemep.2021.100707.

3. A. P. Wibawa, Kurniawan, A. C., Rosyid, H. A., and Salah, A. M. M. "International Journal Quartile Classification Using the K-Nearest Neighbor Method," in 2019 *International Conference on Electrical, Electronics and Information Engineering (ICEEIE)*, Oct. 2019, pp. 336–341, doi: 10.1109/ICEEIE47180.2019.8981413.

4. A. P. Wibawa *et al.*, "Naïve Bayes classifier for journal quartile classification," *Int. J. Recent Contrib. from Eng. Sci. IT*, vol. 7, no. 2, p. 91, 2019, doi: 10.3991/ijes.v7i2.10659.

5. B. van Giffen, D. Herhausen, and T. Fahse, "Overcoming the pitfalls and perils of algorithms: A classification of machine learning biases and mitigation methods," *J. Bus. Res.*, vol. 144, pp. 93–106, May 2022, doi: 10.1016/j.jbusres.2022.01.076.

6. D. Zhang, and S. Lou, "The application research of neural network and BP algorithm in stock price pattern classification and prediction," *Futur. Gener. Comput. Syst.*, vol. 115, pp. 872–879, Feb. 2021, doi: 10.1016/j.future.2020.10.009.

7. Y. Zhang, Y. Wang, X.-Y. Liu, S. Mi, and M.-L. Zhang, "Large-scale multi-label classification using unknown streaming images," *Pattern Recognit.*, vol. 99, p. 107100, Mar. 2020, doi: 10.1016/j.patcog.2019.107100.

8. R. Li, C. Ren, X. Zhang, and B. Hu, "A novel ensemble learning method using multiple objective particle swarm optimization for subject-independent EEG-based emotion recognition," *Comput. Biol. Med.*, vol. 140, p. 105080, Jan. 2022, doi: 10.1016/j.compbiomed.2021.105080.

9. Y. Zhang, G. Cao, B. Wang, and X. Li, "A novel ensemble method for k-nearest neighbor," *Pattern Recognit.*, vol. 85, pp. 13–25, Jan. 2019, doi: 10.1016/j.patcog.2018.08.003.

10. J. Lin, H. Chen, S. Li, Y. Liu, X. Li, and B. Yu, "Accurate prediction of potential druggable proteins based on genetic algorithm and bagging-SVM ensemble classifier," *Artif. Intell. Med.*, vol. 98, pp. 35–47, Jul. 2019, doi: 10.1016/j.artmed.2019.07.005.

11. K. Golalipour, E. Akbari, S. S. Hamidi, M. Lee, and R. Enayatifar, "From clustering to clustering ensemble selection: A review," *Eng. Appl. Artif. Intell.*, vol. 104, p. 104388, Sep. 2021, doi: 10.1016/j.engappai.2021.104388.

12. G. Kaur, "A comparison of two hybrid ensemble techniques for network anomaly detection in spark distributed environment," *J. Inf. Secur. Appl.*, vol. 55, p. 102601, Dec. 2020, doi: 10.1016/j.jisa.2020.102601.

13. S. Kumari, D. Kumar, and M. Mittal, "An ensemble approach for classification and prediction of diabetes mellitus using soft voting classifier," *Int. J. Cogn. Comput. Eng.*, vol. 2, pp. 40–46, Jun. 2021, doi: 10.1016/j.ijcce.2021.01.001.

14. F. Liu, M. Cai, L. Wang, and Y. Lu, "An ensemble model based on adaptive noise reducer and over-fitting prevention LSTM for multivariate time series forecasting," *IEEE Access*, vol. 7, pp. 26102–26115, 2019, doi: 10.1109/ACCESS.2019.2900371.

15. A. B. Shaik, and S. Srinivasan, "A Brief Survey on Random Forest Ensembles in Classification Model," in *Lecture Notes in Networks and Systems*, Singapore: Springer, 2019, pp. 253–260.

16. S. M. Putra, A. P. Wibawa, T. Widiyaningtyas, and I. A. E. Zaeni, "Performance of SVM in Classifying the Quartile of Computer Science Journals," *Proceeding - 2019 5th Int. Conf. Sci. Inf. Technol. Embrac. Ind. 4.0 Towar. Innov. Cyber Phys. Syst. ICSITech 2019*, pp. 13–17, 2019, doi: 10.1109/ICSITech46713.2019.8987453.

17. R. P. Adiperkasa, A. P. Wibawa, I. A. E. Zaeni, and T. Widiyaningtyas, "International Reputable Journal Classification Using Inter-correlated Naïve Bayes Classifier," *Proc. - 2019 2nd Int. Conf. Comput. Informatics Eng. Artif. Intell. Roles Ind. Revolut. 4.0, IC2IE 2019*, pp. 49–52, 2019, doi: 10.1109/IC2IE47452.2019.8940887.

18. E. T. Bekar, P. Nyqvist, and A. Skoogh, "An intelligent approach for data preprocessing and analysis in predictive maintenance with an industrial case study," *Adv. Mech. Eng*, vol. 12, no. 5, p. 168781402091920, 2020, doi: 10.1177/1687814020919207.

19. M. J. Willemink *et al.*, "Preparing medical imaging data for machine learning," *Radiology*, vol. 295, no. 1, pp. 4–15, Apr. 2020, doi: 10.1148/radiol.2020192224.

20. B. Sekeroglu, K. Dimililer, and K. Tuncal, "Student Performance Prediction and Classification Using Machine Learning Algorithms," in *Proceedings of the 2019 8th International Conference on Educational and Information Technology*, Mar. 2019, pp. 7–11, doi: 10.1145/3318396.3318419.

21. I. Cordón, J. Luengo, S. García, F. Herrera, and F. Charte, "Smartdata: Data preprocessing to achieve smart data in R," *Neurocomputing*, vol. 360, pp. 1–13, Sep. 2019, doi: 10.1016/j.neucom.2019.06.006.

22. X. Shi, Y. D. Wong, M. Z.-F. Li, C. Palanisamy, and C. Chai, "A feature learning approach based on XGBoost for driving assessment and risk prediction," *Accid. Anal. Prev.*, vol. 129, pp. 170–179, Aug. 2019, doi: 10.1016/j.aap.2019.05.005.

23. T. Wang, H. Ke, X. Zheng, K. Wang, A. K. Sangaiah, and A. Liu, "Big data cleaning based on Mobile edge computing in industrial sensor-cloud," *IEEE Trans. Ind. Informat.*, vol. 16, no. 2, pp. 1321–1329, 2020, doi: 10.1109/TII.2019.2938861.

24. S. Wang, S. Bi, and Y.-J. A. Zhang, "Locational detection of the false data injection attack in a smart grid: A multilabel classification approach," *IEEE Internet Things J.*, vol. 7, no. 9, pp. 8218–8227, 2020, doi: 10.1109/JIOT.2020.2983911.

25. C. N. Egwim, H. Alaka, O. O. Egunjobi, A. Gomes, and I. Mporas, "Comparison of machine learning algorithms for evaluating building energy efficiency using big data analytics," *J. Eng. Des. Technol.*, Sep. 2022, doi: 10.1108/JEDT-05-2022-0238.

26. S. K. Khare, V. Bajaj, A. Sengur, and G. R. Sinha, "Classification of mental states from rational dilation wavelet transform and bagged tree classifier using EEG signals," in *Artificial Intelligence-Based Brain-Computer Interface*, Cham: Elsevier, 2022, pp. 217–235.

27. A. Belghit, M. Lazri, F. Ouallouche, K. Labadi, and S. Ameur, "Optimization of one versus all-SVM using AdaBoost algorithm for rainfall classification and estimation from multispectral MSG data," *Adv. Sp. Res.*, vol. 71, no. 1, pp. 946–963, 2023, doi: 10.1016/j.asr.2022.08.075.

28. C. Bentéjac, A. Csörgő, and G. Martínez-Muñoz, "A comparative analysis of gradient boosting algorithms," *Artif. Intell. Rev.*, vol. 54, no. 3, pp. 1937–1967, 2021, doi: 10.1007/s10462-020-09896-5.

29. H. Tao, M. Habib, I. Aljarah, H. Faris, H. A. Afan, and Z. M. Yaseen, "An intelligent evolutionary extreme gradient boosting algorithm development for modeling scour depths under submerged weir," *Inf. Sci. (Ny).*, vol. 570, pp. 172–184, Sep. 2021, doi: 10.1016/j.ins.2021.04.063.

30. S. Bergen *et al.*, "A review of supervised learning methods for classifying animal behavioural states from environmental features," *Methods Ecol. Evol.*, vol. 14, no. 1, pp. 189–202, Jan. 2023, doi: 10.1111/2041-210X.14019.

31. Z. Md. Jan, and B. Verma, "Evolutionary classifier and cluster selection approach for ensemble classification," *ACM Trans. Knowl. Discov. Data*, vol. 14, no. 1, pp. 1–18, 2020, doi: 10.1145/3366633.

32. G. Ngo, R. Beard, and R. Chandra, "Evolutionary bagging for ensemble learning," *Neurocomputing*, vol. 510, pp. 1–14, Oct. 2022, doi: 10.1016/j.neucom.2022.08.055.

33. A. Aldrees, H. H. Awan, M. F. Javed, and A. M. Mohamed, "Prediction of water quality indexes with ensemble learners: Bagging and boosting," *Process Saf. Environ. Prot.*, vol. 168, pp. 344–361, Dec. 2022, doi: 10.1016/j.psep.2022.10.005.

34. W. A. Bagwan, and R. S. Gavali, "Delineating changes in soil erosion risk zones using RUSLE model based on confusion matrix for the Urmodi River watershed, Maharashtra, India," *Model. Earth Syst. Environ.*, vol. 7, no. 3, pp. 2113–2126, 2021, doi: 10.1007/s40808-020-00965-w.

35. M. Hasnain, M. F. Pasha, I. Ghani, M. Imran, M. Y. Alzahrani, and R. Budiarto, "Evaluating trust prediction and confusion matrix measures for web services ranking," *IEEE Access*, vol. 8, pp. 90847–90861, 2020, doi: 10.1109/ACCESS.2020.2994222.

36. M. Muntean, and F.-D Militaru, "Metrics for Evaluating Classification Algorithms," in *Smart Innovation, Systems and Technologies*, Singapore: Springer, 2023, pp. 307–317.

21 Opinion Mining on Post-COVID-19 Hybrid Learning

Yulita Salim, Desi Anggreani, Huzain Azis,
Herdianti Darwis, and Purnawansyah
Universitas Muslim Indonesia
Makassar, Indonesia

Gulsun Kurubacak
Anadolu University
Eskişehir, Turkey

21.1 INTRODUCTION: BACKGROUND AND DRIVING FORCES

In December 2019, a global pandemic spread throughout the world. The outbreak was known as COVID-19 [1, 2]. Every country paid attention to the spread of the pandemic [3]. The outbreak caused more than 590 million cases, with 6.43 million deaths and 43 million cases, with 1 million deaths reported in the first 10 months [4]. The World Health Organization's latest case report noted that the Southeast Asia region had 186,000 cases, the Western Pacific 3.3 million, Europe 1.9 million, and the Eastern Mediterranean reported a decline in cases for the second week in a row, with just under 123,000 [5]. The unprecedented rate of spread of COVID-19 created a state of emergency with a profound impact on various sectors.

The affected sector may include the economic crisis, industry, and education [6, 7]. By the end of 2021, the spread of the outbreak decreased. Figure 21.1 showed the latest spread of the COVID-19 outbreak [5]. COVID-19 inpatients at the Steve Biko Academic Hospital (SBAH) reached 466, far less than the 3962 inpatients in the previous year [8], illustrating the decrease of COVID-19 cases entering the recovery process.

The post-pandemic recovery process were carried out by improving the economic crisis, health system, education, and industry [9, 10]. In education, various policies have been issued after the learning and teaching process is considered ineffective by students, teachers, and parents [11]. One of the education policies for the post-COVID-19 recovery period is a hybrid learning method system.

Hybrid learning is a learning system that combines online and offline learning [12, 13]. It fulfills the integrity of the student learning process, which has been carried out online. Face-to-face learning improves the quality of education, yet it does not make students more independent [14]. Hybrid learning maximizes learning outcomes by increasing student participation in distance and face-to-face learning [15].

DOI: 10.1201/9781003331674-21

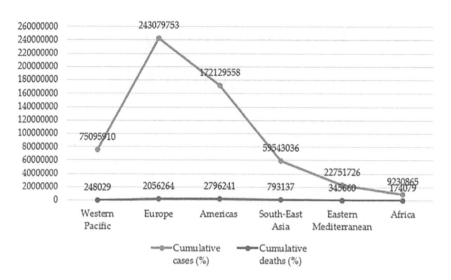

FIGURE 21.1   Spread of the COVID-19 outbreak.

The implementation of hybrid learning receives many public responses, which are varied, ranging from the learning material process and improvement to negative reactions that lead to controversy [16].

Opinion mining is one way to get public feedback. The mining objective is to determine whether the response given by the public is positive, negative, or neutral [17, 18]. It has excellent benefits in various fields as material for evaluation and obtaining ideas in response to an event, statement, or comment [19], and has been implemented in several previous studies. Mujahid [20] conducted research using the Long Short-Term Memory (LSTM) method to mine public opinion regarding implementing online learning during COVID-19. The study indicated that the number of negative opinions, the perceived uncertainty of the institution's opening date, and the rural networking challenges were among students' most worrying topics.

Furthermore, Hasib [21] conducted an opinion-mining analysis of U.S. Airline services using Deep Neural Network (DNN) and Convolutional Neural Network (CNN) methods. This study uses secondary data, consisting of 14640 tweets. The DNN and CNN methods had 91% accuracy in the analysis process. Subsequent research conducted a sentiment analysis to determine public opinion about the COVID-19 vaccines from AstraZeneca/Oxford, Pfizer/BioNTech, and Moderna using the AFINN lexicon to calculate the average daily sentiment from tweets [22]. This study used 701,891 tweet data and found that sentiment regarding Pfizer and Moderna vaccines appeared positive and stable for 4 months. However, the sentiment regarding the AstraZeneca/Oxford vaccine appeared to have turned negative over time.

The research was conducted to analyze opinion mining or sentiment analysis on implementing learning by the hybrid learning method. Unlike previous research, the proposed analysis used the Bidirectional Encoder Representations from Transformers (BERT) method. In addition, the object used was public opinion regarding the hybrid learning method in the recovery process of the post-COVID-19 education sector.

21.2 RESEARCH MATERIAL AND METHODS

The initial process was collecting public opinion data on post-COVID-19 hybrid learning. Data preprocessing is the next step. After the data are processed, it was entered into the opinion mining classification system. BERT was employed in performing the classification. The final stage was to analyze the performance of the BERT method in classifying public opinion. In addition, public opinion was obtained, and the results would answer whether the public's response to hybrid learning was positive or negative. Figure 21.2 shows the research stages.

This study collected real-time data directly from digital social media in August 2022. Several relevant keywords were used in the data collection process, such as Hybrid Learning Post Covid (hybrid learning post covid) and Hybrid Learning Covid (hybrid learning covid). The data collection can be seen in Table 21.1.

The preprocessing stages consisted of cleansing, tokenizing, filtering, stemming, and labeling. Data cleansing was cleaning data, such as deleting duplicate data and removing URLs and tag tags in tweets. Data tokenizing was splitting a sentence into a word. Data filtering was selecting data and retrieving important data in a sentence. Data stemming was normalizing data by forming words into basic words. The final stage of the preprocessing process was data labeling, where the collected tweets were classified into positive and negative polarities. The labeling process made it easier to classify the data into sentiment classification.

The sentiment classification modeling would include data that has gone through the preprocessing stage. BERT was a method for the public opinion mining analysis process regarding hybrid learning. It was a simple method but had a strong structure. BERT would be a two-way representation of labeled and unlabeled datasets, working and collaborating on all layers [23].

The BERT method has two necessary steps, namely pre-training and fine-tuning. Pre-training is a training of an unlabeled model, and fine-tuning was a BERT

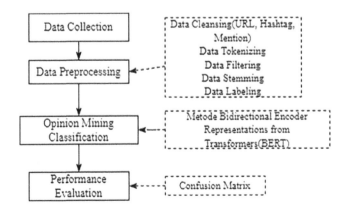

FIGURE 21.2 Research stages.

TABLE 21.1

Data Collection Hybrid Learning Post COVID-19

No.	Data Tweet
1	I'm happy to be able to go to school like years ago even if only a few times because hybrid learning
2	back to school a framework for remote and hybrid learning amid covid mckinsey education
3	healing from covid in education learning with hybrid, Negative
4	rt greg_travis maxjordan_n covid is the single largest killer of children and teachers from diseasen when hybrid learning was off, Negative
5	rt aisha__dani students like workers are preferring hybrid learning due to flexibility post covid in edu definition of hybrid has shi
6	is it better to study online or offline or study hybrid so confused
7	timeshighered uks first professor of hybrid learning says creation of the post shows hybrid and blended learning should be seen as a
8	remote work is here to stay discover methods for setting your team up for success when working remotely or on a hybrid basis with our newest series winning when working in a remote and blended environment
9	today i earned my teach forward best strategies for hybrid remote and blended learning badge im so proud to be celebrating this achievement and hope this inspires you to stayour own microsoftlearn journeynn mslearnbadge
10	hybrid is just a term of convenience that doesnt really define what it is other than that its a combination of two things we somewhat better understand illuminating repoon online learning officers re blended future of online amp ff learning

model initialized with all pre-training parameters, which was then adjusted using the labeled data. In pre-training, the model was trained using unlabeled data to complete various tasks. In fine-tuning, the BERT model was initialized with pre-trained parameters, and all parameters were fine-tuned with data that had labels to complete various Natural Language Processing (NLP) tasks such as text classification, question-answering, and named entity recognition [24, 25]. Figure 21.3 shows the architecture of the BERT method.

This study used the BERT method to classify the negative and positive public opinion. Each incoming data would go through the encoder layer. After going through each encoder, the data would be forwarded to the feed-forward to enter the classification stage. The final result of the process data would be classified into positive and negative [26].

BERT has two models: BERT BASE with 12 transformer blocks, 12 attention layers, and 768 hidden layers, and BERT LARGE, which had more layers than the first model including 24 transformer blocks, 16 attention heads, and 1024 hidden layers. This study used BERT BASE, which is shown in Figure 21.4.

The final stage in this research was the evaluation stage using a confusion matrix. The measures are recall, precision, and accuracy. Recall and precision measure the quantity and quality of the classification. In addition, recall measures how accurately our algorithm can recognize the relevant data. Furthermore, precision is the degree to which identical results are obtained from multiple measurements carried

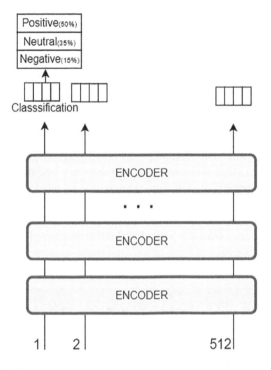

FIGURE 21.3   BERT structure.

out under the same conditions. The degree to which a measurement comes close to reflecting the actual value is known as its accuracy. The accuracy of the formula can be written using Equation (21.1).

$$Accuracy = (TP + TN) / (TP + FP + TN + FN)$$ (21.1)

The precision formula can be written using Equation (21.2).

$$Precision = TP / (TP + FP)$$ (21.2)

The recall formula can be written using Equation (21.3).

$$Recall = TP / (TP + FN)$$ (21.3)

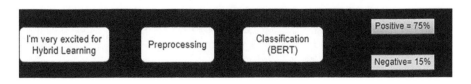

FIGURE 21.4   BERT base.

21.3   OPTION MINING (BERT METHOD) ON POST-COVID-19 HYBRID LEARNING

The data collection process has been carried out, and 531 tweet data related to hybrid learning were obtained. The information would go through the preprocessing data stage. The preprocessing process consisted of cleansing, tokenizing, filtering, stemming, and labeling. Figure 21.5 shows the result of the cleansing stage.

The preprocessing stage of cleansing would delete and clean sentences from URLs, numbers, characters, and punctuation unrelated to the searched keywords, namely hybrid learning. The next step was tokenizing, dividing the text into specific parts. The next stage was converting the data into essential words and removing affixes. Furthermore, the labeling process was to label the data according to their respective classifications. Data with a sentiment Valence Aware Dictionary (VADER) less than 0.5 were categorized into negative categories. In contrast, a sentiment VADER greater than 0.5 was classified as positive. Figure 21.6 shows the results of the preprocessing process at the final stage, namely labeling.

```
0        aisha__dani students like workers are preferri...
1        sasmitasvc addressed as the panelist on the to...
2        sasmitasvc addressed as the panelist on the to...
3        the top five  digital transformation trendsnn ...
4        sasmitasvc addressed as the panelist on the to...
                              ...
527      timeshighered uks first professor of hybrid le...
528      timeshighered uks first professor of hybrid le...
529      timeshighered uks first professor of hybrid le...
530      capdmltd in the age of hybrid work we need hyb...
531      timeshighered uks first professor of hybrid le...
Name: text, Length: 532, dtype: object
```

FIGURE 21.5   Cleansing result.

	text	Vader Sentiment	sentiment
0	aisha__dani students like workers are preferri...	0.5994	Positive
1	sasmitasvc addressed as the panelist on the to...	0.0000	Negative
2	sasmitasvc addressed as the panelist on the to...	0.0000	Negative
3	the top five digital transformation trendsnn ...	0.5994	Positive
4	sasmitasvc addressed as the panelist on the to...	0.0000	Negative

FIGURE 21.6   Result of labeling stage.

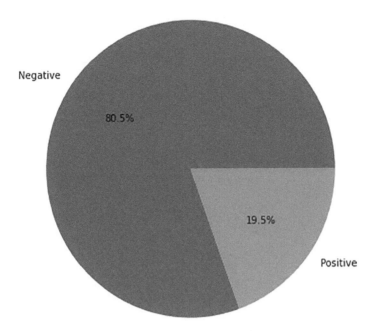

FIGURE 21.7 The pie chart of public opinion.

The labeling process was to label each dataset. Each sentence would be labeled between negative and positive. The overall data show that there were more data classified as negative sentiments than positive. Based on the labeling process, the results showed that in this study, the dataset used 428 data were classified as negative, and 104 were positive. Figure 21.7 shows the results of public opinion regarding implementing hybrid learning.

After passing through the preprocessing stage, the data were sent to the opinion mining method, BERT. In its implementation, the BERT method can be used with the helper library Transformers in the Python programming language. Data processing was carried out using several parameters, including a maximum length of 100; a batch size of 16; a learning rate (Adam) of 2e-5; and epochs of 10, 20, and 30. The analysis process would be carried out repeatedly by looking at the accuracy value of each architecture.

The first analysis was carried out on the model architecture with several epochs of 10. Figure 21.8 shows the results of the accuracy with 10 epochs.

The 10-epoch experiments have results of 96% (0.96) precision, 75% (0.75) recall, and 93% (0.93) accuracy. The accuracy value that reached 93% was high in classifying sentiments. This initial test was the fastest, with lower computation time than other tests. The quick and accurate result indicates that BERT is optimal for sentiment analysis.

The subsequent analysis epoch is 20. The evaluation result of classification with 20 epochs can be seen in Figure 21.9. Experiments with 20 epochs had a precision value of 91%. The obtained precision had a lower value than in the previous test. The recall value was 86%, and the accuracy was 94%. The accuracy obtained in the

	precision	recall	f1-score	support
negative	0.92	1.00	0.96	46
positive	1.00	0.50	0.67	8
accuracy			0.93	54
macro avg	0.96	0.75	0.81	54
weighted avg	0.93	0.93	0.92	54

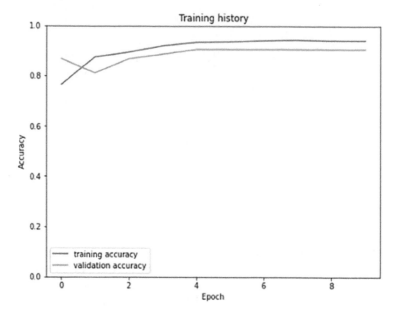

FIGURE 21.8   The classification with 10 epochs.

second test had a higher value than in the previous test. In terms of accuracy, the two experiments carried out had different accuracy values. The highest accuracy value was found in experiments with 20 epochs. In the training history image at 20 epochs, it can be seen that training accuracy and validation accuracy had increased in iterations 1 to 15. Both had the same value in the 15th to 20th iterations. The illustration accuracy of classification with 20 epochs can be seen in Figure 21.9.

Furthermore, experimental analysis was carried out using 30 epochs. The evaluation result of classification with 30 epochs can be seen in Figure 21.10. The 30 epochs obtained an accuracy of 94%. The accuracy values in the second and third tests had the same. The precision value was 97%, and the recall was 81%. The illustration accuracy of classification with 30 epochs can be seen in Figure 21.10. Likewise, in the second experiment, the accuracy value increased compared with the first experiment until it reached 94%. Table 21.2 displays the results of the entire test.

The BERT method was carried out on three test models with different results from each other. From the precision value, the third experiment had advantages over the others, where the precision value reached 97%, whereas in tests 1 and 2, the

	precision	recall	f1-score	support
negative	0.96	0.98	0.97	46
positive	0.86	0.75	0.80	8
accuracy			0.94	54
macro avg	0.91	0.86	0.88	54
weighted avg	0.94	0.94	0.94	54

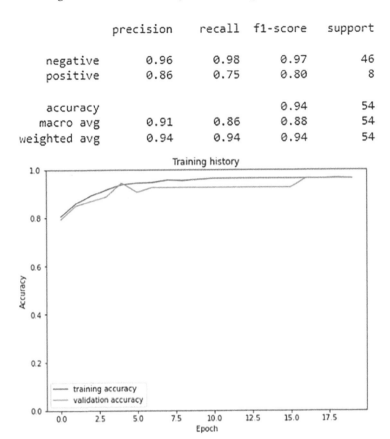

FIGURE 21.9   The classification with 20 epochs.

precision values were only 96% and 91%, respectively. The second test had the lowest precision value compared with the others. The recall value of the second experiment had the best result, reaching 86%. The first test had the lowest recall value (75%). The highest accuracy value was found in the second and third experiments (94%). The lowest accuracy value was in the first experiment, which was 93%.

The testing process shows that the higher the number of epochs used, the higher the accuracy of the classification process. The difference in the accuracy value was low (1%), influenced by the small number of datasets and the unbalanced dataset between negative and positive datasets. Therefore, the BERT method could classify public opinion positively and negatively. Many people had negative views on implementing post-COVID hybrid learning. The percentage of public opinion regarding the policy of the hybrid learning method of 80.5% was negative, and 19.5% was positive. Some examples of negative thoughts were "already used to learning online its hard to enter face to face lectures after COVID hybrid learning recovery covid" and "subsix incredible quote from pediatrician amp aap spokeswomannni dont see us going back to solely remote learning but I worry that."

	precision	recall	f1-score	support
negative	0.94	1.00	0.97	46
positive	1.00	0.62	0.77	8
accuracy			0.94	54
macro avg	0.97	0.81	0.87	54
weighted avg	0.95	0.94	0.94	54

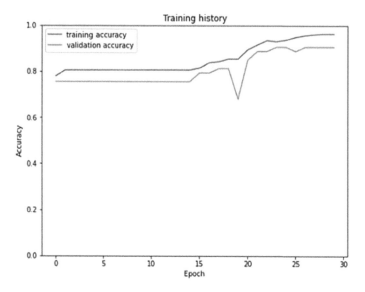

FIGURE 21.10   The classification with 30 epochs.

TABLE 21.2
Testing Result

	10 Epochs	20 Epochs	30 Epochs
Accuracy	0.93	0.94	0.94
Precision	0.96	0.91	0.97
Recall	0.75	0.86	0.81

21.4   CONCLUSION

Based on the analysis and testing of the opinion mining system on the implementation of post-COVID hybrid learning using the BERT method, it can be concluded that the BERT method can perform the opinion mining process following the previous design concept. In the testing phase, the BERT method produces the lowest accuracy value in the first test with an accuracy value of 93%, precision of 96%, and recall of 75%. The highest accuracy value was found in the third test (30 epochs), namely

94% with 97% precision and 81% recall. The analysis process of opinion mining on the implementation of post-COVID hybrid learning using the BERT method finds that much public opinion is classified into negative sentiment, which is 80.5%. In implementing opinion mining with the BERT method, the amount of training data influences the system classification process. The quality of the training data also plays a role. The higher the quality, the more words are stored in the dataset, which may lead to more precise sentiment analysis.

REFERENCES

1. M. Macera, G. De Angelis, C. Sagnelli, and N. Coppola, "Clinical Presentation of COVID-19: Case Series and Review of the Literature," Int. J. Environ. Res. Public Health, vol. 17, no. 14, p. 5062, Jul. 2020, doi: 10.3390/ijerph17145062.
2. R. Lalaoui et al., "What could explain the late emergence of COVID-19 in Africa ?," New Microbes New Infect., vol. 38, p. 100760, 2020.
3. S. Pokhrel, and R. Chhetri, "A Literature Review on Impact of COVID-19 Pandemic on Teaching and Learning," High. Educ. Futur., vol. 8, no. 1, pp. 133–141, Jan. 2021, doi: 10.1177/2347631120983481.
4. N. Fraser, L. Brierley, G. Dey, J. K. Polka, M. Pálfy, and F. Nanni, "Preprinting the COVID-19 pandemic," BioRxiv, pp. 2005–2020, 2020.
5. WHO, "Weekly epidemiological update on COVID-19–10 August 2022," World Health Organization, 2022. https://www.who.int/publications/m/item/weekly-epidemiological-update-on-covid-19---10-august-2022, 2022. [Accessed 18-09-2022].
6. L. Lu, J. Peng, J. Wu, and Y. Lu, "Perceived impact of the COVID-19 crisis on SMEs in different industry sectors: Evidence from Sichuan, China," Int. J. Disaster Risk Reduct., vol. 55, no. 24, p. 102085, 2021.
7. H. S. Munawar, S. I. Khan, F. Ullah, and A. Z. Kouzani, "Effects of COVID-19 on the Australian economy: Insights into the mobility and unemployment rates in education and tourism sectors," Sustainability, vol. 13, no. 20, p. 11300, 2021.
8. F. Abdullah et al., "Decreased severity of disease during the first global omicron variant COVID-19 outbreak in a large hospital in Tshwane, South Africa," Int. J. Infect. Dis., vol. 116, pp. 38–42, 2022.
9. D. J. Barnett, A. J. Rosenblum, K. Strauss-Riggs, and T. D. Kirsch, "Readying for a post-COVID-19 world: The case for concurrent pandemic disaster response and recovery efforts in public health," J. Public Heal. Manag. Pract., vol. 26, no. 4, pp. 310–313, 2020.
10. A. Orîndaru, M. F. Popescu, A. P. Alexoaei, Ştefan C. Căescu, M. S. Florescu, and A. O. Orzan, "Tourism in a post-COVID-19 era: Sustainable strategies for industry's recovery," Sustainability, vol. 13, no. 12, pp. 1–22, 2021.
11. P. Tarkar, "Impact of COVID-19 pandemic on education system," Int. J. Adv. Sci. Technol., vol. 29, no. 9, pp. 3812–3814, 2020.
12. M. B. Cahapay, "Navigating the post-COVID-19 era of 'next normal' in the context of Philippine higher education," ASIA-PACIFIC J. Educ. Manag. Res., vol. 5, no. 3, pp. 57–64, 2021.
13. Q. Li, Z. Li, and J. Han, "A hybrid learning pedagogy for surmounting the challenges of the COVID-19 pandemic in the performing arts education," Educ. Inf. Technol., vol. 26, no. 6, pp. 7635–7655, 2021.
14. B. P. Putri Uleng, M. Mahfuddin, and N. Nurhidayah, "Hybrid learning as an effective learning solution on intensive English program in the new normal era," J. Andi Djemma J. Pendidik., vol. 5, no. 2, p. 56, 2021.

15. C. A. K. Mutmainnah, and Samtidar, "Study of perceptions on hybrid learning in the teaching of English at mtsn 4 bone during the COVID-19 pandemic," *J. Technol. Lang. Pedagog.*, vol. 1, no. 1, pp. 27–37, 2022.

16. A. M. Celestial-Valderama, A. Vinluan, and S. D. Moraga, "Mining students' feedback in a general education course: Basis for improving blended learning implementation," *Int. J. Comput. Sci. Res.*, vol. 5, no. 1, pp. 568–583, 2021.

17. N. C. Dang, M. N. Moreno-García, and F. De la Prieta, "Sentiment analysis based on deep learning: A comparative study," *Electronics*, vol. 9, no. 3, p. 483, Mar. 2020, doi: 10.3390/electronics9030483

18. K. H. Manguri, R. N. Ramadhan, and P. R. Mohammed Amin, "Twitter sentiment analysis on worldwide COVID-19 outbreaks," *Kurdistan J. Appl. Res.*, vol. 5, no. 3, pp. 54–65, 2020.

19. A. Ligthart, C. Catal, and B. Tekinerdogan, *Systematic Reviews in Sentiment Analysis: a Tertiary Study*, vol. 54, no. 7. Springer Netherlands, 2021.

20. M. Mujahid *et al.*, "Sentiment analysis and topic modeling on tweets about online education during COVID-19," *Appl. Sci.*, vol. 11, no. 18, p. 8438, 2021.

21. K. M. Hasib, M. A. Habib, N. A. Towhid, and M. I. H. Showrov, "A Novel Deep Learning based Sentiment Analysis of Twitter Data for US Airline Service," *2021 Int. Conf. Inf. Commun. Technol. Sustain. Dev. ICICT4SD 2021 - Proc.*, pp. 450–455, 2021.

22. R. Marcec, and R. Likic, "Using twitter for sentiment analysis towards AstraZeneca/ Oxford, Pfizer/BioNTech and Moderna COVID-19 vaccines," *Postgrad. Med. J.*, vol. 98, no. 1161, pp. 544–550, 2021.

23. R. Qasim, W. H. Bangyal, M. A. Alqarni, and A. Ali Almazroi, "A fine-tuned BERT-based transfer learning approach for text classification," *J. Healthc. Eng.*, vol. 2022, Article ID 3498123, 2022.

24. R. Saputra, *Implementasi Bidirectional Encoder Representations From Transformers (Bert) Untuk Mendeteksi Hatespeech Dan Abusive Language Pada Twitter Bahasa Indonesia Jurusan Teknik Informatika Uin Suska Riau.* Universitas Islam Negeri Sultan Syarif Kasim Riau, 2022.

25. J. Devlin, M. W. Chang, K. Lee, and K. Toutanova, "BERT: Pre-training of deep bidirectional transformers for language understanding," in *Proc. NAACL HLT*, 2019, Minneapolis, Minnesota, vol. 1, p. 2.

26. E. Kannan, and L. A. Kothamasu, "Fine-tuning BERT based approach for multi-class sentiment analysis on twitter emotion data," *Ing. Des Syst. d'Information*, vol. 27, no. 1, pp. 93–100, 2022.

22 Sentiment Analysis Concerning Indonesian Community Acceptance of COVID-19 Vaccine in Social Media

Aisyah Larasati and Deni Prastyo
Universitas Negeri Malang
Malang, Indonesia

Agus Rachmad Purnama
Universitas Nahdlatul Ulama Sidoarjo
Sidoarjo, Indonesia

22.1 INTRODUCTION

Today information moves very fast; information in one place quickly spreads to all corners of the world and can be accessed easily through various platforms. One of the platforms that have a large mass is social media. Thousands of text data come in and out every few seconds with factual and hoax topics [1]. Therefore, there is a need to extract information from that data so that the information is easy to understand.

Considering social media platforms, Twitter is one of the social media platforms that has an extensive database of information. This platform delivers a great deal of information that is still ambiguous and even completely incomprehensible [2]. Thus, the role of text mining is beneficial in finding or extracting information that has not been clear yet. Text mining has similar properties to data mining, but it focuses on text rather than more structured forms of data. In short, text mining analyzes large amounts of unstructured text data assisted by software that can identify concepts, patterns, topics, keywords, and other attributes in the data [3]. An easy way to implement text mining on big data on Twitter is to use the Application Programming Interface (API) provided by Twitter. We can easily retrieve data from Twitter that will then be processed as needed.

During this pandemic, the most sought after information on the Twitter platform is about the COVID-19 vaccination. The pros and cons color the Twitter page to become trending in the world. Naturally, it has been more than a year since the whole world has been affected by the COVID-19 pandemic. To return the situation to normal as before, of course, vaccines are the right solution. Although it took quite a long time, in the end, some types of vaccines have been accepted by the community.

DOI: 10.1201/9781003331674-22

Regarding the vaccines used by the Indonesian government, six types of vaccines are used: those from Bio Farma, Astra Zeneca, Sinopharm, Moderna, Pfizer-BioNTech, and Sinovac BioTech [4]. The use of various types of vaccines has sparked controversy in the community. Of course, the COVID-19 vaccine controversy continues to be discussed on social media with all the pros and cons [5].

For this reason, it is necessary to carry out a data analysis process to make understanding the pattern of public opinion on the COVID-19 vaccine easier. Furthermore, the information can be used by related institutions, organizations, and companies for different purposes.

Data analysis processes on Twitter commonly carried out include data retrieval (crawling), preprocessing, and data analysis (sentiment). The output of the process is information that has been patterned and grouped. However, the challenge in developing a classification model is determining the method. Each algorithm model is only fit for specific data distribution and may cause bias if its use is generalized. So, this research focuses on optimizing algorithms suitable for public opinion problems related to the COVID-19 vaccine.

22.2   LITERATURE REVIEW

Text mining is extracting patterns from several patterns by identifying interesting ones. It aims to find information or something that is not yet known and cannot be written. The text mining process is the same as data mining, yet with different inputs. The first stage in text mining is data retrieval, which is continued by preprocessing before classification [6]. Social media is the biggest source for text mining databases. Twitter is a massive platform for sharing information and having the possibility to analyze. Twitter is a website owned and operated by Twitter Inc., which offers a social network in the form of microblogging that allows users to send and read tweets [6]. A microblog is one type of online communication tool where users can update the status of their opinion on a matter concerning personal problems experienced or problems that are currently trending. Tweets are written text displayed on a user's profile page that can be written in up to 140 characters. Twitter has the advantage of providing an excellent API. When viewed from the official Twitter page, an API is a way for computers to talk to each other to order and deliver something. In this study, data was taken from Twitter about Indonesian people's acceptance of the COVID-19 vaccine.

Part of people's perception of social media activity is how they are getting interaction based on their opinion. Sentiment analysis, or opinion mining, is the process of extracting, processing, analyzing, and understanding textual data to obtain the sentiment information in a text opinion sentence. This analysis focuses on processing opinions that contain polarity, which has various sentiment values (positive, negative, and neutral). Sentiment analysis is used to obtain information from a dataset or opinion tendencies toward a problem, whether they tend to have negative, positive, or neutral opinions [7]. Based on that, a database from sentiment analysis can be used to people's tendency of their status on social media.

As a part of artificial intelligence, machine learning can create accurate predictions by dealing with the biggest data text. This chapter focuses on developing a

Support Vector Machine (SVM) and Neural Network (NN) to obtain optimal performance based on optimization parameters. SVM is a supervised machine learning classification method that predicts classes based on models or patterns from the training process results. Classification is done by looking for a hyperplane or dividing line that separates one class from another [8]. NN is a computational-based artificial NN adapted from the human neural system [9]. SVM and NN create tendency prediction, which is useful to the mapping information.

22.3   RESEARCH METHODOLOGY

The basis of experimental research is one form of response related to the acceptance of the Indonesian people of the COVID-19 vaccine. This research focuses on public sentiment through keywords or keywords obtained from Twitter about the Indonesian Public Acceptance of the COVID-19 Vaccine. The flow of this research is described in the following sections.

22.3.1   BUSINESS UNDERSTANDING

Sentiment analysis in this study aims to determine the response of the Indonesian people regarding government programs related to COVID-19 vaccination. Through this approach, it is hoped that it can become a reference regarding the performance of government programs to optimize the evaluation of policies made by the government through feedback provided by the community in the form of opinions [2]. Data analysis based on opinion classification into sentiment will produce some appropriate decisions as a source of information in making decisions [10].

22.3.2   DATA UNDERSTANDING, CRAWLING, AND PREPROCESSING

The COVID-19 vaccine program, classified as a new government program, creates pros and cons in the community behind the procurement and process. To find out the pros and cons in the community, it is necessary first to know the public's opinion more specifically based on their emotions, commonly called sentiment [6]. The platform for gathering public opinion is social media, including Twitter [11]. The data crawling occurred on April 20, 2021, or 3 months after the vaccination program phase 1 was announced by the Indonesian government [12]. The crawled data are 2500 raw data with only one variable tweet text, as presented in Figure 22.1.

Crawling is a way to collect various types of data on Twitter through the Twitter API. Crawling conducted by Jupyter Notebook with Tweepy library (query for the retrieved data from Twitter API is "Vaksin COVID-19") explicitly focused on Bahasa and Indonesian regions without duplication (that means without retweeting). Limitation data was based on the limitation of the API ordered; Twitter gave access to only past weeks of data (Up to 7–9 days of historical tweets). Data from using the JSON file, converting data into tabular data like Figure 22.2, needed to be manipulated in another process.

	Tweet
0	Walau Sudah Vaksin\nIngat Covid-19 Belum Berakhir \n\nAyoo....\nSelalu patuhi 5M :\n1. Memakai Masker\n2. Mencuci Tangan... https://t.co/komE7pCWjl
1	Thailand Akan Miliki Vaksin COVID-19 Buatan Dalam Negeri Pada 2024 https://t.co/YopyYKvG3k
2	Warga Kotawaringan Barat sehat dengan vaksin COVID-19. https://t.co/9YSbL1WFZJ
3	Walau Sudah Vaksin\nIngat Covid-19 Belum Berakhir \n\nAyoo....\nSelalu patuhi 5M :\n1. Memakai Masker\n2. Mencuci Tangan... https://t.co/AOssaK3Q1H
4	Bagi warga Surabaya yang membutuhkan vaksin booster pertama dan kedua untuk nakes, terdapat pfizer yang tersedia ha... https://t.co/JHPjWy0IPR
...	...
1671	[SALAH] AIDS jenis baru yang merupakan hasil dari pencampuran COVID-19, vaksin, dan Cacar Monyet atau Monkeypox\n\nBe... https://t.co/Cd29hVo892
1672	KAKANWIL KEMENKUMHAM JATENG, A. YUSPAHRUDDIN : Puluhan Narapidana Rutan Salatiga Disuntik Vaksin Covid-19\nhttps://t.co/kpv9S5fx7f
1673	Vaksin Influenza mengaktifkan tindak balas imun yang spesifik terhadap Influenza manakala vaksin COVID-19 mengaktif... https://t.co/TNFlrnC5rF
1674	Halo, teman-teman ada yang butuh Penerjemahan Tersumpah (Sworn Translation) oleh Penerjemah Tersumpah untuk dokumen... https://t.co/1R72tVkeD1
1675	Buka setiap hari kerja mulai pukul 08.00 Wib Gerai vaksin Polsek Teluknaga Tetap utamakan protokol kesehatan covid... https://t.co/IpXC7xhJyg

FIGURE 22.1   Twitter text data.

User Name	Description_user	Location	Tweet	Likes	Retweet
InhuSat	Melindungi, mengayomi dan melayani	NaN	Walau Sudah Vaksin\nIngat Covid-19 Belum Berakhir \n\nAyoo....\nSelalu patuhi 5M :\n1. Memakai Masker\n2. Mencuci Tangan... https://t.co/komE7pCWjl	0	0
VIVAcoid	NaN	NaN	Thailand Akan Miliki Vaksin COVID-19 Buatan Dalam Negeri Pada 2024 https://t.co/YopyYKvG3k	2	0
SuntiksJr	Vaksin untuk semua orang.	NaN	Warga Kotawaringan Barat sehat dengan vaksin COVID-19. https://t.co/9YSbL1WFZJ	0	0
JovendraYadi	ulang tahun	NaN	Walau Sudah Vaksin\nIngat Covid-19 Belum Berakhir \n\nAyoo....\nSelalu patuhi 5M :\n1. Memakai Masker\n2. Mencuci Tangan... https://t.co/AOssaK3Q1H	0	0
detik_jatim	Baca berita di https://t.co/dViBxMnBDj yo rek	Kota Surabaya, Jawa Timur	Bagi warga Surabaya yang membutuhkan vaksin booster pertama dan kedua untuk nakes, terdapat pfizer yang tersedia ha... https://t.co/JHPjWy0IPR	0	0

FIGURE 22.2   Tabular data from API.

Sentiment analysis, part of text mining, requires special stages because it is unstructured data [13]. The steps in preprocessing this study's data include case folding, removing characters, stemming, translation, and stop word removal [14].

22.3.3   SENTIMENT ANALYSIS OPTIMIZATION

The text data of a collection of opinions are analyzed to obtain conclusions about the topic. At this stage, we use the text blob to know the polarity. It can be seen from the polarity to find out the sentiment of positive, negative, or neutral values. If the polarity is greater than 0, the sentiment is positive, 0 means neutral, and less than 0 means negative.

The classification algorithms used in sentiment are SVM and NN. We use sklearn library at the development stage and GridSearchCV library for parameter setting. The ROC performance evaluates the best model. ROC is used because it has a higher level of sensitivity and specificity, so it is appropriate for unbalanced label data [15]. At the same time, the validation stage of the algorithm uses 10 K-Fold to get the ideal performance [16]. Parameters that will be used in this research include SVM using gamma, C, and kernel, and NN parameters are momentum, alpha, and hidden layer.

22.4   EXPERIMENTAL RESULT

The research is divided into five steps, with requirements from each step. The first step is crawling data, preprocessing data in Bahasa, translating it into English, and creating labeling, and the final step is modeling using machine learning.

22.4.1   MODELING STAGES

Machine learning modeling is applied to classification algorithms in sentiment analysis using Anaconda software with a Jupyter module and Python 3 programming. This research will result in experiments from testing the classification algorithm to producing the best performance value based on the ROC value. Thus, in the final stage of the study, it will be concluded that the best model for classifying sentiment toward public opinion regarding the COVID-19 vaccine will be established.

SMOTE handles unbalancing data by resampling data based on ROC value. SMOTE using 0.8 SMOTE strategy ratio and 0.9 undersampling ratios. Splitting data to have a good learning model is done using 0.8 splitting data for training data and 0.2 for testing data. Model validation is done based on K-fold with the default K number 10 K-fold.

22.4.2   SENTIMENT RESULT

The results of the preprocessing text show that 2500 initial data were turned into data with high noise characteristics [17]. The noise consists of text with emoticons, characters, link websites, and other noise. The step for preprocessing data based on reduction fits the second stage in Figure 22.3. The crawled data are the Twitter raw data without retweet status. Remove duplication stage filters duplications based on username repetition with the same tweet. The clean data are 1100 and have 1490 data duplication data.

Text data are divided into opinion and fact data categories because sentiment research only focuses on opinion processing [6]. This study retrieved 1010 text data from Twitter, producing 339 opinion data and 671 data containing facts. Facts on the tweets occur because many online news media use Twitter to spread news, so tweets lead to facts [18]. Based on factual data is not used, and neutral data is classified as factual, so polarity equal to 0 will be eliminated [19]. Fifteen of 339 data are classified as factual, data are ready for modeling, and analysis is 324.

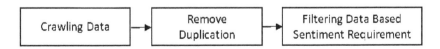

FIGURE 22.3   Sentiment analysis stage.

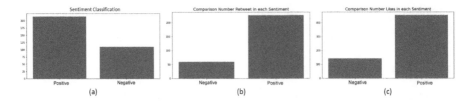

FIGURE 22.4   Sentiment value: (a) sentiment classification, (b) number retweeted, (c) number of likes.

The 324 opinion texts resulted in 214 (66.04%) positive sentiments and 110 (33.95%) negative sentiments. Figure 22.4(a) indicates that the data label is unbalanced. Therefore, the proper metric to evaluate the model's performance is the ROC score [15]. Comparing numbers of retweets and likes also has unbalanced data, as seen in Figure 22.4(b) and (c).

Figure 22.5 shows the words cloud labeling from the text based on the value of polarity and subjectivity. The results of positive sentiment produce some frequent words: the emergence of the Omicron variant, pride in the vaccination program, and the belief that vaccines can protect against COVID-19. Most negative sentiments talk about increasing vaccine acceleration and complaints about socialization and the effect of vaccination. In addition, there are still some public sentiments that are still afraid of vaccines and some cases about illegal vaccination certification.

Figure 22.6 describes the relationship of the word to each sentiment. The description can display a more detailed visualization of the sentiment. The results of the association in the positive group, such as the implementation of vaccines, are closely related to the word antigen and swab and are strong that vaccines are urgent. It also shows that the word coronavirus is related to the words launched and record. The association for negative words such as inflammation and heart disease is related to the 8-year-old kid. The relationship shows that the application of the vaccines still harms specific age groups. The word vaccine is related to the word panicked for the people with immunization.

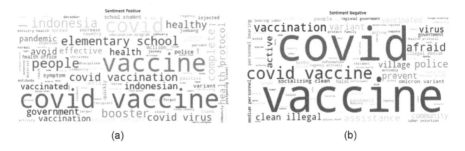

FIGURE 22.5   Words cloud-based sentiment: (a) positive sentiment and (b) negative sentiment.

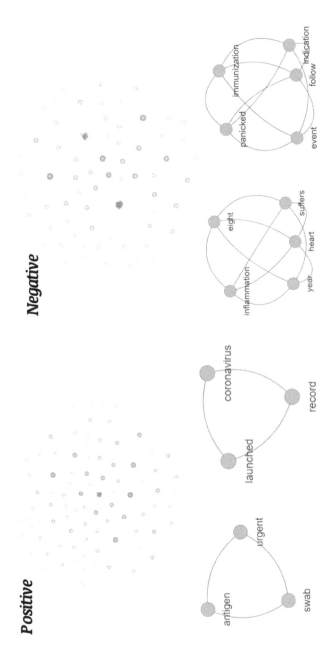

FIGURE 22.6 World association-based sentiment.

TABLE 22.1

Parameters and Levels of NN

Variable	Level
Hidden layer sizes	10, 20, 30, 40
Alpha	0.01, 0.1, 0.5, 1
Momentum	0.2, 0.4, 0.8, 1

22.4.3 NEURAL NETWORK ALGORITHM

The NN algorithm uses three parameters: hidden layer sizes, alpha, and momentum. Each parameter has four levels, as in Table 22.1.

The ROC score (Figure 22.7) concludes that the increase in learning rate or alpha value leads to a performance decline. The model runs faster and causes weight oscillations. The increased size of hidden layers may cause overfitting. In contrast, underfitting may happen when hidden layer sizes are at the smallest level [9].

As described in Figure 22.7, the performance of the NN parameters shows that the best learning rate or alpha parameter is level 0.01 with an ROC value above 0.845. Momentum, which functions as a process to shorten learning [9], has the best value when the level is 1.0 with an ROC of 0.845. The best number of hidden layer sizes is 30, with an ROC of 0.845. NN has the top five biggest combinations, resulting in Table 22.2.

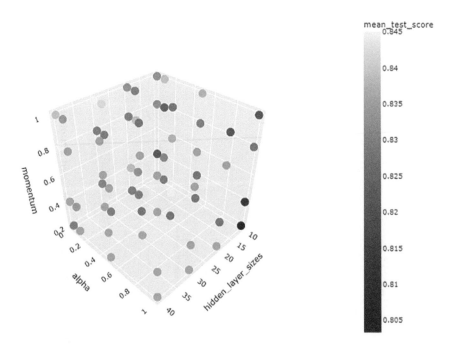

FIGURE 22.7   Performance of NN parameters against ROC score.

TABLE 22.2

Top 5 Best Parameters of NN

Hidden Layer Size	Alpha	Momentum	Mean ROC Score
30	0.01	1	0.8450
30	0.1	1	0.8417
10	0.01	0.2	0.8383
10	0.5	1	0.8367
30	0.01	0.2	0.8350

The result of the experimental research from NN is random combination performance, or whatever stagnant performance is based on Figure 22.7. Table 22.2 points out the best combination of ROC from the hidden layer and alpha parameters (30, 0.01) with an ROC value of 0.845. The best combination of the hidden layer and momentum is (30, 1). A combination of momentum parameters and alpha is (1, 0.01). This combination indicates that the performance tends to increase with the smallest alpha, the highest moment of the hidden layer, and momentum.

The best combination values are alpha, hidden layer, and momentum parameters (0.01, 1, 30), with the ROC model value of 0.845 (84.5%). The lowest ROC is obtained from the combined value of alpha, hidden layer, and momentum parameters (10, 1, 0.2) with an ROC of 0.803 (80.3%). In conclusion, this study shows that the best parameter combination in the sentiment model with the NN algorithm is maximizing the hidden layer value and choosing a small learning rate value to reduce the time consumption and overfitting. The maximal performance of training is 1.00, and 0.713 for the data testing.

22.4.4 SUPPORT VECTOR MACHINE ALGORITHM

The SVM algorithm uses a hyperplane to separate its classes. This algorithm requires supporting parameters such as kernel, C, and gamma to improve model performance [20]. Experiments on the SVM model use these three parameters, each of which has three levels, as shown in Table 22.3.

The ROC of the polynomial kernel parameter has the worst performance compared with the linear kernel and radial basis function (RBF) due to the model's sensitivity to data noise [21]. Gamma is a parameter sensitive to the kernel's use [22]. The highest impact parameter on ROC is when the C (cost) is equal to 0.1 and 10.

TABLE 22.3

Parameters and Levels of SVM

Variable	Levels
Kernels	RBF, Poly, Linear
C	0.1, 1, 10
Gamma	10, 1, 0.1

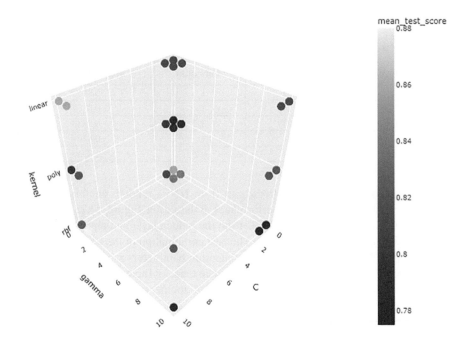

FIGURE 22.8 Performance of SVM parameters against ROC score.

The best performance of the gamma parameter, shown in Figure 22.8, is at level 1 with an ROC value of 0.88. The kernel parameter produces the best model when using the RBF kernel. Meanwhile, the C parameter is at level 10.

The combination parameter between the kernel and cost increased the polynomial kernel, as described in Table 22.4, is better than shown in Figure 22.8. The RBF and linear parameters still use the Cost as a parameter level, as described in Figure 22.8. The best value on the RBF parameter is with a cost of 1 with an ROC value of 0.88. While the use of the gamma parameter has decreased in the RBF kernel because the use of these two parameters is very sensitive to performance [22], the best value is at the level of gamma 1 and kernel polynomial.

TABLE 22.4
Top Five Best Parameters of SVM

C	Gamma	Kernel	Mean ROC Score
10	1	RBF	0.8800
10	10	Linear	0.8567
0.1	1	RBF	0.8367
10	0.1	RBF	0.8200
0.1	10	Polynomial	0.8167

TABLE 22.5

Comparison Model

Algorithm	Best Parameters	ROC
NN	Alpha: 0.01 Hidden layer: 30 Momentum: 1.0	0.845
SVM	Kernels: 'RBF' Cost: 10 Gamma: 1	0.880

Combining the C and gamma parameters produces the same graph at the C with level 1. The best combination is obtained at the C parameter level 10 and gamma 1 with RBF kernel. Using gamma produces the same value in the linear kernel but varies in the RBF kernel [22]. The combination of gamma and C parameters experienced an increasing trend, with the best value of ROC of 0.88 at gamma level 1 and C at 10. The performance of SVM optimization, with K = 10, reached 0.88, within the range of 1.00 for data training and 0.723 for data testing.

22.4.5 COMPARISON OF MODELS

A further development is to find the best model for classifying sentiment on public opinion regarding the COVID-19 vaccine, as described in Table 22.5.

The results show that the SVM model performs best with an ROC value of 0.880 (88%) in classifying public opinion sentiments regarding the COVID-19 vaccine. The result overcomes the ROC of other previous studies in Twitter sentiment analysis: accuracy of up to 70% [23]; accuracy around 70% to 81% [24]; and precision, recall, and F1 values for most classes exceeded 80% [25]. Thus, compared with other existing studies on sentiment analysis, the model resulting from this study has already had a good level of performance in terms of ROC score.

22.5   CONCLUSION

The sentiment model aims to determine the characteristics of emotions in text data. People especially use sentiment to evaluate programs (i.e., the government's program). The algorithm comparison needs to be done empirically to determine model performance differences. An optimization algorithm must be done to compare the classification performance.

Sentiment research using NN and SVM determines the characteristics of public opinion regarding the COVID-19 vaccine program. The SVM becomes the algorithm with the best performance, with an ROC score of 88%. The optimum results cannot be separated from the optimization method using experiments from various levels in each algorithm. In model development, not all parameters in the model move linearly. In the development of model optimization, it is necessary to experiment with all parameters to determine the characteristics of the model and the data used.

REFERENCES

1. F. Rahutomo, I. Y. R. Pratiwi, and D. M. Ramadhani, "Eksperimen naïve bayes pada deteksi berita hoax berbahasa Indonesia," *J. Penelit. Komun. Dan Opini Publik*, vol. 23, no. 1, Jul. 2019, doi: 10.33299/jpkop.23.1.1805.

2. O. Alqaryouti, N. Siyam, A. Abdel Monem, and K. Shaalan, "Aspect-based sentiment analysis using smart government review data," *Appl. Comput. Inform.*, Jul. 2020, doi: 10.1016/j.aci.2019.11.003.

3. S. A. Salloum, et al., "Mining social media text: Extracting knowledge from facebook," *Int. J. Comput. Digit. Syst.*, vol. 6, no. 2, pp. 73–81, Mar. 2017, doi: 10.12785/IJCDS/060203.

4. "Penetapan Jenis Vaksin untuk Pelaksanaan Vaksinasi Corona Virus Desease 2019 (COVID-19)," Kementerian Kesehatan Republik Indonesia, Jakarta, Nomor HK.01.07/MENKES/9680/2020.

5. Universitas Islam Indonesia, "Vaksinasi sebagai Solusi Penyelesaian Pandemi," *Vaksinasi sebagai Solusi Penyelesaian Pandemi*. https://www.uii.ac.id/vaksinasi-sebagai-solusi-penyelesaian-pandemi/

6. T. Carpenter, and T. Way, "Tracking sentiment analysis through Twitter." In *Proceedings of the International Conference on Information and Knowledge Engineering (IKE)* (p. 1). The Steering Committee of The World Congress in Computer Science, Computer Engineering and Applied Computing (WorldComp), 2012.

7. D. Hazarika, G. Konwar, S. Deb, and D. J. Bora, "Sentiment analysis on Twitter by using TextBlob for natural language processing," *ICRMAT* vol. 24, pp. 63–67, 2020. doi: 10.15439/2020KM20.

8. A. Larasati, A. M. Hajji, and A. N. Handayani. "Preferences analysis of engineering students on choosing learning media using support vector machine (SVM) model." In *2nd International Conference on Vocational Education and Training (ICOVET 2018)*, pp. 57–59. Atlantis Press, Malang, Indonesia, 2019.

9. M. Badrul, "Optimasi neural network dengan algoritma genetika untuk prediksi hasil pemilukada," *Bina Insani ICT Journal* vol. 3, no. 1, pp. 229–242, 2016.

10. T. S. Dandibhotla, and Dr. V. V. Bulusu, "Obtaining feature- and sentiment-based linked instance RDF data from unstructured reviews using ontology-based machine learning," *Int. J. Technol.*, vol. 6, no. 2, p. 198, Apr. 2015, doi: 10.14716/ijtech.v6i2.555.

11. V. N. Patodkar, and I. R. Sheikh, "Twitter as a corpus for sentiment analysis and opinion mining," *IJARCCE*, vol. 5, no. 12, pp. 320–322, 2016, doi: 10.17148/IJARCCE.2016.51274.

12. Kementerian Kesehatan, "Petunjuk Teknis Pelaksanaan Vaksinasi dalam Rangka Penanggulangan Pandemi Corona Virus Disease 2019 (COVID-19)," Kementerian Kesehatan Republik Indonesia, NOMOR HK.02.02/4/1/2021.

13. D. S. Vijayarani, and J. Ilamathi, "Preprocessing techniques for text mining - an overview," *International Journal of Computer Science & Communication Networks* 5, no. 1 (2015): 7–16.

14. S. Mujilahwati, "Pre-processing text mining pada data Twitter," *Semin. Nas. Teknol. Inf. dan Komun.*, 2016, no. Sentika, 2089–9815, 2016.

15. M. Sokolova, N. Japkowicz, and S. Szpakowicz, "Beyond accuracy, F-score and ROC: A family of discriminant measures for performance evaluation," in A. Sattar and B. Kang, Eds. *AI 2006: Advances in Artificial Intelligence*, vol. 4304, Berlin, Heidelberg: Springer Berlin Heidelberg, 2006, pp. 1015–1021. doi: 10.1007/11941439_114.

16. D. Berrar, "Cross-validation," in *Encyclopedia of Bioinformatics and Computational Biology*, Elsevier, 2019, pp. 542–545. doi: 10.1016/B978-0-12-809633-8.20349-X.

17. L. V. Subramaniam, S. Roy, T. A. Faruquie, and S. Negi, "A survey of types of text noise and techniques to handle noisy text," in *Proceedings of The Third Workshop on*

Analytics for Noisy Unstructured Text Data - AND '09, Barcelona, Spain, 2009, p. 115. doi: 10.1145/1568296.1568315.

18. N. A. Paramastri, and G. Gumilar, "Penggunaan Twitter Sebagai Medium Distribusi Berita dan News Gathering Oleh Tirto.Id," *J. Kaji. Jurnalisme*, vol. 3, no. 1, p. 18, 2019, doi: 10.24198/jkj.v3i1.22450.

19. R. Xia, F. Xu, J. Yu, Y. Qi, and E. Cambria, "Polarity shift detection, elimination and ensemble: A three-stage model for document-level sentiment analysis," *Inf. Process. Manag*, vol. 52, no. 1, pp. 36–45, 2016, doi: 10.1016/j.ipm.2015.04.003.

20. A. A. Abdillah, and S. Suwarno, "Diagnosis of diabetes using support vector machines with radial basis function kernels," *Int. J. Technol*, vol. 7, no. 5, p. 849, 2016, doi: 10.14716/ijtech.v7i5.1370.

21. N. R. Feta, and A. R. Ginanjar, "Komparasi fungsi kernel metode support vector machine untuk pemodelan klasifikasi terhadap penyakit tanaman kedelai," *BRITech, Jurnal Ilmiah Ilmu Komputer, Sains Dan Teknologi Terapan* 1, no. 1 (2019): 33–39.

22. I. S. Al-Mejibli, J. K. Alwan, and D. H. Abd, "The effect of gamma value on support vector machine performance with different kernels," *Int. J. Electr. Comput. Eng. IJECE*, vol. 10, no. 5, p. 5497, 2020, doi: 10.11591/ijece.v10i5.pp5497-5506.

23. T. Hendrawati, and C. P. Yanti, "Analysis of Twitter users sentiment against the COVID-19 outbreak using the backpropagation method with Adam optimization," *J. Electr. Electron. Inform*, vol. 5, no. 1, p. 1, 2021, doi: 10.24843/JEEI.2021.v05.i01.p01.

24. M. Rezwanul, A. Ali, and A. Rahman, "Sentiment analysis on Twitter data using KNN and SVM," *Int. J. Adv. Comput. Sci. Appl.*, vol. 8, no. 6, 2017, DOI: 10.14569/IJACSA.2017.080603.

25. I. Surjandari, R. A. Wayasti, Z. Zulkarnain, E. Laoh, A. M. Masbar Rus, and I. Prawiradinata, "Mining public opinion on ride-hailing service providers using aspect-based sentiment analysis," *Int. J. Technol*, vol. 10, no. 4, p. 818, 2019, doi: 10.14716/ijtech.v10i4.2860.

23 Graph Clustering for Social Media Listening during COVID-19

Esther Irawati Setiawan, Joan Santoso,
Julius Sugianto, Alvin Sucita, Michael Tenoyo,
Mitchell Arthur, and Willyanto Dharmawan
Institut Sains dan Teknologi Terpadu Surabaya
Surabaya, Indonesia

23.1 INTRODUCTION

The novel coronavirus (COVID-19) pandemic had hurt society by restricting social activities and causing mental health problems [1–3] because people had to prioritize safety over economic activity [4]. Indonesian people could comply with this, as COVID-19 was a genuine and irreversible threat. However, people whose livelihoods depend on the informal economy became uncertain about how to meet their daily necessities [5], because most Indonesians work in the informal sector and depend on economic relationships between social groupings [6].

Sentiment analysis on the COVID-19 reported negative sentiments from fear, frustration, and hatred as the form of the negative impact of the pandemic [7]. Another study debates various topics and promotes the implementation of high-scale restrictions on social activity [8]. The use of social media as a means of communication between people has increased [9]. There was also a significant increase in social media use, impacting business marketing strategies [10]. Because of the pandemic, people have turned to the Internet and social media as a source of information.

Social Network Analysis (SNA) exists to inform the public relationships between events that occur in the community, and the information that appears during this pandemic can be analyzed using the SNA technique in the form of a weighted graph [11]. In Saraswathi et al. [12], the authors employed SNA to investigate the COVID-19 outbreak in Karnataka, India, and to evaluate SNA's potential as a tool for outbreak monitoring and control.

Thus, several multidisciplinary approaches with machine learning on COVID-19 data have increased [13]. Along with social media posts, false material about the COVID epidemic also increased and needs to be debunked by a fact-checker on social media such as Twitter [7, 14]. Using Natural Language Processing (NLP) and machine learning classifiers, the sentiment analysis of

DOI: 10.1201/9781003331674-23

tweets produced by Indian residents was performed and results showed that most Indian population supports the government during a coronal mass ejection [15]. Spam posts also need to be identified by network analysis to obtain valuable insights [16].

The hashtag #*dirumahsaja* (stay at home) was popularized on social media to help the community cope and overcome the pandemic situation as quickly as possible to avoid economic blows [17]. As a result, we analyzed hashtags associated with the #*dirumahsaja* hashtag further to analyze the community response to the lockdown initiative and to comprehend the impact of the stay-at-home campaign to determine what efforts could be made to mitigate the negative effects during the new normal era. We aim to analyze the social network Instagram using one main topic to be chosen and to know the issues on Instagram during the pandemic with graph clustering.

23.2 SOCIAL NETWORK ANALYSIS (SNA)

A social network is a social structure consisting of a set of social actors (e.g., individuals or organizations), a collection of dyad ties, and other social interactions between actors. Interacting with strangers on the Internet will create a social network. The depiction and definition of structured data about the relationship between members in the network are called SNA.

The use of SNA in network evaluation began in the early to mid-90s [18]. SNA was used in several network evaluations, including finding leaders [19], public health [20], and assessing interdisciplinary research collaborations [21]. Monitoring people's mentions and questions on social media has become a critical issue that needs to be considered. The social media listening technique is one of the most effective strategies for finding out what people talk about [22]. In Hsu et al. [23], the authors collected at least 1000 documents, information, and definition that described positive or negative statement syntax features, such as with the weights to quantify substances scores and used the tree line graph to provide a comparative analysis of the condition of two or more products that have been analyzed and compared with the value per unit weight.

A network is generally a one-mode network where, for example, an actor is connected to another actor. However, in a complex network, some networks can be categorized as bipartite networks or two-network modes, where the nodes on the network are divided into two groups, namely X and Y, and connections that can occur are connections between different groups (group X can connect with group Y, but group X cannot connect with group X which others, and vice versa). Some examples of bipartite networks that are often found are actors with movie titles. From this bipartite network, it can be changed to one-network mode, namely by projecting it based on X or Y. If based on X, a one-network mode will be formed, which contains the relationship between group X with weights obtained from the number of similarities Y connected from those two groups of X.

There are various metrics for analyzing social networks, such as centrality, community detection, and clique. The idea of centrality is used simultaneously in a variety of applications. Centrality is an essential part of the complex network that affects the habits of dynamic processes such as synchronization and the spread of epidemics. It can carry important information from complex systems in an organization. Centrality in this chapter is divided into four types according to their respective uses. Betweenness centrality finds how often nodes become bridges connecting one node with another. Degree centrality could find the number of friends a node has; the node with the most friends is the node with the most impact and the highest position. Closeness centrality measures the closeness between one user and another, and Betweenness centrality is used to calculate the weight of each node based on how many nodes are traversed based on the shortest path. Eigenvector centrality quantifies the influence of a node within a network. It assigns relative scores to all nodes in the network based on the principle that connections to high-scoring nodes contribute more to the score of the node being analyzed than connections to low-scoring nodes with equal weight [24].

Betweenness centrality is calculated based on Equation (23.1) where $\sigma st(v)$ is the shortest trajectory of s and t passing through the vertex v, and σst is the total shortest trajectory from s to t.

$$CB(v) = \frac{\sigma st(v)}{\sigma st} \tag{23.1}$$

Closeness centrality is used to find the closest node to another node in a network to obtain information more efficiently. The formula used to find the closeness of centrality is as displayed in Equation (23.2), where N is the number of nodes in the network and $d(ni, nj)$ is the sum of the shortest paths from node i to node j.

$$CC(ni) = \frac{[N-1]}{\Sigma d(ni, nj)} \tag{23.2}$$

Degree centrality is used to find the number of nodes connected directly to other nodes. The formula used to find the degree of centrality is displayed in Equation (23.3), where $d(ni)$ is the number of interactions that the ni node has with other nodes.

$$CD(ni) = d(ni) \tag{23.3}$$

A clique is a complete subgraph of a given graph or group of people in which each person is directly connected to another person. "Maximum" means that no other nodes can be added to the clique. The littlest clique that can be found consists of two actors.

Using a forest fire case in Indonesia, we can summarize and extract patterns from specific cases using social media listening, as in this study [22], which used Instagram hashtags as a data source and analyzed the social interaction within the context of a forest fire. The analysis used graph clustering to obtain an information summary.

23.3 METHOD

This section explains how to listen to social media for conversations about hashtag *#dirumahsaja*. As displayed in Figure 23.1, the proposed method consists of five main phases, i.e., Instagram data acquisition, layouting, social media listening with community detection, labeling, and visualization.

23.3.1 DATA ACQUISITION AND PREPROCESSING

The first stage in preprocessing is feature extraction to prepare the features necessary to build a network. Some unnecessary features will be discarded, such as shortcodes, display_url, loc_id, loc_name, loc_lat, loc_lon, and taken_at_timestamp. The next step is to collect what hashtags are used in each post and then save them into a variable in the form of an array. In the end, the final dataset consists of the id, which is the post's id; hashtag_list, which is the list of the post's hashtag; user_id, which is the owner_id of the post; and the user_name, which is the owner_name of the post.

In the node and edge initialization, nodes and edges are created based on variables that have been processed and used to build a network. The nodes used come from all hashtags in the dataset, and the edge comes from the connections between hashtags in each post. Figure 23.2 displays the nodes obtained from this step and Figure 23.3 shows the edges acquired from the social media posts.

23.3.2 GRAPH LAYOUTING

The next step, graph layouting, is done on the network so that it looks neater and can be appropriately analyzed logically using the default method of the NetworkX library, namely the spring layout. Spring Layout is a function owned by NetworkX that uses the Fruchterman-Reingold force-directed algorithm in laying its nodes. This algorithm simulates a force-directed representation of a network whose edge is considered an object that attracts its nodes. In contrast, the node is considered a rejecting object, sometimes called the anti-gravity force.

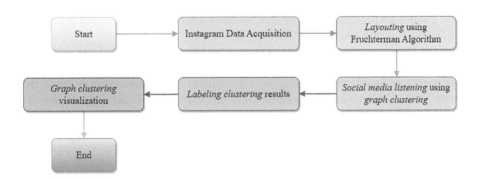

FIGURE 23.1 Research framework.

'motivasibisnis'
'motivasisukses'
'belajarbisnisdigital'
'motivasipengusaha'
'dirumahajadulu'
'workfromhome'
'kerjadarirumah'
'kerjadirumah'
'janeellenbusiness'
'bisnisjaneellen'
'usahasampingan'
'usahaonlineshop'

FIGURE 23.2   Node examples.

['stayathome', 'covid19']
['stayathome', *'jagajarak'*]
['stayathome', 'fashion']
['stayathome', *'fashionwanita'*]
['stayathome', 'newnormal']

FIGURE 23.3   Edge examples.

The simulation used k to determine the distance between the nodes. The scale and center also determine the size and location after re-scaling at the end of the simulation. Figure 23.4 displays the resulting graph using the spring layout method.

23.3.3   GRAPH CLUSTERING

Graph clustering is the grouping of data in the form of graphs. Two different forms of grouping can be performed on the graph data. Vertex clustering seeks to group nodes from the graph into densely connected regional groups based on edge weight or edge distance. The second form of graph clustering treats graphs as objects to be grouped and clusters those objects based on similarity. In this proposed framework, the grouping will be based on variable variables that have been processed previously using the Louvain community method.

The Louvain community method is used to detect communities from a network by maximizing the value of modularity of each community, where its modularity measures quality from a node to its community. This evaluates how dense the node's relationship with its community is compared with other networks at random. Louvain community detection is a method of extracting communities from an extensive network created by Blondel et al, [25]. of the University of Louvain. The method is a clever optimization method and seems to run in time in the number of nodes on the network.

$$O\left(n \cdot \log^2 n\right) \tag{23.4}$$

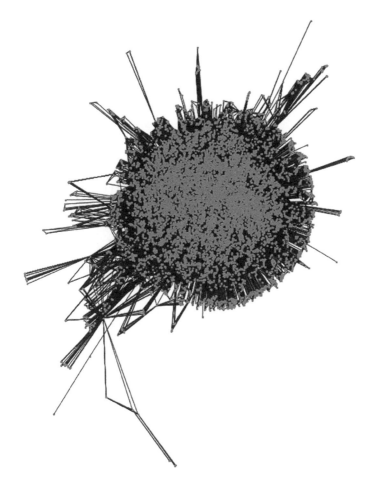

FIGURE 23.4   Layouting results.

23.3.4   CLUSTER SORTING

The next step sorts the clusters formed using the degree centrality of the cluster members. Table 23.1 displays the clustering result data. The last step is displaying a graph of clustering results using the Louvain community method, as visualized in Figure 23.5.

23.4   RESULTS AND ANALYSIS

Based on the nodes and relations obtained with Scrapy, we could display the nodes with top centralities in Table 23.1. The hashtag #indonesia has the highest degree, eigenvector, and closeness centrality, #newnormal has a pretty high closeness centrality, and the highest score for the betweenness centrality as most #dirumahsaja post is associated with the #newnormal campaign.

TABLE 23.1
Centralities from Nodes

Degree		Eigenvector		Betweenness		Closeness	
Hashtag	Centrality	Hashtag	Centrality	Hashtag	Centrality	Hashtag	Centrality
"indonesia"	0.083	"indonesia"	0.086	newnormal"	0.005	"indonesia"	0.506
"newnormal"	0.066	"lfl"	0.069	indonesia"	0.005	"newnormal"	0.502
"staysafe"	0.06	"staysafe"	0.067	hiring"	0.003	"staysafe"	0.499
"lfl"	0.058	"newnormal"	0.066	onlineshop"	0.003	"lfl"	0.497
"jakarta"	0.050	"likeforlikes"	0.062	JagaJarak"	0.002	"jakarta"	0.495
"likeforlikes"	0.049	"jakarta"	0.057	staysafe"	0.002	"jagajarak"	0.494
"jagajarak"	0.039	"tiktok"	0.051	BelajarOnline"	0.002	"likeforlikes"	0.494
"workfromhome"	0.038	"fff"	0.047	jakarta"	0.002	"workfromhome"	0.492
"tiktok"	0.038	"jagajarak"	0.047	pengusahamuda"	0.002	"tiktok"	0.492
"wfh"	0.037	"lfl 🖤"	0.047	"kerjadarirumah"	0.002	"wfh"	0.4913187164879858

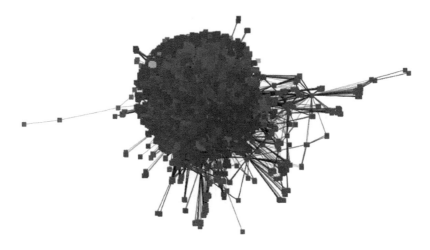

FIGURE 23.5   Graph clustering results.

Table 23.2 displays cluster labeling with degree centrality compared with eigenvector, betweenness, closeness, and count of nodes.

This analysis succeeded in conducting social media listening for issues. From 6742 rows of data obtained, 17305 nodes and 2,222,405 edges were obtained. Using the Louvain community detection method, 160 communities were found. Eigenvector centrality is a measure of the influence of a node in a network. It assigns relative scores to all nodes in the network based on the concept that connections to high-scoring nodes contribute more to the score of the node in question than equal connections to low-scoring nodes. Based on several experiments, it is shown that our analysis defines seven clusters on several topics, which are complementary hashtag; social media and entertainment; work at home; random video hashtag; hashtag related to our subject location, i.e., Surabaya; lifestyle at home; and Honda product owner hashtag. Table 23.2 shows several top-related nodes with each topic in the cluster, i.e., for the work-at-home topics, several topics appear, such as *dirumahjadulu*, workfromhome, *bisnisonline*, *kerjadirumah*, and *kerjadarirumah*, which are several tags or nodes that show the lifestyle of Indonesians during the COVID-19 pandemic. Our constructed graph for the analysis consisting of 17,305 nodes and 2,222,405 edges and the network parameters is displayed in Table 23.3.

There are also several network parameters that can be obtained from our graph, i.e., diameter of the network is 8, the radius of the network is 4, the mean path length is about 5768.667, the mean of number of neighbors is about 30.967, and the network's density is 0.00178 with a clustering coefficient of about 0.913.

We conduct the most closeness and betweenness by the degree of most central node in the networks. We can obtain that the node with the highest value of degree centrality is "indonesia" with a value of 0.083, the highest value of closeness centrality is shown on node "*dirumahsaja*" with a value of 0.911, and the highest value of betweenness centrality is on "indonesia" with a value of 0.5061. This analysis shows that the most discussed topic in the pandemic era was work from home in Indonesia.

TABLE 23.2

Cluster Results

Category	Node	Degree	Eigenvector	Betweenness	Closeness	Count
Complementary hashtags	lfl	0.058137	0.069189	0.001506	0.497130	198
	likeforlikes	0.049006	0.062294	0.000965	0.493793	203
	Lfl ❤	0.035714	0.046571	0.000589	0.489098	113
	fff	0.035425	0.047468	0.000509	0.490442	129
	like4likes	0.031727	0.046333	0.000788	0.490485	141
	likeforfollow	0.028895	0.043701	0.000911	0.490787	101
	followforfollowback	0.024387	0.038257	0.000220	0.487081	61
	likeforlike	0.019822	0.030181	0.000476	0.487024	32
Social media and entertainment	tiktok	0.038141	0.051036	0.000826	0.491910	131
	instagram	0.027797	0.042615	0.000311	0.488485	83
	tiktokindo	0.014679	0.025012	0.000278	0.482248	56
	youtube	0.013754	0.019178	0.000119	0.482915	40
	video	0.010691	0.016887	0.000036	0.479806	38
Work at home	dirumahajadulu	0.040684	0.046852	0.001439	0.492473	2086
	workfromhome	0.038315	0.045921	0.001162	0.492357	2148
	bisnisonline	0.0305013	0.035294	0.001232	0.490127	109
	kerjadirumah	0.018840	0.024523	0.000206	0.485980	2090
	kerjadarirumah	0.016990	0.021000	0.001658	0.486445	2038
	motivasibisnis	0.012020	0.016972	0.000150	0.481708	2029
	bisnisdarirumah	0.011153	0.014941	0.000062	0.481625	12
Random video hashtags	indonesia	0.083218	0.086442	0.004658	0.506102	310
	bandung	0.025659	0.039861	0.000315	0.488955	47
	dagelan	0.015546	0.024449	0.000113	0.483890	45
	literasi30detik	0.015257	0.022196	0.000177	0.482456	35
	motivasi	0.015257	0.021803	0.000204	0.482220	32

(Continued)

TABLE 23.2 (Continued)

Cluster Results

Category	Node	Degree	Eigenvector	Betweenness	Closeness	Count
Random video hashtags (Continued)	literasi	0.014621	0.021052	0.000089	0.482581	29
	tangerang	0.014390	0.017699	0.000792	0.481542	43
	storywa	0.014216	0.021057	0.000151	0.482401	17
	indovidgram	0.014216	0.018247	0.000092	0.481003	36
	motivasihidup	0.011327	0.019952	0.000284	0.483583	17
Hashtags related to Surabaya	surabaya	0.028837	0.038634	0.001564	0.489798	91
	jawatimur	0.008437	0.014953	0.000039	0.479751	19
	kulinersurabaya	0.006299	0.011876	0.000023	0.479326	25
	infosurabaya	0.005490	-	0.000010	-	17
	banggasurabaya	0.004739	-	0.000007	-	12
Lifestyle at home	dirumahaja	0.279993	0.234128	0.050585	0.568866	3205
	hidupsehat	0.011674	0.014816	0.000126	0.480865	67
	instafood	0.009593	0.015424	0.000047	0.480562	36
	dirumahsajadulu	0.007975	0.014059	0.000040	0.480879	13
	kesehatan	0.007686	0.017232	0.000030	0.481459	7
	alami	0.006704	0.011788	0.000018	0.478820	66
	cantikalami	0.005259	0.010053	0.000171	0.478369	5
	makanankekinian	0.005143	-	0.000009	-	10
Honda product owner hashtag	dirumahsaja	0.9185784	0.539172	0.851597	0.910779	7099
	honda	0.004334	-	0.000007	-	11
	vintage	0.002196	-	-	-	5
	aktivitasdirumah	0.001676	-	-	-	2
	c50	0.001676	-	-	-	4
	hondas90z_owner	0.001676	-	-	-	4

TABLE 23.3

Network Parameters

Node Attribute	Range	Mean
Outdegree	0–15,895	30.95775787344698
Indegree	0–15,895	30.95775787344698
Degree	0–15,895	30.95775787344698
Betweenness	0–0.851	0.00006
Harmonic Closeness	0–16425.33	8027.469878372092
Eccentricity	4–8	4.97659635943369

During our analysis, there are some findings that shows three vertices whose centrality scores differ (e.g., high betweenness but medium closeness) and explain from their position in the network why this happens (Table 23.4).

The results from Table 23.4 show that the proximity score is higher than other centralities. The proximity score is higher than other centrality scores because even though these nodes can quickly reach other nodes, they do not have an important role in bridging a cluster with other clusters and do not have many edges or degrees that are directly connected to those nodes.

Nodes that have a high degree of centrality indicate that they have many connections, are popular with other nodes, or have made many transactions. On the other hand, if the degree of centrality of a node is low, the node does not have many connections, is not popular, or performs few transactions. The degree centrality information helps find nodes that have the most information or individuals that can quickly connect to the wider network. A node that has high closeness centrality indicates that it can affect all nodes in the network quickly. Conversely, if the closeness centrality of a node is low, the node's influence on all nodes in the network is weak. Closeness centrality information helps find the best nodes to influence the entire network quickly. Nodes that have high betweenness centrality indicate that nodes hold authority, play an important role over different clusters in the network, or they are on the periphery of the two clusters. On the other hand, if the betweenness centrality of the node is low, the influent node is only in one cluster in the network. Betweenness centrality information helps to find nodes that affect the flow of a system. In the Batak culture of North Sumatra, Indonesia, the phrase *anik panggoaran* is used. The first-born child, who is customarily expected

TABLE 23.4

Noise and Abnormality in Network Graph

Node	Degree	Betweennness	Closeness
anakpanggoaran	16331/17304	17304/17304	5687/17304
anakpanggoaranku	16330/17304	17303/17304	5686/17304
anakbaik	16329/17304	17302/17304	5685/17304

to assume significant duties within the family and community, is referred to. The word *panggoaran*, which translates to "holder" or "caretaker," describes the belief that the first-born child is expected to uphold the family's traditions and values as well as look after their parents and younger siblings. The significance of the family and community in Batak society is reflected in this cultural idea. This information is shown as an abnormality from our graph analysis in social media. This result is considered as noise and outliers from our analysis because there is no relationship between this topics and the pandemic situation.

23.5 CONCLUSION

This study discussed the lifestyle of Indonesians during the COVID-19 pandemic. We analyzed the graph from social media and our graph consists of 17,305 nodes and 2,222,405 edges. Based on the clustering results, the seven largest hashtag categories were acquired, i.e., social media and entertainment, working at home, random video hashtags, hashtags related to Surabaya, lifestyle at home, hashtags of Honda product owners, and complementary hashtags. It can be seen that during a stay-at-home campaign, the posts are related to how to adapt by working at home. This can also be seen on the cluster result shown in Table 23.2. With this analysis, we can see the habit of our community during the pandemic; it also can be used by the government to obtain information that circulates quickly in the community. In the future, this analysis can also open new opportunities for further research development in the field of social analysis using live data crawling to use data that is up to date. It is also possible that this research is helpful in sectors other than information needs for the government including content creators, business owners, and others.

REFERENCES

1. "How Does COVID Affect Mental Health?" Columbia University Irving Medical Center. Jul. 2021, [Online]. Available: https://www.cuimc.columbia.edu/news/how-does-covid-affect-mental-health (accessed October 25, 2022).
2. J. Torales, M. O'Higgins, J. M. Castaldelli-Maia, and A. Ventriglio, "The outbreak of COVID-19 coronavirus and its impact on global mental health," *Int. J. Soc. Psychiatry*, vol. 66, no. 4, pp. 317–320, Jun. 2020, doi: 10.1177/0020764020915212.
3. H. Syafri, E. Sangadji, and R. R. M. Utami, "Impact analysis of the large-scale social restrictions (PSBB) policy implementation in Jakarta," *Journal of Indonesian Health Policy and Administration*, vol. 5, no. 2, pp. 57–60, May 2020, doi: 10.7454/ihpa.v5i2.4056.
4. A. Gaduh, R. Hanna, G. Kreindler, and B. Olken, "Lockdown and Mobility in Indonesia," Harvard University, 2020. https://histecon.fas.harvard.edu/climate-loss/indonesia/index.html (accessed October 26, 2022)
5. M. A. Novaldi, and D. Hidayat, "Public perception of large scale social restrictions," *BASKARA: Journal of Business and Entrepreneurship*, vol. 3, no. 1, pp. 35–45, 2020.
6. H. Andriani, "Effectiveness of large-scale social restrictions (PSBB) toward the new normal era during COVID-19 outbreak: A mini policy review," *Journal of Indonesian Health Policy and Administration*, vol. 5, no. 2, pp. 61–65, May 2020, doi: 10.7454/IHPA.V5I2.4001.

7. K. Saini, D. K. Vishwakarma, and C. Dhiman, "Sentiment Analysis of Twitter Corpus related to COVID-19 induced Lockdown," *ICSCCC 2021 - International Conference on Secure Cyber Computing and Communications*, pp. 465–470, May 2021, doi: 10.1109/ICSCCC51823.2021.9478112.

8. A. M. Tri Sakti, E. Mohamad, and A. A. Azlan, "Mining of opinions on COVID-19 large-scale social restrictions in Indonesia: Public sentiment and emotion analysis on online media," *Journal of Medical Internet Research.*, vol. 23, no. 8, p. e28249, 2021.

9. "Keeping Our Services Stable and Reliable During the COVID-19 Outbreak | Meta." https://about.fb.com/news/2020/03/keeping-our-apps-stable-during-COVID-19/ (accessed October 25, 2022).

10. "Significant Social Media Usage Increase Under COVID-19 For Businesses." https://www.insil.com.au/post/significant-increase-in-social-media-usage-under-COVID-19-heres-what-that-means-for-businesses/ (accessed October 25, 2022).

11. R. Liu, S. Feng, R. Shi, and W. Guo, "Weighted graph clustering for community detection of large social networks," *Procedia Comput Sci.*, vol. 31, pp. 85–94, 2014.

12. S. Saraswathi, A. Mukhopadhyay, H. Shah, and T. S. Ranganath, "Social network analysis of COVID-19 transmission in Karnataka, India," *Epidemiol Infect.*, vol. 148, p. e230, 2020, doi: 10.1017/S095026882000223X.

13. "Worldwide Access to Indonesian National Research on COVID-19: Indonesia's Scientific Contribution to National, Regional and Global Pandemic Response." https://www.who.int/indonesia/news/detail/09-08-2021-worldwide-access-to-indonesian-national-research-on-COVID-19-indonesia-s-scientific-contribution-to-national-regional-and-global-pandemic-response (accessed November 09, 2022).

14. A. Pramiyanti, I. D. Mayangsari, R. Nuraeni, and Y. D. Firdaus, "Public perception on transparency and trust in government information released during the COVID-19 pandemic," *Asian Journal for Public Opinion Research.*, vol. 8, no. 3, pp. 351–376, 2020.

15. P. Gupta, S. Kumar, R. R. Suman, and V. Kumar, "Sentiment analysis of lockdown in India during COVID-19: A case study on Twitter," *IEEE Transactions on Computational Social Systems*, vol. 8, no. 4, pp. 939–949, 2021, doi: 10.1109/TCSS.2020.3042446.

16. E. I. Setiawan, C. P. Susanto, J. Santoso, S. Sumpeno, and M. H. Purnomo, "Preliminary study of spam profile detection for social media using Markov clustering: Case study on Javanese people," *20th International Computer Science and Engineering Conference: Smart Ubiquitos Computing and Knowledge, ICSEC 2016*, Feb. 2017, doi: 10.1109/ICSEC.2016.7859942.

17. Z. Qodir, V. P. Pratiwi, M. Hidayati, and H. Jubba, "The #dirumahaja as a people movement on Twitter," *Jurnal Ilmu Komunikasi*, vol. 19, no. 2, Desember, pp. 233–248, 2022.

18. M. M. Durland, and K. A. Fredericks, "An introduction to social network analysis," *New Dir Eval.*, vol. 2005, no. 107, pp. 5–13, 2005, doi: 10.1002/EV.157.

19. B. Hoppe, and C. Reinelt, "Social network analysis and the evaluation of leadership networks," *The Leadership Quarterly*, vol. 21, no. 4, pp. 600–619, 2010, doi: 10.1016/J.LEAQUA.2010.06.004.

20. D. A. Luke, and J. K. Harris, "Network Analysis in Public Health: History, Methods, and Applications," *Annual Review of Public Health*, vol. 28, pp. 69–93, Mar. 2007, doi: 10.1146/ANNUREV.PUBLHEALTH.28.021406.144132.

21. V. A. Haines, J. Godley, and P. Hawe, "Understanding interdisciplinary collaborations as social networks," *American Journal of Community Psychology*, vol. 47, no. 1–2, pp. 1–11, 2011, doi: 10.1007/S10464-010-9374-1.

22. T. Chumwatana, and I. Chuaychoo, "Using social media listening technique for monitoring people's mentions from social media: A case study of Thai airline industry,"

2017 2nd International Conference on Knowledge Engineering and Applications, ICKEA 2017, pp. 103–106, Dec. 2017, doi: 10.1109/ICKEA.2017.8169910.

23. T. C. Hsu, D. M. Chang, H. J. Lee, and C. Y. Hsu, "Using social listening to evaluate opinion research for social network brand community," *Proceedings – 2nd International Conference on Trustworthy Systems and Their Applications, TSA 2015*, pp. 30–35, Nov. 2015, doi: 10.1109/TSA.2015.16.

24. P. Bonacich, "Some unique properties of eigenvector centrality," *Social Networks*, vol. 29, no. 4, pp. 555–564, 2007, doi: 10.1016/J.SOCNET.2007.04.002.

25. V. D. Blondel, J.-L. Guillaume, R. Lambiotte, and E. Lefebvre, "Fast unfolding of communities in large networks," J. Stat. Mech. Theory Exp., vol. 2008, no. 10, p. P10008, Oct. 2008, doi: 10.1088/1742-5468/2008/10/P10008